THE PSYCHOLOGY OF OBESITY

THE PSYCHOLOGY
OF OBESITY

Dynamics and Treatment

Edited by

NORMAN KIELL

Professor, Psychological Services Center
Department of Student Affairs and Services
Brooklyn College
Brooklyn, New York

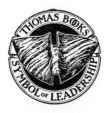

CHARLES C THOMAS · PUBLISHER
Springfield · Illinois · U.S.A.

Published and Distributed Throughout the World by

CHARLES C THOMAS • PUBLISHER

BANNERSTONE HOUSE

301-327 East Lawrence Avenue, Springfield, Illinois, U.S.A.

© *1973, by* CHARLES C THOMAS • PUBLISHER

ISBN 0-398-02685-8

Library of Congress Catalog Card Number: 72-8847

With THOMAS BOOKS *careful attention is given to all details of
manufacturing and design. It is the Publisher's desire to present books
that are satisfactory as to their physical qualities and artistic possibilities
and appropriate for their particular use.* THOMAS BOOKS *will be true
to those laws of quality that assure a good name and good will.*

Printed in the United States of America

C-1

FOR GLADYS AND AARON

Flectere si nequeo superos, Acheronta movebo

Contributors

Pauline Austin Adams, Ph.D.
John L. Bernard, Ph.D.
Carol G. Bruner, B.A.
Robert G. Burnight, Ph.D.
Gustav Bychowski, M.D.
Frank Carrera III, M.D.
Ida Lou Coley, O.T.R.
Frank A. Dinello, Ph.D.
Johanna T. Dwyer, D.Sc.
Milton H. Erickson, M.D.
Jacob J. Feldman, Ph.D.
Helen H. Glaser, M.D.
Myron L. Glucksman, M.D.
Phillip B. Goldblatt, M.D.
Harry Gottesfeld, Ph.D.
Frederick W. Hanley, M.D.
Mary B. Harris, Ph.D.
Jules Hirsch, M.D.
J. M. C. Holden, M.R.C. Psych.
U. P. Holden, B.A.
Herbert Holt, M.D., Ph.D.
Eric J. Kahn, M.D.
William S. Kroger, M.D.
Ruth M. Lapi, M.D.

A. Russell Lee, M.D.
Dorothy G. Levin, P.S.W.
Veronica Liederman, M.A.
Robert S. McCully, Ph.D.
George L. Maddox, Ph.D.
Parker G. Marden, Ph.D.
Jean Mayer, Ph.D., D.Sc.
Myer Mendelson, M.D.
Mary E. Moore, M.D.
Susan Nathan, Ph.D.
Sidnor B. Penick, M.D.
Dorothy Pisula, Ph.D.
Hortense Powdermaker, Ph.D.
Ronald S. Reivich, M.D.
Rene A. Ruiz, Ph.D.
Stanley J. Schachter, Ph.D.
J. Trevor Silverstone, M.D.
E. James Stanley, M.D.
Richard B. Stuart, D.S.W.
Albert J. Stunkard, M.D.
David W. Swanson, M.D.
Charles Winick, Ph.D.
Janet P. Wollersheim, Ph.D.

Introduction

THIS volume attempts to delineate the best efforts of practitioners of various disciplines—psychoanalysts, psychiatrists, psychologists, internists, sociologists, demographers, anthropologists, and nutritionists—to solve the puzzle of obesity. While the experts have long understood the emotional bases of obesity, it is only within the last few years that inroads have been made in developing effective treatment procedures.

The "consuming passion" is a mysterious one. It has been, as Churchill put it in another context, a riddle wrapped in a mystery inside an enigma. Therapies still resist solutions although, as the behavior modification approach demonstrates, there is legitimate cause for optimism. To compound the problems, the proliferation of scientific information from research has resulted in an information gap among investigators as well as between doctors seeking to apply their knowledge on their patients. This gap is strikingly revealed in Stunkard's paper on the newer therapies. Although the behavior therapists have been working on obesity for a decade with far greater successful results than any other modality used, it is just now that psychiatry is becoming aware of the technique. Such parochialism is to be regretted. This book can, perhaps, serve as a bridge for it contains papers which present a variety of disciplines and subdisciplines, ranging from the traditional Freudian approach to behavior modification.

The essays indicate the complexities of the problem as well as the complexities of people; there is no single or simple answer to obesity. Whatever is ultimately discovered concerning obesity and the behavior of the obese will probably come about through a synthesis of theories involving multivariate disciplines. What is needed is a paradigm, a new key with which to decode the problems the investigator faces with the obese. With the discovery of a new paradigm, all the previous propositions, hypotheses, and theories will probably have to be profoundly changed, or at least modified. Perhaps behavior therapy has the key.

At this time, obesity is best viewed as having multiple causes: metabolic, neurological, psychological, and socioeconomic. Thus it is like many other disorders in medicine and especially those in psychiatry; an exact cause-and-effect relationship and pathophysiology is unknown.[1] The simplistic aphorism of Brillat-Savarin, "Tell me what you eat, and I will tell what you are," is too pat for credulity.

Although the field is relatively muddled, it is not the purpose of this volume to resolve the confusion or speciously inject order or clarity or connection where there is none. Without the help of systematic research—rigorously conducted to include control and experimental groups, adequate specifications of the independent variables with details of treatment procedures and replicability—the solution will continue to escape us. At present, with the exception of the behavior therapy approach, we have largely an accumulation of beliefs and dogmatically held preconceptions that are mostly irrefutable, unrepeatable, yet omnisciently interpretative. Further, dangerous jujus and gimcrack panaceas in dieting crop up regularly to lure the obese sufferer to illusory cures.

A definition of obesity is obviously desirable, but one that is precise and generally accepted does not exist.[2] The term obesity is derived from the Latin *obesus,* meaning to devour, and has many definitions, principally stated in terms of relationship between skeletal size and body weight.[3] Thus, Pargman[4] states that females who exceeded the upper limit of their appropriate weight range, according to the Metropolitan Life Insurance Company's *Desirable Weights of 1959,* were considered obese; males were classified as obese if they exceeded their appropriate weight by 20 per cent. MacBryde[5] defines obesity as that bodily state in which there is excessive accumulation of fat in both the relative and absolute sense. Becker[6] says that obesity is a state of having more weight than is consistent with the bodily build. On the other hand, Bychowski[7] observes that obesity is a somatic manifestation of a personality disturbance, as does Bruch.[8] Sperling states overeating and excessive gratification of oral instincts in reality are common; thus, she does not consider obesity a psychosomatic disorder but would place it, together with drug addicts and alcoholics, in the category of impulse-ridden characters.

However obesity may be defined, there is now general agreement that persistence in overeating has its basis in unresolved emotional problems and that the overeating serves as a substitute for other satisfactions. This finding is comparatively recent. One of the roadblocks to the understanding of obesity has been the failure to acknowledge the psychological aspects involved. The mind-body dichotomy that permeated so much of pre-Freudian medical thinking, and is still clung to by doctors more comfortable with the palpable soma than the spooky psyche is much in evidence when it comes to obesity. The traditional medical view blames the failure of the obese to diet simply on the inability to control food intake, a view that is as helpful as stating that alcoholics can not control their liquor consumption. But a more enlightened outlook perceives the adipose person as the victim of social and unconscious forces which compel him to persist in a repetitive, self-destructive pattern.

A recent editorial in the *Journal of the American Medical Association*[9] emphasizes the need to utilize psychology in the treatment program for adiposity.

Obesity is a major public health problem in America today. The Build and Blood Pressure Study of 1959 conducted by the Society of Actuaries reveals that over 30 per cent of adult Americans between the ages of 40 and 60 are more than 20 per cent overweight (Statistical Bulletin 41, January-April, 1960). These individuals have a greater than 40 per cent chance of dying in any given year from heart disease, greater than a 30 per cent chance of dying from coronary artery disease, a greater than 50 per cent death rate from cerebrovascular disease as well as an increased death rate from many other diseases. The data are undeniable, as is the fact that weight reduction will reduce the hazard of death from these causes. Unfortunately, only a small number of obese patients are unable to lose weight successfully, and an even smaller number are able to maintain the weight loss. Despite further recognition that obesity is a vocational and social disability, there is only limited understanding of the pathophysiology of this disorder and even less application of physiologic principles to weight reduction.

The final goal of the many therapeutic maneuvers which have been proposed to induce weight loss in obese individuals is induction of negative caloric balance to produce a significant decrease in total body fat. However, change in total body fat is not readily measured by either physician or patient, and one must rely on measurements of change in total body weight. It has long been recognized that the weight loss induced by a restricted caloric diet may exceed or be less than that anticipated from the caloric deficit provided. Total fasting is an excellent illustration of this phenomenon. Bloom,[10] who originally introduced fasting as a treatment for obesity, called attention to the fact that weight loss in fasting patients was greater than that which could be explained on a caloric basis. For example, a fat loss of 1.5 lb/day (0.7 kg) represents a calorie loss of approximately 6,100 calories. Subsequently, several investigators clearly demonstrated that the major portion of the weight loss induced by short-term fasting is water and protein. More recently, Ball and associates[11] studied obese patients during three consecutive thirty-two-day periods during which each patient fasted for sixteen days and then began an 800-calorie diet for sixteen days before again fasting. The major component of the weight loss during each starvation period was not fat but water and protein. The periods of calorie restriction which followed each starvation were characterized by minimal change in body weight, rapid reaccumulation of previously lost water and nitrogen, and continued loss of body fat. Confirming the observations of others that intermittent fasting will induce a net loss of body weight, these investigators also demonstrated that fat loss during short-term intermittent fasting is not greater than that recorded in the following periods of intermittent caloric restriction. The inability of obese individuals to accelerate fat loss in response to this therapeutic maneuver is intriguing, but at this time is unexplained.

Treatment of obesity is often a frustrating task. Consequently, the plethora of "treatments" that are published each year by physicians and laymen is not surprising. Unfortunately, most of these regimens are directed toward accelerating weight loss which is not necessarily the same as accelerating fat loss. Recognition of this discrepancy, coupled with the realization that the problems of the obese are not restricted to the area of caloric intake, begins to establish a foundation upon which to approach this disorder.

Studies published from several different laboratories would indicate that obese individuals respond to their environment in a manner which is quite different from that of people of normal weight. Obese individuals are frequently hostile, frustrated, and often severely depressed. The goal of weight loss is seen as a panacea to alleviate the multiple problems in their psychosocial and vocational lives. Weight reduction per se frequently causes these feelings to surface so that the thinned obese individuals find adjusting to their feeling extremely difficult and control of weight almost impossible. Clearly, achievement of weight loss should not be utilized as the sole end-point for therapy, but rather *treatment of the basic underlying emotional problems must be incorporated into the treatment program* (italics added).

Thus, obesity is presented as a disturbance of the whole person, with due recognition to the importance of psychological intervention. But one of the tragic themes running through most of the thirty articles in this collection is the frustration of treating the obese. The search persists. The proper therapeutic approach, wrote Bruch as long ago as 1948, is not through drugs or endocrine products, and not so much through diets as through an understanding and treatment of the emotional problems of the obese, their frustrations and anxieties. It was just fifty years ago that psychoanalytic psychology asserted that the compulsive need for eating went beyond meeting merely physiological needs and signified, rather, unrealized emotional drives.[12] At first, psychoanalysts tended to interpret all psychosomatic phenomena as if they were forms of conversion hysteria—a defense against unconscious wishes.

As practitioners gained more experience with obese patients, greater understanding developed. Soon there seemed to be as many theories concerning the dynamics and etiology of obesity as there were therapists. Reeve[13] attributed obesity to a sadomasochistic defensive system. According to Blazer,[14] the obese character is a stock character: the core of the problem is that the compulsive eater unconsciously has given up the struggle to preserve a nonderogatory attitude toward himself. Rascovsky[15] felt that the family environment of the obese child is characterized by an overprotecting and domineering mother who stimulates in an exaggerated fashion the relation of dependence on the child. Hammar[16] reported that even in the case of clinical problems which are generally regarded as constitutional in origin, there is evidence that modeling after the parents sometimes plays a major part in establishing the dysfunction. Lemieux and Martel[17] found that overeating by adolescents is a deficiency in emotional maturity.

Overeating has been most generally explicated as an activity to reduce anxiety caused by emotional conflicts. While not denying the presence of anxiety in obese patients, Holland and Ward[18] suggest that it is possible that those emotional conflicts upset physical homeostasis not through their effects of emotions such as anxiety, but rather through their effect upon a more basal level of central nervous system functioning, the midbrain or pain-pleasure level of functioning. The newer research findings of Penick and Stunkard[19] has attracted considerable attention. They have developed evidence that obesity is a disease of multiple etiology involving social factors, situational determinants, physiology of adipose tissue, disturbance of body image, and the effectiveness of behavioral measures for the control of obesity.

The few random studies just cited give a mere glimpse into the vast amount of work done in the field of obesity and psychiatry. Its attraction to investigators will continue as long as the problems persist and as long as the efforts to unravel the significances of the known factual data remain barren. The basic questions raised by Berblinger[20] need answers: Does the tendency to lose or gain weight reflect psychiatric illness? Is obesity the result of psychological trauma or a unified need? Does a change in one's body image lead to shifts in one's self-concept and self-esteem? Does weight gain have a conscious or unconscious purpose in an interpersonal situation?

Many psychiatrists have shown remarkably little interest in obesity.[21] Most physicians regard obesity as a sin and treat fat patients with disdain,[22] or chivvy them with a dietary admonishment. Until only recently, clinical psychologists let the experimentalists preempt the field. Behavior therapy has greatly expanded our knowledge of obesity, providing explanations that have important implications for effective diet control measures.[23-29] While its practitioners are hopeful, skeptics claim this approach may cure the symptom but not uncover the unconscious factors which lie behind the overeating. Thus, it is contended, behavior therapy may be a useful tool for special situations but does not yet provide the answers.

The use of aversion therapy, operant techniques, learning theory, drug therapy, group therapy, and the others generally prove the lack of efficiency of any one single method. While it is true that advances in medical and psychological knowledge have brought about increased understanding by the specialists, the ordinary individual suffering from the disorder still is likely to run the gamut of various therapeutic measures, managing to lose a few pounds but inevitably regaining them.

The articles in this volume speak for themselves. Written by some of the foremost authorities in the field, they cover the pantheon of problems manifest in the overweight and the obese. They range from discussions of dynamics and etiology to body image and self-concept, psychosocial factors, the varieties of techniques and therapies, including individual, group, and hypnosis, with children, adolescents, adults, and psychotics, to dieting and psychometrics. The idea of diversity in consideration of obesity permeates the book and is clearly illustrated by the journals from which the readings have been taken. They include such varied publications as the *Journal of the American Academy of Child Psychiatry, Psychosomatics, Clinical Pediatrics, Journal of Health and Social Behavior, Journal of Abnormal Psychology, Diseases of the Nervous System, Behaviour Research and Therapy,*

and the *Journal of Medical Education*. If obesity is to be approached holistically, then the diverse illustrations in this book should prove useful to
all interested in the problem.

NORMAN KIELL

January 6, 1972

REFERENCES

1. Swanson, D. W. and Dinello, F. A.: Severe obesity as a habitual syndrome. *Arch Gen Psychiat*, 22:120-127, 1970.
2. Macdonald, I.: Trends in the treatment of obesity. *Guy's Hosp Rep*, 119:329-336, 1970.
3. Kennedy, W. A. and Foreyt, J. P.: Control of eating behavior in an obese patient by avoidance conditioning. *Psychol Rep*, 22:571-576, 1968.
4. Pargman, D.: The incidence of obesity among college students. *J School Health*, 39:621-627, 1969.
5. MacBryde, I.: Obesity. *Proceedings of the Royal Society of Medicine*, 57:103-107, 1964.
6. Becker, B. J.: The obese patient in group psychoanalysis. *Amer J Psychother*, 14:322-337, 1960.
7. Bychowski, G.: On neurotic obesity. *Psychoanal & Psychoanal Rev*, 37:301-319, 1950.
8. Bruch, H.: Obesity. *Ped Clinics No Amer*, 613-627, 1958.
9. Editorial: *JAMA*, 211:492-493, 1970.
10. Bloom, W. L.: Fasting as an introduction to the treatment of obesity. *Metabolism*, 8:214-220, 1959.
11. Ball, M. F., Canary, J. J. and Kyle, L. H.: The tissue changes during intermittent starvation and calorie restriction as treatment for severe obesity. *Arch Intern Med*, 125:62-68, 1970.
12. Coriat, I. H.: Sex and hunger. *Psychoanal Rev*, 8:375-381, 1921.
13. Reeve, G. H.: Psychological factors in obesity. *Amer J Orthopsychiat*, 12:674-678, 1942.
14. Blazer, A.: The obese character: Psychodynamics and psychotherapy as an adjunct to medical management. *Int Rec Med*, 164:24-30, 1951.
15. Rascovsky, A.: Notas sobre la psicogénesis de la obesidad. *Prensa Medicale Argentina*, 15:1735-1739, 1948.
16. Hammar, S. L.: A study of adolescent obesity. In A. Bandura and R. H. Walters (Eds.), *Social Learning and Personality Development*, New York, Holt, Rinehart & Winston, 1964, 71.
17. Lemieux, R. and Martel, A.: L'obésité de la puberté. *Laval Médical*, 13:60-73, 1948.
18. Holland, B. C. and Ward, R. S.: Homeostasis and psychosomatic medicine. In S. Arieti (Ed.), *American Handbook of Psychiatry*, Vol. 3, New York, Basic Books, 1966, 344-361.
19. Penick, S. B. and Stunkard, A. J.: Newer concepts of obesity. *Med Clinics No Amer*, 54:745-754, 1970.
20. Berblinger, K. W.: Obesity—Psychologic stress: A cause or result. *Psychiat Opin*, 7:31-36, 1970.
21. Rubin, T. I.: Obesity: An addiction, incurable but controllable. *Roche Rep Frontiers of Psychiat*, 1(17):1-2, 8, 1971.

22. Kurland, H. D.: Obesity: An unfashionable problem. *Psychiat Opin,* 7:20-24, 1970.
23. Schachter, S.: Obesity and eating. *Science,* 16:751-756, 1968.
24. Schachter, S.: Some extraordinary facts about obese humans and rats. *Am Psychol,* 26:129-144, 1971.
25. Stuart, R. B.: Behavioral control of overeating. *Behav Res & Ther,* 5:357-365, 1967.
26. Stuart, R. B.: A three-dimensional program for the treatment of obesity. *Behav Res & Ther,* 9:177-186, 1971.
27. Harris, M. B.: Self-directed program for weight control: A pilot study. *J Abn Psychol,* 74:263-270, 1969.
28. Harris, M. B. and Bruner, C. G.: A comparison of a self-centered and a contract procedure for weight control. *Behav Res & Ther,* 9:347-354, 1971.
29. Wollersheim, J. P.: Effectiveness of group therapy based upon learning principles in the treatment of obese women. *J Abn Psychol,* 76:462-474, 1970.

Acknowledgments

I T is a pleasure to give acknowledgment and thanks to the twenty-seven editors and publishers in whose journals these articles originally appeared and to the forty-seven authors who wrote them. Their kindness in granting me permission to reproduce their work is deeply appreciated. The listing is congruent with the order of the articles as they appear in the book.

Penick, S. B. and Stunkard, A. J.: Newer concepts of obesity. *Medical Clinics of North America*, 54:745-754, 1970.

Schachter, S.: Some extraordinary facts about obese humans and rats. *American Psychologist*, 26:129-144, 1971. Copyright 1971, American Psychological Association.

Stunkard, A. J. and Mendelson, M.: Obesity and body image: Characteristics of disturbance in the body image of some obese persons. *American Journal of Psychiatry*, 123:1296-1300, 1967. Copyright 1967, the American Psychiatric Association.

Glucksman, M. L. and Hirsch, J.: The perception of body size. The response of obese patients to weight reduction. *Psychosomatic Medicine*, 31:1-7, 1969.

Goldblatt, P. B., Moore, M. E., and Stunkard, A. J.: Social factors in obesity. *Journal of the American Medical Association*, 192:1039-1044, 1965.

Silverstone, J. T.: Psychosocial aspects of obesity. *Proceedings of the Royal Society of Medicine*, 61:371-375, 1968.

Powdermaker, H.: An anthropological approach to the problems of obesity. *Bulletin of the New York Academy of Medicine*, 36:285-295, 1960. By permission of the Co-executors of the Estate of Hortense Powdermaker.

Maddox, G. L. and Liederman, V.: Overweight as a social disability with medical implications. *Journal of Medical Education*, 44:214-220, 1969.

Burnight, R. G. and Marden, P. G.: Social correlates of weight in an aging population. *Milbank Memorial Fund Quarterly*, 45:75-92, 1967.

Kahn, E. J.: Obesity in children: Identification of a group at risk in a New York ghetto. *Journal of Pediatrics*, 77:771-774, 1970. Copyrighted by The C. V. Mosby Co., St. Louis, Mo.

Carrera, F.: Obesity in adolescence. *Psychosomatics*, 8:342-349, 1967.

Nathan, S. and Pisula, D.: Psychological observations of obese adolescents during starvation treatment. *Journal of the American Academy of Child Psychiatry*, 9:722-740, 1970.

Stanley, E. J., Glaser, H. H., Levin, D. G., Adams, P. A. and Coley, I. L.: Overcoming obesity in adolescence. *Clinical Pediatrics*, 9:29-36, 1970.

Bychowski, G.: On neurotic obesity. *Psychoanalytic Review*, 27:301-319, 1950.

Lee, A. R.: Clinical symposium: Psychological and physiological aspects of marked obesity in a young adult female. *Journal of the Hillside Hospital*, 29:203-231, 1955.

Stuart, R. B.: A three-dimensional program for the treatment of obesity. *Behaviour Research and Therapy*, 9:177-186, 1971.

Holt, H. and Winick, C.: Group psychotherapy with obese women. *Archives of General Psychiatry,* 5:64-76, 1961. Copyright 1961, 1971.

Wollersheim, J. P.: Effectiveness of group therapy based upon learning principles in the treatment of obese women. *Journal of Abnormal Psychology,* 76:462-474, 1970. Copyright by the American Psychological Association.

Kroger, W. S.: Systems approach for understanding obesity: Management by behavioral modification through hypnosis. *Psychiatric Opinion,* 7:7-19, 1970.

Erickson, M. H.: The utilization of patient behavior in the hypnotherapy of obesity: Three case reports. *American Journal of Clinical Hypnosis,* 3:112-116, 1960.

Hanley, F. W.: The treatment of obesity by individual and group hypnosis. *Canadian Psychiatric Association Journal,* 12:549-551, 1967.

Dwyer, J. T., Feldman, J. J. and Mayer, J.: The social psychology of dieting. *Journal of Health and Social Behavior,* 11:269-287, 1970.

Swanson, D. W. and Dinello, F. A.: Therapeutic starvation in obesity. *Diseases of the Nervous System,* 30:669-674, 1969.

Harris, M. B. and Bruner, C.: A comparison of self-control and a contract procedure for weight control. *Behaviour Research and Therapy,* 9:347-354, 1971.

McCully, R. S., Glucksman, M. L., and Hirsch, J.: Nutrition imagery in the Rorschach materials of food-deprived, obese patients. *Journal of Projective Techniques and Personality Assessment,* 32:375-382, 1968. Copyright by the *Journal of Personality Assessment.*

Gottesfeld, H.: Body and self-cathexis of super-obese patients. *Journal of Psychosomatic Research,* 6:177-183, 1962. Copyright by Maxwell International Microforms Corp.

Reivich, R. S., Ruiz, R. A., and Lapi, R. M.: Extreme obesity—psychiatric, psychometric and psychotherapeutic. *Journal of the Kansas Medical Society,* 67:134-140, 146, 1966.

Holden, J. M. C. and Holden, U. P.: Weight changes with schizophrenic psychosis and psychotropic drug therapy. *Psychosomatics,* 11:551-561, 1970.

Bernard, J. L.: Rapid treatment of gross obesity by operant techniques. *Psychological Reports,* 23:663-666, 1968.

Contents

Chapter

I
DYNAMICS AND ETIOLOGY

II
BODY IMAGE

III
PSYCHOSOCIAL FACTORS

IV
CHILDHOOD AND ADOLESCENT OBESITY

X
PSYCHOSES

THE PSYCHOLOGY OF OBESITY

I
DYNAMICS AND ETIOLOGY

1

Newer Concepts of Obesity

Sidnor B. Penick
AND
Albert J. Stunkard

RECENT research on obesity has done far more than merely advance our understanding of this condition. In distinction to most earlier research in the field, it has provided information upon which it may be possible for the first time to construct effective treatment programs. This is welcome news, for careful study of the results of treatment for obesity have revealed that "most obese persons will not enter treatment; of those who do, most will not lose weight; and of those who lose weight, most will regain it."[19]

The traditional medical view ascribes these failures quite simply to an inability of obese persons to control their food intake—an observation approximately as helpful as that which ascribes alcoholism to an inability to control alcohol intake. The traditional response of physicians has been similar—frustration and even anger.

Newer research findings have provided support for the concept that obesity is a disease of multiple etiology. Evidence has been developed of a) the influence of social factors upon the prevalence of obesity, b) the influence of situational determinants upon overeating, c) distinctive characteristics of the physiology of adipose tissue, d) the determinants of disturbance in the body image of some obese persons, and e) the effectiveness of behavioral measures for the control of obesity.

SOCIAL CLASS AND OBESITY

Within the very recent past a series of studies have documented precisely a heretofore suspected determinant of obesity: social class. To a remarkable degree the prevalence of obesity in the general population is under the control of social factors. The most carefully studied is probably socioeconomic status, as defined by education and occupation. In at least three urban populations in the United States and Great Britain, socioeconomic status is inversely related to the prevalence of obesity, particularly in women, and often to a surprising degree.

The first dramatic evidence of the influence of social factors came from the Midtown Manhattan study, a comprehensive survey of the epidemiology of mental illness. Subjects consisted of 1660 adults, between the ages of twenty and fifty-nine, selected by stratified random sampling so that their social class distribution approximated that of a far larger area. Subjects were divided into three weight categories, "obese," "normal," and "thin," by measures whose validity seems acceptable. Socioeconomic status was rated through an interview by a simple score based upon occupation, education, weekly income, and monthly rent, and these scores were divided into "low," "medium," and "high."

There was a marked inverse relationship between the prevalence of obesity and socioeconomic status. Data show that the prevalence of obesity among women of lower socioeconomic status was 30 per cent, falling to 16 per cent among those of middle status, and to only 5 per cent in the upper status group. The prevalence of obesity in the lower class was thus six times that found in the upper class! And when socioeconomic status was divided into twelve classes, as the richness of the data permitted, the difference between the lowermost and uppermost social classes became even greater, from a low of less than 2 per cent in the uppermost to a high of 37 per cent in the lowermost class.

Among men, the differences between social classes were similar, but of lesser degree. Men of lower socioeconomic status, for example, showed a prevalence of obesity of 32 per cent as contrasted with a prevalence of 16 per cent among upper-class men.

One notable feature of this study was that it was designed to permit causal inferences about the influence of social factors. Earlier studies, which had demonstrated associations between socioeconomic status and psychiatric disorders, had been unable to go beyond these correlations to any statements about cause. The Midtown study, however, ascertained not only the socioeconomic status of the respondent at the time of the study, but also that of his parents when he was eight years old. Although a subject's schizophrenia, or obesity, might conceivably influence his own social class, his disability in adult life could not have influenced that of his parents. Therefore, associations between the social class of the respondent's parents and his disability can be viewed as causal. The preceding data show that such associations were almost as powerful as those between the social class of the respondents and their obesity!

The influence of socioeconomic status on the prevalence of obesity was confirmed by two recent studies. One, from London, found an inverse relationship between social class and obesity, although the differences were less marked than in Manhattan.[14] The second, carried out by Hinkle *et al.* on the executives of the Bell Telephone system, was designed to determine the effect of socioeconomic status and social mobility upon the incidence of coronary heart disease. In dramatic contrast to expectations, it was found that socioeconomic status and upward social mobility were *inversely* related to coronary heart disease.[4] These findings were the opposite of the stereotype of coronary disease as the consequence of the drive for achievement and the pressures of responsibility. Examination of the data revealed that obesity was also inversely correlated with status, in part explaining the distribution of coronary heart disease.

SITUATIONAL DETERMINANTS OF OVEREATING

As sociology has demonstrated the impact of environment in a broad sense upon human obesity, experimental social psychology has been able to pinpoint specific situations in which immediate environment exerts an impact. Recent studies have demonstrated the surprising degree to which the eating behavior of obese people is under environmental control.

These studies, by Stanley Schachter and his students,[13] might be said to take their theme from the title of an old paper by Neal Miller,[9] "Decreased hunger and increased food intake in hypothalamic obese rats." In this remarkably prescient study, Miller described for the first time the peculiar feeding behavior of rats made obese by hypothalamic lesions. The cardinal feature of this behavior was that obese rats overate when food was freely available, but when an impediment was placed in the way of their eating, food intake not only decreased, but actually decreased to a far lower level than that of control rats without hypothalamic lesions. Furthermore, it seemed to make little difference what kind of impediment was used. Motivation to work for food was impaired by every task that was devised. These tasks included lifting the covers to food cages, lever pressing for food, accepting the discomfort of crossing an electrified grid, or tolerating dilution of their food with quinine. These studies exploded traditional views of "hunger" as a unitary phenomenon. Hunger as defined by food intake can be quite a different matter from hunger as defined by motivation to work for food.

Study of behavior of hypothalamic obese animals suggests that behavior is characterized by an impairment in the mechanism of satiety, and probably also by an impairment in the drive to eat, as measured in standard experimental situations.[3, 9] This view of the food intake of hypothalamic obese animals has proved congenial to clinicians who have dealt with obese persons. A characteristic complaint is an inability to stop eating once they have started, and it is the exceptional obese person who presents a picture of voracious overeating, or a desire for food which drives him in the way that a desire for narcotics drives the addict, or the need for a drink drives the alcoholic. Until the work of Schachter, however, such characterizations had been based largely upon self reports, and the problem had not been approached experimentally. To a large degree this failure had been based upon the great difficulty in getting obese persons to approximate their usual food intake when they entered a laboratory or, indeed, any controlled environment. Instead, most obese persons undereat and lose weight when they enter a hospital, even when access to food is unrestricted and when they are encouraged to maintain their body weight temporarily. The "impediment" in this situation is observation of eating behavior by medical personnel. In years of study of obese persons under a variety of conditions, we have observed only one in the act of overeating.

An ingenious experiment by Nisbett[11] assessed in man the behavior described by Miller for hypothalamic obese rats—relative overeating when food was freely available and relative undereating when an impediment was placed in their way. Subjects, who were male university students, were invited to participate in an experiment which was presented to them as an investigation of certain physiological variables. They were told that in order to obtain accurate baselines, it was essential that they not eat after 9:00 AM on the day of the test. Appointments were made for early afternoon hours so that the minimum period of food deprivation was four hours. Bogus recording electrodes were attached to the subjects, and they performed a monitoring task for approximately thirty minutes. At the end of this period the experimenter announced that the experiment was over, disengaged the subjects from their electrodes, and led them into another room "to fill out some final questionnaires."

The new experimental room contained a refrigerator, a chair, and a table on which were a bottle of soda and either one roast beef sandwich or three roast beef sandwiches. While the subject sat down, the experimenter said casually, "Since you skipped lunch for the experiment, we would like to give you lunch now. You can fill out the questionnaires while you eat. There are dozens more sandwiches in the refrigerator, by the way; have as many as you want." The experimenter asked the subject to check by his office on the way out, and then left, shutting the door behind him.

The procedure was designed to reduce any possible self-consciousness on the part of the overweight subjects in a number of ways. First, the experimenter was absent while the subject ate, and the meal was completely private. The subject could assume that he would not be interrupted because he was to go to the experimenter's office when he was through. Second, the subject was told that there were dozens of sandwiches in the refrigerator and could assume that if he were to take one or two they would not be missed. Third, the subject was given no reason to believe that the experimenter had any interest in how many sandwiches he ate.

Food intake of the obese persons paralleled that of the obese rats. When provided relatively unlimited access to food (under the three-sandwich condition), the obese persons ate considerably more than did their normal weight controls. When the impediment of taking additional food from the refrigerator was introduced in the one-sandwich condition, however, the food intake of the obese subjects fell considerably below that of the controls. This simple and striking experiment is probably the first direct demonstration in man of a kind of eating behavior characteristic of a wide variety of experimentally obese animals.

PHYSIOLOGIC STUDIES OF ADIPOSE TISSUE

A series of classic studies by Hirsch and his colleagues have established that the fundamental characteristics of adipose tissue are determined early in life.[5, 6, 12] The state of nutrition of a rat during its first three weeks of life, for example, determines the subsequent character of its adipose tissue and even its future size. Overfeeding during this critical period produces a highly cellular adipose tissue, whereas undernutrition results in tissue with an abnormally low number of adipose tissue cells. With increasing age, adipose tissue progressively loses its ability to grow by cellular hyperplasia, and by adult life, any increase in body fat is accomplished by an increase in cell size, not by an increase in cell number. The marked obesity produced in adult rats by hypothalamic lesions, for example, was achieved solely by increased cell size, with no change in the number of adipose tissue cells.

The development of a convenient needle biopsy of human adipose tissue has permitted the extension of these studies to human obesity. Results are entirely consistent with those from lower animals. For example, there was little difference in the metabolism of fat samples obtained from obese and nonobese subjects. Furthermore, serial studies of obese subjects during weight reduction revealed that the loss in body fat resulted entirely from a decrease in the size of adipose tissue cells, and not from a decrease in the number of these cells.

The latter findings may explain the carbohydrate intolerance of obese persons, and the restoration of carbohydrate tolerance following weight loss, for the *in vitro* insulin sensitivity of adipose tissue depends upon the size of the cells and not upon their number. In any given sample of adipose tissue, the larger the cells, the less responsive the sample is to insulin. And it is precisely the size of cells and not their number which is decreased in weight reduction.

This work has important implications for our understanding of obesity in man. The fact that cell number does not change in adult life implies a critical period in man, as in the rat, during which the number of adipose tissue cells is established for life. Persons who become obese during this period, perhaps in infancy, perhaps in childhood, may do so through hyperplasia of adipose tissue cells, in contrast to those who become obese in adult life. If this is the case, one would expect them to experience a greater difficulty in weight reduction, for they would be dealing with the double burden of an increased number and an increased size of adipose tissue cells. A person with adult-onset obesity could return to a normal weight simply by emptying his adipose tissue cells of their excessive load of fat. One suffering from juvenile-onset obesity, on the other hand, might be able to achieve a similar degree of weight loss only by decreasing the fat content of his excessive number of adipose tissue cells to an abnormally low concentration.

Clinical experience accords well with these predictions. Juvenile-onset obesity is more resistant to treatment than obesity beginning in adult life. And, as noted below, such persons seem more vulnerable to psychological complications of obesity. Recognition of these factors may help us set more realistic treatment goals for persons with juvenile-onset obesity, decreasing the frustration of the physician and, more importantly, of his patients.

DISTURBANCES IN BODY IMAGE

A distinctive kind of disturbance in body image is one of the very few psychopathological characteristics specific to obesity. These disturbances, which affect only some obese persons, appear to be persistent, unaffected by weight reduction, even of long duration, and relieved only by psychotherapy—often not even then.

A study of seventy-four randomly selected obese persons revealed disturbances in three aspects of the body image of some of these persons.[18] Interestingly, other obese persons were entirely free of this disorder. The disturbances were noted in a) view of the self: many patients were revolted by the sight of their bodies and were almost unable to look into a mirror; some avoided activities such as shopping for fear of catching glimpses of themselves in store windows; b) self-consciousness in general: many obese persons harbored an intense self-consciousness and even misconceptions of how others viewed them; they sometimes seemed to feel that nothing ever happened to them except in some kind of (usually derogatory) relationship to their weight; c) self-consciousness in relation to the opposite sex: these disturbances ranged from avoidance and inhibitions to hateful devaluation of the opposite sex.

One of the most surprising aspects of the body image disturbance was the age of onset. Disturbances occurred almost exclusively among persons who had become obese during childhood or adolescence. Table 1-I shows that not one of forty subjects with adult-onset obesity showed a severe body image disturbance, while such disturbances were found in fully half of those with onset of obesity in childhood or adolescence, the so-called "juvenile obese."

TABLE 1-I

DEGREE OF BODY IMAGE DISTURBANCE ACCORDING TO AGE OF
ONSET OF OBESITY IN SEVENTY-FOUR PERSONS

Onset Category	Severe	Mild	None
Juvenile	17	8	9
Adult	0	10	30

$\chi^2 = 19.44$, df = 2, p < .001.

Further study of juvenile obese subjects strongly suggested that adolescence constituted a kind of critical period for the development of these disturbances in body image, and that the disorder was largely confined to persons who were obese during these impressionable years. This presumption strengthens the argument for the prevention of obesity in childhood, and for prompt treatment of children who become obese. The difficulty of this latter task is well documented by a further finding of this study. In a group of nearly 2000 children followed for a period of thirty years, the odds against an obese child becoming a normal weight adult were 4 to 1; for those who did not reduce during adolescence they were more than 28 to 1!

An intriguing experimental study of disturbances in body image of obese persons was carried out by means of a projector with a distorting lens which could be manipulated to make pictures of the subjects seem leaner or fatter than they were. Six severely obese adults were studied during a period of several months hospitalization for weight reduction. At the beginning of the study, all six patients slightly underestimated their actual size. As weight loss proceeded, however, they began to overestimate their actual size, and this trend continued throughout the period of weight loss. Their estimations of the body size of other persons showed no such distortions. These findings suggest that the internalized image of the body size of these patients was relatively fixed, and could not be altered as rapidly as the actual change in body configuration.

IMPLICATIONS FOR TREATMENT

The newer research findings have two implications for therapy. There is a strong probability that obese persons, particularly those with early onset of obesity, suffer from a metabolic disorder. Nevertheless, their food intake is determined to a considerable degree by environmental factors. Appropriate use of these findings could be effective in the control of food intake by obese persons.

The traditional medical model could well be considered an inappropriate use of these findings. This model defines an authoritarian role for the physician, who prescribes a diet and appetite-depressing medication. The patient loses weight, if at all, in large part to please the doctor and to meet his expectations. When the relationship is terminated or attenuated, the patient discontinues the diet and regains weight.

Systematic application of the principles of the new field of the experimental analysis of behavior (behavior therapy) may help the physician design programs more suited to the needs of the obese patient. Recent reviews of the field are commended to the reader.[7, 20] Stuart has reported results which appear better than any yet reported in the medical literature.[16] However, controlled studies with longer follow-up periods must be carried out.

Stuart has published details of his program, which consists, initially, of

twelve to fifteen sessions of thirty minutes each, occurring three times a
week. Subsequent treatment sessions occurred as needed, usually at intervals of two weeks for the next three months, followed by sessions on a
planned monthly basis, as well as "maintenance" session as needed.

Daily records of food intake and body weight were kept by each patient.
These records were notable for their great detail. For example, the food
intake record listed the time, nature, quantity, and circumstances of all
food and fluid intake, while the weight record consisted of weights recorded four times a day—before breakfast, after breakfast, after lunch, and before bedtime. Initial efforts were directed primarily toward helping the patient gain control over the time and circumstances of his eating, rather than
toward weight loss. For example, a measure introduced early into the treatment consisted of interrupting the meal for a predetermined period of time,
usually two or three minutes, gradually increased to five minutes. The patient was instructed to put down his utensils and merely sit in his place at
the table for this period of time. The rationale of this maneuver was to give
the patient, as early as possible, an experience of control over one aspect of
his eating, however small, and to learn that eating was a response which
could be broken down into components which could be successfully mastered. Another early device was an attempt to make eating a "pure experience," paired with no other activity such as reading, listening to the radio,
watching television, or talking with friends. The rationale of this maneuver was to keep eating separate from any other behavior which might induce
eating to continue as a conditioned response to the occurrence of the other
behavior. Only after a variety of such techniques of self-control had been
mastered did weight loss become a major focus of treatment.

Stuart treated patients individually. The possibility of utilizing group
methods for teaching behavioral controls of eating raises the hope of multi-
plying the effectiveness of a potentially effective technique. Recently evidence has been obtained that group therapy of obesity is superior to individual therapy, under a variety of treatment conditions.[8] Furthermore,
there is a strong reason to believe that major assistance in the control of
obesity is available from patient self-help groups. Very recently a study of
such a group (Take Off Pounds Sensibly—TOPS) has revealed that the
average results obtained by twenty-two chapters compare favorably with
those achieved by medical management, and that the results of the most effective chapters rank with the very best results in the medical literature.[17]

SUMMARY

Research on obesity has recently produced new evidence for the influence
of both metabolic and behavioral factors in its etiology. Both kinds of factors have therapeutic significance. In the metabolic area, evidence that the

total fat cell content of adipose tissue may be determined early in life may help to set more realistic goals for the notoriously difficult treatment of persons suffering from juvenile-onset obesity. Recent behavioral discoveries may have more positive therapeutic consequences. Three such discoveries are the marked influence of social factors on the prevalence of obesity, the large effect of situational determinants on the eating behavior of obese persons, and the surprising effectiveness reported by one study on the behavioral management of obesity. These findings give reasonable grounds for hope of improvement in our traditionally poor results of treatment for obesity.

REFERENCES

1. Glucksman, M. L. and Hirsch, J.: The response of obese patients to weight reduction. III. The perception of body size. *Psychosom Med*, 31:1, 1969.
2. Goldblatt, P. B., Moore, M. E. and Stunkard, A. J.: Social factors in obesity. *JAMA*, 192:1039, 1965.
3. Graff, H. and Stellar, E.: Hyperphagia, obesity and finickiness. *J Comp Physiol Psychol*, 55:418, 1962.
4. Hinkle, L. E., Jr.: Occupation, education and coronary heart disease. *Science*, 161: 238, 1968.
5. Hirsch, J. and Knittle, J. L.: Cellularity of obese and nonobese human adipose tissue. *Fed Proc*, 1969.
6. Knittle, J. L. and Hirsch, J.: Effect of early nutrition on the development of rat epididymal fat pads: Cellularity and metabolism. *J Clin Invest*, 47:2091, 1968.
7. Krasner, L. and Ullmann, L. P. (Ed.): *Research in Behavior Modification*. New York, Holt, Rinehart and Winston, 1965.
8. Louden, A. M. and Schreiber, E. D.: A controlled study of the effects of group discussions and an anorexiant in outpatient treatment of obesity with attention to the psychological aspects of dieting. *Ann Int Med*, 65:80, 1966.
9. Miller, M. E., Bailey, C. J. and Stevenson, J. A. F.: Decreased hunger and increased food intake in hypothalamic obese rats. *Science*, 112:256, 1950.
10. Moore, M. E., Stunkard, A. J. and Srole, L.: Obesity, social class, and mental illness. *JAMA*, 181:962, 1962.
11. Nisbett, R. E.: Determinants of food intake in obesity. *Science*, 159:1254, 1968.
12. Salons, L. B., Knittle, J. L. and Hirsch, J.: Role of adipose cell size and adipose tissue insulin sensitivity in the carbohydrate intolerance of human obesity. *J Clin Invest*, 47:153, 1968.
13. Schachter, S.: Obesity and eating. *Science*, 161:751, 1968.
14. Silverstone, J. T., Gordon, R. P. and Stunkard, A. J.: Social factors in obesity in London. *The Practitioner*, 202:682, 1969.
15. Srole, L., *et al.*: *Mental Health in the Metropolis. Midtown Manhattan Study*. New York, McGraw-Hill Book Co., Inc., 1962.
16. Stuart, R. B.: Behavioral control of overeating. *Behav Res Ther*, 5:357, 1967.
17. Stunkard, A. J., Levine, H. and Fox, S.: A study of a patient self-help group for obesity. Proceedings Eighth International Congress of Nutrition, Prague, 1969 (in press).
18. Stunkard, A. J. and Burt, V.: Obesity and the body image. II. Age at onset of disturbances in the body image. *Am J Psychiat*, 123:1443, 1967.

19. Stunkard, A. and McLaren-Hume, M.: Results of treatment for obesity. A review of the literature and report of a series. *Arch Int Med*, 102:79, 1959.
20. Ullmann, L. P. and Krasner, L. (Eds.): *Case Studies in Behavior Modification*. New York, Holt, Rinehart and Winston, 1965.
21. Blohmke, M., Depner, R., Koschorreck, B. and Stelzer, O.: Uebergewichtigkeit bei berufstätigen Frauen in Abhängigkeit ausgewählter biologischer und sozialer Faktoren. Arbeitsmedizin, Sozialmedizin, *Arbeitshygeiene*, 4:190, 1969.

2

Some Extraordinary Facts About Obese Humans and Rats

STANLEY J. SCHACHTER

SEVERAL years ago, when I was working on the problem of the labeling of bodily states, I first became aware of Stunkard's[34] work on obesity and gastric motility. At that time, my students and I had been working on a series of studies concerned with the interaction of cognitive and physiological determinants of emotional state.[27] Our experiments had all involved manipulating bodily state by injections of adrenalin or placebo and simultaneously manipulating cognitive and situational variables that were presumed to affect a subject's interpretation of his bodily state. In essence, these experiments had demonstrated that cognitive factors play a major role in determining how a subject interprets his bodily feelings. Precisely the same set of physiological symptoms—an adrenaline-induced state of sympathetic arousal—could be interpreted as euphoria, or anger, or anxiety, or indeed as no emotional state at all, depending very largely on our cognitive and situational manipulations. In short, there is not an invariant, one-to-one relationship between a set of physiological symptoms and a psychological state.

This conclusion was based entirely on studies that manipulated bodily state by the exogenous administration of adrenalin or some other agent. My interest in Stunkard's research was generated by the fact that his work suggested that the same conclusion might be valid for endogenous physiological states. In his study, Stunkard had his subjects do without breakfast and come to his laboratory at 9:00 AM. They swallowed a gastric balloon, and for the next four hours, Stunkard continuously recorded stomach contractions. Every fifteen minutes, he asked his subjects, "Do you feel hungry?" They answered "Yes" or "No," and that is all there was to the study. He has then a record of the extent to which stomach contractions coincide with self-reports of hunger. For normally sized subjects, the two coincide closely. When the stomach contracts, the normal subject is likely to report hunger; when the stomach is quiescent, the normal subject is likely to say that he does not feel hungry. For the obese, on the other hand, there is little correspondence between gastric motility and self-reports of hunger. Whether or not the obese subject describes himself as hungry seems to have almost

15

nothing to do with the state of his gut. There are, then, major individual differences in the extent to which this particular bodily activity—gastric motility—is associated with the feeling state labeled "hunger."

To pursue this lead, we[31] designed an experiment in which we attempted to manipulate gastric motility and the other physiological correlates of food deprivation by the obvious technique of manipulating food deprivation so that some subjects had empty stomachs and others full stomachs before entering an experimental eating situation. The experiment was disguised as a study of taste, and subjects had been asked to do without the meal (lunch or dinner) that preceded the experiment.

When a subject arrived, he was, depending on condition, either fed roast beef sandwiches or fed nothing. He was then seated in front of five bowls of crackers, presented with a long set of rating scales and told, "We want you to judge each cracker on the dimensions (salty, cheesy, garlicky, etc.) listed on these sheets. Taste as many or as few of the crackers of each type as you want in making your judgments; the important thing is that your ratings be as accurate as possible."

The subject then tasted and rated crackers for 15 minutes, under the impression that this was a taste test, and we simply counted the number of crackers that he ate. There were, of course, two types of subjects: obese subjects (from 14% to 75% overweight) and normal subjects (from 8% underweight to 9% overweight).

To review expectations: If it is correct that the obese do not label as hunger the bodily states associated with food deprivation, then this manipulation should have no effect on the amount eaten by obese subjects; on the other hand, the eating behavior of normal subjects should directly parallel the effects of the manipulation on bodily state.

It will be a surprise to no one to learn that normal subjects ate considerably fewer crackers when their stomachs were full of roast beef sandwiches than when their stomachs were empty. The results for obese subjects stand in fascinating contrast. They ate as much, in fact slightly more, when their stomachs were full as when they were empty. Obviously, the actual state of the stomach has nothing to do with the eating behavior of the obese.*

In similar studies[28, 29] we have attempted to manipulate bodily state by manipulating fear and by injecting subjects with epinephrine. Both manipulations are based on Cannon's[4] and Carlson's[5] demonstrations that both the state of fear and the injection of epinephrine will inhibit gastric motility and increase blood sugar—both peripheral physiological changes associated

---

* The obese subject's failure to regulate when preloaded with sandwiches or some other solid food has now been replicated three times. Pliner's recent work,[21] however, indicates that the obese will regulate, though not as well as normals, when preloaded with liquid food.

with low hunger. These manipulations have no effect at all on obese subjects, but do affect the amounts eaten by normal subjects.

It seems clear that the set of bodily symptoms the subject labels "hunger" differs for obese and normal subjects. Whether one measures gastric motility as Stunkard did, or manipulates motility and the other physiological correlates of food deprivation, as I assume my students and I have done, one finds, for normal subjects, a high degree of correspondence between the state of the gut and eating behavior and, for obese subjects, virtually no correspondence.

Whether or not they are responsive to these particular visceral cues, the obese *do* eat, and the search for the cues that trigger obese eating occupied my students' and my attention for a number of years. Since the experimental details of this search have been published, and I believe are fairly well known, I will take time now only to summarize our conclusions—eating by the obese seems unrelated to any internal, visceral state, but is determined by external, food-relevant cues such as the sight, smell, and taste of food. Now, obviously, such external cues to some extent affect anyone's eating behavior. However, for normals these external factors clearly interact with internal state. They may affect what, where, and how much the normal eats, but chiefly when he is in a state of physiological hunger. For the obese, I suggest, internal state is irrelevant, and eating is determined largely by external cues.

As you may know, there have been a number of experiments testing this hypothesis about the external sensitivity of the obese. To convey some feeling for the nature of the supporting data, I will describe two typical experiments. In one of these, Nisbett[18] examined the effects of the sight of food. He reasoned that if the sight of food is a potent cue, the externally sensitive, obese person should eat just as long as food is in sight, and when, in effect, he has consumed all of the available cues, he should stop and make no further attempt to eat. In contrast, the amounts eaten by a normal subject should depend on his physiological needs, not on the quantity of food in sight. Thus, if only a small amount of food is in sight but the subject is given the opportunity to forage for more, the normal subject should eat more than the obese subject. In contrast, if a large amount of food is in sight, the obese should eat more than the normal subject.

To test these expectations, Nisbett provided subjects, who had not eaten lunch, with either one or three roast beef sandwiches. He told them to help themselves and, as he was leaving, pointed to a refrigerator across the room and said, "There are dozens more sandwiches in the refrigerator. Have as many as you want." His results are presented in Table 2-I. As you can see, obese subjects ate significantly more than normals when presented with three sandwiches, but ate significantly less than normals when presented with only one sandwich.

TABLE 2-I

EFFECT OF QUANTITY OF VISIBLE FOOD ON AMOUNTS EATEN

Subjects	No. Sandwiches	
	One	Three
Normal	1.96	1.88
Obese	1.48	2.32

Note: From Nisbett (1968a).

In another study, Decke[6] examined the effects of taste on eating. She reasoned that taste, like the sight or smell of food, is essentially an external cue. Good taste, then, should stimulate the obese to eat more than normals, and bad taste, of course, should have the reverse effect.

In a taste test context, Decke provided her subjects with either a decent vanilla milkshake or with a vanilla milkshake plus quinine. The effects of this taste manipulation are conveyed in Table 2-II where obese subjects drank more than normals when the milkshake was good and drank considerably less when the milkshake had been laced with quinine.

Now, anyone who sees Decke's milkshake data and who is familiar with physiological psychology will note that this is precisely what Miller, Bailey, and Stevenson[16] found and what Teitelbaum[35] found in the lesioned hyperphagic rat. For those of you who are unfamiliar with this preparation, let me review the facts about this animal. If you make bilateral lesions in the ventromedial nuclei of the hypothalamus, you are likely to get an animal that will eat prodigious amounts of food and will eventually achieve monumental weight—a creature of nightmares. This has been demonstrated for rats, cats, mice, monkeys, rabbits, goats, dogs, and sparrows. Classic descriptions of these preparations portray an animal that immediately after the operation staggers over to its food hopper and shovels in food. For several weeks, this voracious eating continues, and there is, of course, very rapid weight gain. This is called the dynamic phase of hyperphagia. Finally, a plateau is reached, at which point the animal's weight levels off, and its food intake drops to a level only slightly above that of the normal animal. This is called the static phase. During both the static and the dynamic stages, the

TABLE 2-II

EFFECT OF TASTE ON EATING

Subjects	Ounces Consumed in	
	Good Taste	Bad Taste
Normal	10.6	6.4
Obese	13.9	2.6

Note: From Decke (1971).

lesioned animal is also characterized as markedly inactive, and as irascible, emotional, and generally bitchy.

Now it turns out that though the lesioned animal is normally a heavy eater, if you add quinine to its food it drastically decreases its intake to levels far below that of a normal animal's whose food has been similarly tainted. On the other hand, if to its normal food you add dextrose, or lard, or something that is apparently tasty to a rat, the lesioned animal increases its intake to levels considerably above its regular intake and above the intake of a control rat whose food has also been enriched.

The similarity of these facts about the finickiness of the lesioned rat to Decke's findings in her milkshake experiment is, of course, striking, and many people[18, 20] have pointed to this and other similarities between our data on obese humans and the physiologist's data on the obese rat. In order to determine if there was anything more to this than an engaging, occasional resemblance between two otherwise remotely connected sets of data, Judith Rodin and I decided to treat the matter dead seriously and, where possible, to make a point-for-point comparison of every fact we could learn about the hypothalamic, obese rat with every fact we could learn about the obese human. Before describing the results of our work, I would like, however, to be sure that you are aware of the areas of my expertise. I am not a physiological psychologist. Though I am pretty sure that I have eaten a hypothalamus, I doubt that I have ever seen one. When I say something like "bilateral lesions of the ventromedial nuclei of the hypothalamus," you can be sure that I've memorized it. I make this personal confession because of the dilemma that Rodin, also a physiological innocent, and I faced in our work. Though we couldn't have succeeded, we attempted to read *every-thing* about the ventromedial lesioned rat. If you've ever made this sort of attempt, you may have been seized by the same despair as were we when it sometimes seemed as if there were no such thing as a fact that *someone* had not failed to confirm. (I include in this sweeping generalization, by the way, the apparent fact that a ventromedial lesion produces a hyperphagic, obese animal.[22, 24]) And it sometimes seemed as if there were no such thing as an experiment which *someone* had not failed to replicate. Since I happen to have spent my college physics lab course personally disproving most of the laws of physics, I cannot say that I find this particularly surprising, but if one is trying to decide what is the fact, it is a depressing state of affairs. In our own areas of expertise, this probably isn't too serious a problem. Each of us in our specialties knows how to evaluate a piece of work. In a field in which you are not expert, you simply cannot, except in the crudest of cases, evaluate. If several experimenters have different results, you just don't know which to believe. In order to cope with this dilemma, Rodin and I decided to treat each of our facts in batting average terms. For each fact, I will inform you of the number of studies that have been concerned with the fact and the proportion of these studies that work out in a given direction. To be included in the batting average, we required only that a study present all or a substantial portion of its data, rather than report the author's impressions or present only the data of one or two presumably representative cases. I should also note that in all cases we have relied on the data and not on what the experimenter said about the data. It may seem silly to make this point explicit, but it is the case that in a few studies, for some perverse reason, the experimenter's conclusions simply have nothing to do with his data. Finally, I should note that in all comparisons of animal and human data, I will consider the data only for animals in the static phase of obesity, animals who, like our human subjects, are already fat. In general, however, the results for dynamic and static animals are quite similar.

As a shorthand method of making comparisons between studies and species, I shall throughout the rest of this article employ what we can call a Fat to Normal (F/N) ratio in which we simply get an index by dividing the magnitude of the effect for fat subjects by the magnitude of the effect for normal control subjects. Thus, if in a particular study the fat rats ate an average of 15 gm of food and normal rats ate 10 gm, the F/N ratio would be 1.50, indicating that the fat rats ate 50 per cent more food than normal rats.

To begin our comparisons, let us return to the effects of taste on eating behavior. We know that fat human beings eat more of a good-tasting food than do normal human beings and that they eat less of bad-tasting food than do normals. The physiologists have done almost identical experiments to ours, and in Line 1 of Table 2-III we can compare the effects of good-tasting food on lesioned animals and on men. You will notice on the left that Rodin and I found six studies on lesioned animals, in this case largely rats. Batting average: five of the six studies indicate that lesioned, static, obese animals eat more of a good-tasting food than do their normal controls. The average F/N ratio for these six studies is 1.45, indicating that fat rats on the average eat 45 per cent more of good-tasting food than do normal rats. On the right side of the table, you can see that there have been two human studies, and that both of these studies indicate that fat humans eat more of good-tasting food than do normal humans. The average F/N ratio for humans is 1.42, indicating that fat humans eat 42 per cent more of good-tasting food than do normally sized humans.[*]

---

[*] The technically informed reader undoubtedly will wish to know precisely which studies and what data are included in Tables 2-III and 2-IV. There are so many studies involved that, within the context of this paper, it is impossible to supply this information. Dr. Rodin and I are preparing a monograph on this work which will, of course, provide full details on such matters.

TABLE 2-III

EFFECTS OF TASTE ON EATING

Condition	Animals		Humans	
	Batting Average	Mean F/N	Mean F/N	Batting Average
Good food	5/6	1.45	1.42	2/2
Bad food	3/4	.76	.84	1/2

Note: F/N = Fat to normal ratio.

Incidentally, please keep in mind throughout this exercise that the left side of each table will always contain the data for lesioned animals, very largely rats, that have been abused by a variety of people named Epstein, and Teitelbaum, and Stellar, and Miller, and so on. The right side of each table will always contain the data for humans, mostly Columbia College students, nice boys who go home every Friday night, where, I suppose, they too are abused by a variety of people named Epstein, and Teitelbaum, and Stellar, and Miller.

In Line 2 of Table 2-III, we have the effects of bad taste on consumption. For both animals and men, in all of these studies bad taste was manipulated by the addition of quinine to the food. There are four animal studies; three of the four indicate that fat animals eat less than normal animals, and the average F/N ratio is .76. There are two human studies: one of the two indicates that fats eat considerably less bad food than normals; the other indicates no significant difference between the two groups, and the mean F/N ratio for these two studies is .84. For this particular fact, the data are more fragile than one would like, but the trends for the two species are certainly parallel.

To continue this examination of parallel facts: the eating habits of the lesioned rats have been thoroughly studied, particularly by Teitelbaum and Campbell.[37] It turns out that static obese rats eat on the average slightly, not considerably, more than normal rats. They also eat fewer meals per day, eat more per meal, and eat more rapidly than do normal animals. For each of these facts, we have parallel data for humans. Before presenting these data, I should note that for humans, I have, wherever possible, restricted myself to behavioral studies, studies in which the investigators have actually measured how much their subjects eat. I hope no one will be offended, I assume no one will be surprised, if I say that I am skeptical of the self-reports of fat people about how much they eat or exercise.* For those of you who feel that this is high-handed selection of studies, may I remind you of Stunkard's famous chronic fat patients who were fed everything that,

---

* In three of four such self-report studies, fat people report eating considerably less food than do normals.

in interviews, they admitted to eating daily, and who all steadily lost weight on this diet.

Considering first the average amount eaten per day when on ad-lib feeding of ordinary lab chow or pellets, you will note in Line 1 of Table 2-IV that consistently static obese rate eat somewhat (19%) more than do their normal counterparts. The data for humans are derived from all of the studies I know of in which eating is placed in a noshing, or ad-lib, context; that is, a bowl of ordinary food, usually nuts or crackers, is placed in the room, the experiment presumably has nothing to do with eating, and the subject is free to eat or not, as he chooses, just as in a rat in its cage. In two of the three experiments conducted in this context, obese subjects eat slightly more than do normals; in the third experiment, the two groups eat precisely the same number of crackers. For both humans and rats, then, the fat subject eats only slightly more than the normal subject.

Turning next to the number of meals per day, we note on Line 2 of Table 2-IV that for both rats and humans, fatter subjects consistently eat fewer meals per day. (A rat meal is defined by Teitelbaum and Campbell[37] as "any burst of food intake of at least five pellets separated by at least five minutes from any other burst [p. 138].") For humans, these particular data are based on self-report or interview studies, for I know of no relevant behavioral data. In any case, again the data for the lesioned rat and the obese human correspond very closely indeed.

From the previous two facts, it should, of course, follow that obese subjects will eat more per meal than normal subjects, and, as can be seen in Line 3 of Table 2-IV, this is the case for both lesioned rats and obese humans. The data for rats are based on two experiments that simply recorded the amount of food eaten per eating burst. The data for humans are based on all experiments in which a plate of food, usually sandwiches, is placed before a subject, and he is told to help himself to lunch or dinner.

Our final datum on eating habits is the speed of eating. Teitelbaum and Campbell[37] simply recorded the number of pellets their animals ate per minute. Since there is nothing else to do when you are sitting behind a

TABLE 2-IV

EATING HABITS

| | Animals | | Humans | |
Variable	Batting Average	Mean F/N	Mean F/N	Batting Average
Amount of food eaten ad lib	9/9	1.19	1.16	2/3
No. meals per day	4/4	.85	.92	3/3
Amount eaten per meal	2/2	1.34	1.29	5/5
Speed of eating	1/1	1.28	1.26	1/1

Note: F/N = Fat to normal ratio.

one-way screen watching a subject eat, Nisbett[19] (data not reported in paper) recorded the number of spoonfuls of ice cream his subjects ate per minute. The comparison of the two studies is drawn in Line 4 of Table 2-IV, where you will note an unsettling similarity in the rate at which lesioned rats and obese humans outspeed their normal counterparts.*

All told, then, in the existing literature, Rodin and I found a total of six items of behavior on which it is possible to make rather precise comparisons between lesioned rats and obese humans. These are mostly nonobvious facts, and the comparisons drawn between the two sets of experiments do not attempt to push the analogies beyond the point of common sense. I do not think there can be much debate about pellets versus spoonfuls of ice cream consumed per minute as equivalent measures of eating rate. For all six facts in the existing literature, the parallels between the species are striking. What the lesioned, fat rat does, the obese human does.

In addition to these facts, we identified two other areas of behavior in which it is possible to draw somewhat more fanciful, though still not ridiculous, comparisons between the species. These are the areas of emotionality and of activity. Though there has been little systematic study of emotionality, virtually everyone who has worked with these animals agrees that the lesioned animals are hyperexcitable, easily startled, overemotional, and generally bitchy to handle. In addition, work by Singh[32] and research on active avoidance learning do generally support this characterization of the lesioned animal as an emotional beast.

For humans, we have two experiments from which it is possible to draw conclusions about emotionality. In one of these,[31] we manipulated fear by threat of painful electric shock. On a variety of rating scales, fat subjects acknowledge that they were somewhat more frightened and anxious than did normal subjects. In a second experiment, Rodin[25] had her subjects listen to an audio tape while they were working at either a monitoring or a proofreading task. The tapes were either neutral (requiring the subject to think about either rain or seashells) or emotionally charged (requiring the subject to think about his own death or about the bombing of Hiroshima). The emotionally charged tapes produced dramatic differences between subjects. On a variety of rating scales, the obese described themselves as considerably more upset and disturbed than did normal subjects; they reported more palpitations and changes in breathing rate than did normals; and performance, at either the proofreading or monitoring tasks, deteriorated dramatically more for obese than for normal subjects. Again, then, the data are consistent, for both the lesioned animal and the obese human seem to react more emotionally than their normal counterparts.

---

* Fat rats do not drink more rapidly than do normals. There are no comparable data for humans.

Finally, on activity, numerous studies using stabilimeter cages or activity wheels have demonstrated that the lesioned animal is markedly less active than the normal animal. This is not, I should add, a totally trivial fact indicating only that the lesioned animal has trouble moving his immense bulk around the cage, for the dynamic hyperphagic rat—who though not yet fat, will be—is quite as lethargic as his obese counterpart. On the human side, Bullen, Reed, and Mayer[3] have taken movies of girls at camp during their scheduled periods of swimming, tennis, and volleyball. They categorize each camper for her degree of activity or exertion during these periods, and do find that the normal campers are more active than are the obese girls.

All told, then, Rodin and I found a total of eight facts, indicating a perfect parallel between the behavior of the lesioned rat and the obese human. We have, so far, found no fact on which the two species differ. Now all of this has proved such an engaging exercise that my students and I decided to play "real" scientist, and we constructed a matrix. We simply listed every fact we could find about the lesioned animals and every fact we could find about obese humans. I have told you about those facts for which parallel data exist. There are, however, numerous holes in the matrix—facts for rats for which no parallel human data have yet been collected, and vice versa. For the past year, we have been engaged in filling in these holes —designing for humans, experiments that have no particular rhyme or reason except that someone once did such an experiment on lesioned rats. For example, it is a fact that though lesioned rats will outeat normal rats when food is easily available, they will not lift a paw if they have to work to get food. In a Skinner box setup, Teitelbaum[36] finds that at FR1, when one press yields one pellet, fat lesioned rats outpress normal. As the payoff decreases, however, fat rats press less and less until at FR256, they do not manage to get a single pellet during a twelve-hour experimental session, whereas normal rats are still industriously pressing away. Similarly, Miller *et al.*[16] found that though lesioned rats ate more than normal controls when an unweighted lid covered the food dish, they ate less than did the controls when a 75 gm weight was fastened to the lid. They also found that the lesioned rats ran more slowly down an alley to food than controls did and pulled less hard when temporarily restrained by a harness. In short, fat rats will not work to get food.

Since there was no human parallel to these studies, Lucy Friedman and I designed a study in which, when a subject arrived, he was asked simply to sit at the experimenter's desk and fill out a variety of personality tests and questionnaires. Besides the usual student litter, there was a bag of almonds on the desk. The experimenter helped herself to a nut, invited the subject to do the same, and then left him alone with his questionnaires and nuts for fifteen minutes. There were two sets of conditions. In one, the nuts had shells on them; in the other, the nuts had no shells. I assume we agree that eating nuts with shells is considerably more work than eating nuts with no shells.

The top half of Table 2-V presents for normal subjects the numbers who do and do not eat nuts in the two conditions. As you can see, shells or no shells has virtually no impact on normal subjects. Fifty-five per cent of normals eat nuts without shells, and 50 per cent eat nuts with shells. I am a little self-conscious about the data for obese subjects, for it looks as if I were too stupid to know how to fake data. I know how to fake data, and where I to do so, the bottom half of Table 2-V certainly would not look the way it does. When the nuts have no shells, 19 of 20 fat subjects eat nuts. When the nuts have shells on them, one out of twenty fat subjects eats. Obviously, the parallel to Miller's and the Teitelbaum's rats is perfect. When the food is easy to get at, fat subjects, rat or human, eat more than normals; when the food is hard to get at, fat subjects eat less than normals.

Incidentally, as a casual corollary of these and other findings, one could expect that, given acceptable food, fat eaters would be more likely than normals to choose the easiest way of eating. In order to check on this, Lucy Friedman, Joel Handler, and I went to a large number of Chinese and Japanese restaurants, categorized each patron as he entered the restaurant as obese or normal, and then simply noted whether he ate with chopsticks or with silverware. Among Occidentals, for whom chopsticks can be an ordeal, we found that almost five times the proportion of normal eaters ate with chopsticks as did obese eaters—22.4 per cent of normals and 4.7 per cent of the obese ate with chopsticks.

In another matrix-hole-filling experiment, Patricia Pliner[21] has demonstrated that obese humans, like lesioned rats, do not regulate food consumption when they are preloaded with solids but, again like the rats, do regulate when they are preloaded with liquids.

In addition to these experiments, we are currently conducting studies on

TABLE 2-V

EFFECT OF WORK ON THE EATING BEHAVIOR OF
NORMAL AND FAT SUBJECTS

| | | Number Who |
Nuts Have	Eat	Don't Eat
Normal subjects		
Shells	10	10
No shells	11	9
Fat subjects		
Shells	1	19
No shells	19	1

pain sensitivity and on passive versus active avoidance learning—all designed to fill in more holes in our human-lesioned rat matrix. To date,
we have a total of twelve nonobvious facts in which the behaviors of lesioned rats parallel perfectly the behaviors of obese humans. Though I
cannot believe that as our matrix-hole-filling experiments continue, this
perfect parallelism will continue, I submit that even now these are mind-
boggling data. I would also submit, however, that we have played this en-
chanting game just about long enough. This is, after all, science through
analogy—a sport I recommend with the same qualifications and enthusiasms
with which I recommend skiing—and it is time that we asked what on earth
does it all mean? To which at this point I can only answer ruefully that I
wish to God I really knew.

On its most primitive level, I suppose that I would love to play doctor
and issue pronouncements such as, "Madam, you have a very sick hypothalamus." And, indeed, I do know of one case of human obesity[23] accompanied by a precisely localized neoplasm that destroyed the ventromedial
hypothalamus. This is an astonishing case study, for the lady reads like a
lesioned rat—she ate immense amounts of food, as much as 10,000 calories
a day, grew impressively fat and was apparently a wildly emotional creature
given to frequent outbursts of laughing, crying, and rage. Now I am not, of
course, going to suggest that this lady is anything but a pathological extreme. The only vaguely relevant study I know of is a morphological study[14]
of the hypothalami of genetically obese mice, an animal whose behavior
also resembles the lesioned rat's, which found no structural differences between obese and normal mice.

Mrosovsky[17] has been developing a more sober hypothesis. Comparing
the hibernator and the ventromedial lesioned rat, Mrosovsky has been
playing much the same analogical game as have I, and he, too, has noted
the marked behavioral similarities of his two species to the obese human.
He hypothesizes that the unlesioned, obese animal, rodent or human, has a
ventromedial hypothalamus that is functionally quiescent. Though I would
be willing to bet that when the appropriate biochemical and electrophysio-
logical studies are done, Mrosovsky will be proven correct, I do not believe
that this is a fact which is of fundamental interest to psychologists. Most of
us, I suspect, have long been convinced, psychodynamics notwithstanding,
that there is *something* biologically responsible for human obesity, and to
be able suddenly to point a finger at an offending structure would not really
put us much ahead. After all, we've known about the adrenal medulla and
emotion for more than fifty years, and I doubt that this particular bit of
knowledge has been of much help in our understanding of aggression, or
fear, or virtually any other emotional state.

If it is true that the ventromedial hypothalamus is functionally quiescent, for us the question must be, for what function, psychologically speaking, is it quiescent? What processes, or inputs, or outputs are mediated by this particular structure? Speculation and theorizing about the functions of this area have tended to be cautious and modest. Essentially, two suggestions have been made—one that the area is a satiety center, and the other that the area is an emotionality center. Both Miller[15] and Stellar[33] have tentatively suggested that the ventromedial area is a satiety center—that in some fashion it monitors the signals indicating a sufficiency of food and inhibits the excitatory (Eat! Eat!) impulses initiated in the lateral hypothalamus. This inhibitory-satiety mechanism can account for the hyperphagia of the lesioned animals and, consequently, for their obesity. It can also account for most of the facts that I outlined earlier about the daily eating habits of these animals. It cannot by itself, however, account for the finickiness of these animals, nor can it, as I believe I can show, account for the apparent unwillingness of these animals to work for food. Finally, this hypothesis is simply irrelevant to the demonstrated inactivity and hyperemotionality of these animals. This irrelevance, however, is not critical if one assumes, as does Stellar, that discrete neural centers, also located in the ventromedial area, control activity and emotionality. The satiety theory, then, can account for some, but by no means all, of the critical facts about eating, and it has nothing to say about activity or emotionality.

As a theoretically more ambitious alternative, Grossman[9, 10] has proposed that the ventromedial area be considered the emotionality center and that the facts about eating be derived from this assumption. By definition, Grossman's hypothesis accounts for the emotionality of these animals, and his own work on active avoidance learning certainly supports the emotionality hypothesis. I must confess, however, that I have difficulty in understanding just why these emotional animals become fat. In essence, Grossman assumes that "lesions in or near the VMH sharply increase an animal's affective responsiveness to apparently all sensory stimuli [p. 1]." On the basis of this general statement, he suggests that "the 'finickiness' of the ventromedial animal might then reflect a change in its affective response to taste." This could, of course, account for the fact that lesioned animals eat more very good-tasting food and less very bad-tasting food than do normals. However, I simply find it hard to believe that this affective hypothesis can account for the basic fact about these animals—that for weeks on end, the lesioned animals eat grossly more of ordinary, freely available lab chow.

Grossman[10] attributes the fact that lesioned animals will not work for food to their "exaggerated response to handling, the test situation, the deprivation regimen, and the requirement of having to work for their daily bread [p. 358]." I suppose all of this is possible, I simply find it farfetched.

At the very least, the response to handling and to the deprivation regime should be just as exaggerated whether the reinforcement schedule is FR1 or FR256 and the lesioned animals do press more than the normals at FR1.

My skepticism, however, is irrelevant, and Grossman may be correct. There are, however, at least two facts with which, it seems to me, Grossman's hypothesis cannot cope. First, it would seem to me that an animal with an affective response to food would be likely to eat more rather than less often per day, as is the fact. Second, it is simply common sense to expect that an animal with strong "affective responsiveness to all sensory stimuli" will be a very active animal indeed, but the lesioned animal is presumably hypoactive.

None of the existing theories, then, can cope with all of the currently available facts. For the remainder of this article, I am going to try my hand at developing a hypothesis that I believe can cope with more of the facts than can the available alternatives. It is a hypothesis that derives entirely from our work on human obesity. I believe, however, that it can explain as many of the facts about ventromedial-lesioned rats as it can about the human obese. If future experimental work on animals proves this correct, it would certainly suggest that science by analogy has merits other than its entertainment value.

The gist of our findings on humans is that the eating behavior of the obese is under external, rather than internal, control. In effect, the obese seem stimulus-bound. When a food-relevant cue is present, the obese are more likely to eat and to eat a great deal than are normals. When such a cue is absent, the obese are less likely to try to eat or to complain about hunger. Though I have not, in this article, developed this latter point, there is evidence that, in the absence of food-relevant cues, the obese have a far easier time fasting than do normals, while in the presence of such cues, they have a harder time fasting.[8]

Since it is a little hard to believe that such stimulus-binding is limited to food-relevant cues, for some time now my students and I have been concerned with the generalizability of these facts. Given our starting point, this concern has led to some rather odd little experiments. For example, Judith Rodin, Peter Herman, and I have asked subjects to look at slides on which are portrayed thirteen objects or words. Each slide is exposed for five seconds, and the subject is then asked to recall what he saw. Fat subjects recall more objects than do normal subjects. The experiment has been replicated, and this appears to be a reliable phenomenon.

In another study, Rodin, Herman, and I compared fat and normal subjects on simple and on complex or disjunctive reaction time. For simple reaction time, they are instructed to lift their finger from a telegraph key as soon as the stimulus light comes on. On this task, there are no differences between obese and normal subjects. For complex reaction time, there are two stimulus lights and two telegraph keys, and subjects are instructed to lift their left finger when the right light comes on and lift their right finger when the left light comes on. Obese subjects respond more rapidly and make fewer errors. Since this was a little hard to believe, this study was repeated three times, each time with the same results. The obese are simply better at complex reaction time than are normals. I do not pretend to understand these results, but they do seem to indicate that, for some reason, the obese are more efficient stimulus or information processors.

At this stage, obviously, this is shotgun research which, in coordination with the results of our eating experiments, seems to indicate that it may be useful to more generally characterize the obese as stimulus-bound and to hypothesize that any stimulus, above a given intensity level, is more likely to evoke an appropriate response from an obese than from a normal subject.

Our first test of implications of this hypothesis in a noneating setting is Rodin's[25] experiment on the effects of distraction on performance. She reasoned that if the stimulus-binding hypothesis is correct, distracting, irrelevant stimuli should be more disruptive for obese than for normal subjects when they are performing a task requiring concentration. Presumably, the impinging stimulus is more likely to grip the attention of the stimulus-bound obese subject. To test this guess, she had her subjects work at a simple proofreading task. In one condition, the subjects corrected proof with no distractions at all. In the three other conditions, they corrected proof while listening to recorded tapes that varied in the degree to which they were likely to grip a subject's attention, and therefore distract him. The results show that the obese are better at proofreading when undistracted but their performance seriously deteriorates as they are distracted until, at extreme distraction, they are considerably worse than normals. Rodin finds precisely the same pattern of results, by the way, in a similar study in which she uses the complex reaction time task I have already described rather than the proofreading task. For humans, then, there is evidence, outside of the eating context, to support the hypothesis.

Let us return to consideration of the ventromedial lesioned animal and examine the implications of the hypothesis that any stimulus, above a given intensity level, is more likely to evoke an appropriate response from a lesioned than from an intact animal. This is a hypothesis which is, in many ways, similar to Grossman's hypothesis and, on the face of it, would appear to be vulnerable to exactly the same criticisms as I have leveled at his theory. There are, however, crucial differences that will become evident as I elaborate this notion. I assume it is self-evident that my hypothesis can explain the emotionality of the lesioned animals and, with the exception of meal frequency—a fact to which I will return—can account for virtually all of our facts about the daily eating habits of these animals. I will, therefore, begin consideration of the hypothesis by examining its implications for those facts that have been most troubling for alternative formulations and by examining those facts that seem to most clearly contradict my own hypothesis.

Let us turn first to the perverse and fascinating fact that though lesioned animals will outeat normals when food is easily available, they simply will not work for food. In my terms, this is an incomplete fact which may prove only that a remote food stimulus will not evoke a food-acquiring response. It is the case that in the experiments concerned with this fact, virtually every manipulation of work has covaried the remoteness or prominence of the food cue. Food at the end of a long alleyway is obviously a more remote cue than food in the animal's food dish. Pellets available only after 256 presses of a lever are certainly more remote food stimuli than pellets available after each press of a lever. If the stimulus-binding hypothesis is correct, it should be anticipated that, in contrast to the results when the food cue is remote, the lesioned animal will work harder than the normal animal when the food stimulus is prominent and compelling. Though the appropriate experiment has not yet been done on rats, to my delight I have learned recently that such an experiment has been done on humans by William Johnson,[12] who independently has been pursuing a line of thought similar to mine.

Johnson seated his subject at a table, fastened his hand in a harness, and, to get food, required the subject for twelve minutes to pull, with his index finger, on a ring that was attached by wire to a seven-pound weight. He received food on a VR50 schedule, that is, on the average, a subject received a quarter of a sandwich for every fifty pulls of the ring. Obviously, this was moderately hard work.

To vary stimulus prominence, Johnson manipulated food visibility and prior taste of food. In "food visible" conditions, he placed beside the subject one desirable sandwich covered in a transparent wrap. In addition, as the subject satisfied the VR requirements, he placed beside him quarter sandwiches similarly wrapped. In "food invisible" conditions, Johnson followed exactly the same procedures, but wrapped the sandwiches in white, nontransparent shelf paper. Subjects, of course, did not eat until they had completed their twelve minutes of labor.

As a second means of varying cue prominence, half of the subjects ate a quarter of a very good sandwich immediately before they began work. The remaining subjects ate a roughly equivalent portion of plain white bread.

I have arranged the conditions along the dimension of food cue prominence, ranging from no prominent food cues to two prominent food cues, that is, the subjects ate a quarter sandwich and the food was visible. As you can see, the stimulus prominence manipulations have a marked effect on the obese, for they work far harder when the food cues are prominent and compelling than when they are inconspicious. In contrast, cue prominence has relatively little effect on normal subjects.

Please note also that these results parallel Miller's and Teitelbaum's results with lesioned rats. When the food cues are remote, the obese human works less hard for food than the normally sized human. The fact that this relationship flips when the cues are prominent is, of course, a delight to me, and wouldn't it be absorbing to replicate this experiment on lesioned rats?

Let us turn next to the fact that lesioned rats are hypoactive. If ever a fact were incompatible with a hypothesis, this one is it. Surely an animal that is more responsive to any stimulus should be hyperactive, not hypoactive. Yet, this is a most peculiar fact—for it remains a fact only because one rather crucial finding in the literature has been generally overlooked and because the definition of activity seems restricted to measures obtained in running wheels or in stabilimeter-type living cages.

Studies of activity have with fair consistency reported dramatically less activity for lesioned than for normal rats. With one exception, these studies report data in terms of total activity per unit time, making no distinction between periods when the animal room was quiet and undisturbed and periods involving the mild ferment of animal-tending activities. Gladfelter and Brobeck,[7] however, report activity data separately for the "forty-three-hour period when the constant-temperature room was dark and quiet and the rats were undisturbed" and for the "five-hour period when the room was lighted and the rats were cared for [p. 811]." During the quiet time, these investigators find precisely what almost everyone else does—lesioned rats are markedly less active. During the animal-tending period, however, lesioned animals are just about as active as normal animals. In short, when the stimulus field is relatively barren and there is little to react to, the ventromedial animal is inactive; when the field is made up of the routine noises, stirrings, and disturbances involved in tending an animal laboratory, the lesioned animal is just about as active as the normal animal.

Though this is an instructive fact, it hardly proves my hypothesis, which specifies that above a given stimulus intensity the lesioned animal should be *more* reactive than the normal animal. Let us then ask—is there any evidence that lesioned animals are more active than normal animals? There is, if you are willing to grant that specific activity such as lever pressing or avoidance behavior are as much "activity" as the gross, overall measures obtained in stabilimeter-mounted living cages.

In his study of activity, Teitelbaum[36] has distinguished between random and food-directed activity. As do most other investigators, he finds that in their cages, lesioned rats are much less active than are normals. During a twelve-hour stint in a Skinner box, however, when on an FR1 schedule, the lesioned animals are more active; that is, they press more than do normals. Thus, when the food cue is salient and prominent, as it is on an FR1 schedule, the lesioned animal is very active indeed. And, as you know, when the food cue is remote, as it is on an FR64 or FR256 schedule, the lesioned animal is inactive.

Since lever pressing is activity in pursuit of food, I suppose one should be cautious in accepting these data as support for my argument. Let us turn, then, to avoidance learning where most of the experiments are unrelated to food.

In overall batting average terms,* no area could be messier than this one, for in three of six studies, lesioned animals are better and in three worse at avoidance than normals. However, if one distinguishes between passive and active avoidance, things become considerably more coherent.

In active avoidance studies, a conditioned stimulus such as a light or buzzer precedes a noxious event such as electrifying the floor grid. To avoid the shock, the animal must perform some action such as jumping into the nonelectrified compartment of a shuttle box. In three of four such studies, the lesioned animals learn considerably more rapidly than do normal animals. By this criterion, at least, lesioned animals are more reactive than normal animals.† Parenthetically, it is amusing to note that the response latencies of the lesioned animal are smaller[9] than those of the normal animal, just as in our studies of complex reaction time, obese humans are faster than normal humans.

In contrast to these results, lesioned animals do considerably worse than normal animals in passive avoidance studies. In these studies, the animal's water dish or the lever of a Skinner box are electrified so that if, dur-

---

* Of all the behavioral areas so far considered, avoidance learning is probably the one for which it makes least sense either to adopt a batting average approach or to attempt to treat the research as a conceptually equivalent set of studies. Except in this area, the great majority of experiments have used, as subjects, rats with electrolytically produced lesions. In the avoidance learning area, the subjects have been mice, rats, and cats; the lesions are variously electrolytically produced, produced by gold thioglucose injections, or are "functional" lesions produced by topical application of atropine or some other agent.

† Reactive, yes, but what about activity in the more primitive sense of simply moving or scrambling about the experimental box? Even in this respect, the lesioned animals appear to outmove the normals, for Turner, Sechzer, and Liebelt[38] report the following:

The experimental groups, both mice and rats, emitted strong escape tendencies prior to the onset of shock and in response to shock. Repeated attempts were made to climb out of the test apparatus. This group showed much more vocalization than the control group. . . . In contrast to the behavior of the experimental animals, the control animals appeared to become immobilized or to "freeze" both before and during the shock period. Thus, there was little attempt to escape and little vocalization (p. 242).

ing the experimental period, the animal touches these objects he receives a shock. In both of the studies we have found on passive learning, the lesioned animals do considerably worse than normal animals. They either press the lever or touch the water dish more than do normals and accordingly are shocked far more often. Thus, when the situation requires a response if the animal is to avoid shock, the lesioned animal does better than the normal animal. Conversely, if the situation requires response quiescence if the animal is to avoid shock, the lesioned animal does far worse than the normal animal. This pair of facts, I suggest, provides strong support for the hypothesis that beyond a given stimulus intensity, the lesioned animal is more reactive than the normal animal. I would also suggest that without some variant of this hypothesis, the overall pattern of results on avoidance learning is incoherent.

All in all, then, one can make a case of sorts for the suggestion that there are specifiable circumstances in which lesioned animals will be more active. It is hardly an ideal case, and only an experiment that measures the effects of systematically varied stimulus field richness on gross activity can test the point.

These ruminations on activity do suggest a refinement of the general hypothesis and also, I trust, make clear why I have insisted on inserting that awkward phrase "above a given intensity level" in all statements of the hypothesis. For activity, it appears to be the case that the lesioned animal is less active when the stimulus is remote and more active when the stimulus is prominent. This is a formulation which I believe fits almost all of the available data, on both animals and men, remarkably well. It is also a formulation which for good ad-hoc reasons bears a striking resemblance to almost every relevant set of data I have discussed.

For human eating behavior, virtually every fact we have supports the assertion that the obese eat more than normals when the food cue is prominent and less when the cue is remote. In Johnson's study of work and cue prominence, the obese do not work as hard as normals when there are no prominent food cues, but work much harder when the food cues are highly salient. In Nisbett's one-sandwich and three-sandwich experiment, the obese subjects eat just as long as food cues are prominent, that is, the sandwiches are directly in front of the subject, but when these immediate cues have been consumed, they stop eating. Thus, they eat more than normals in the three-sandwich condition and less in the one-sandwich condition. We also know that the obese have an easy time fasting in the absence of food cues and a hard time in the presence of such cues, and so on.

About eating habits we know that the obese eat larger meals (what could be a more prominent cue than food on the plate?), but eat fewer meals (as they should if it requires a particularly potent food cue to trigger an eating response). Even the fact that the obese eat more rapidly can be easily derived from this formulation.

For rats, this formulation in general fits what we know about eating habits, but can be considered a good explanation of the various experimental facts only if you are willing to accept my reinterpretation, in terms of cue prominence, of such experiments as Miller *et al.'s*[16] study of the effects of work on eating. If, as would I, you would rather suspend judgment until the appropriate experiments have been done on lesioned rats, mark it down as an engaging possibility.

Given the rough state of what we know about emotionality, this formulation seems to fit the data for humans and rats about equally well. The lesioned rats are vicious when handled and lethargic when left alone. In the Rodin[25] experiment which required subjects to listen to either neutral or emotionally disturbing tapes, obese subjects described themselves (and behaved accordingly) as less emotional than normals when the tapes were neutral and much more emotional than normals when the tapes were disturbing.

All in all, given the variety of species and behaviors involved, it is not a bad ad-hoc hypothesis. So far there has been only one study deliberately designed to test some of the ideas implicit in this formulation. This is Lee Ross's[26] study of the effects of cue salience on eating. Ross formulated this experiment in the days when we were struggling with some of the data inconsistent with our external-internal theory of eating behavior (see Schachter[28]). Since the world is full of food cues, it was particularly embarrassing to discover that obese subjects ate less frequently than normals. Short of invoking denial mechanisms, such a fact could be reconciled with the theory only if we assumed that a food cue must be potent in order to trigger an eating response in an obese subject—the difference between a hot dog stand two blocks away and a hot dog under your nose, savory with mustard and steaming with sauerkraut.

To test the effects of cue prominence, Ross simply had his subjects sit at a table covered with a variety of objects among which was a large tin of shelled cashew nuts. Presumably, the subjects were there to take part in a study of thinking. There were two sets of experimental conditions. In high-cue-saliency conditions, the table and the nuts were illuminated by an unshaded table lamp containing a 40-watt bulb. In low-saliency conditions, the lamp was shaded and contained a 7½-watt red bulb. The measure of eating was simply the difference in the weight of the tin of nuts before and after the subject thought his experimentally required thoughts. The results bear a marked resemblance to our theoretical curves.

So much for small triumphs. Let us turn now to some of the problems of this formulation. Though I do not intend to detail a catalog of failings, I would like to make explicit some of my discomforts.

1. Though there has been no direct experimental study of the problem, it seems to be generally thought that the lesioned rat is hyposexual, which, if true, is an unexpected contradiction for a theory which postulates superreactivity. It is the case, however, that gonadal atrophy is frequently a consequence of this operation.[1, 11] Possibly, then, we should consider sexual activity as artifactually quite distinct from either gross activity or stimulus-bound activity such as avoidance behavior.

2. I am made uncomfortable by the fact that the obese, both human and rat, eat less bad food than do normals. I simply find it difficult to conceive of nonresponsiveness as a response. I suppose I could conceptually avoid this difficulty, but I cannot imagine the definition of response that would allow me to cope with both this fact and with the facts about passive avoidance. I take some comfort from the observation that of all of the facts about animals and humans, the fact about bad taste has the weakest batting average. It may yet turn out not to be a fact.

3. Though the fact that obese humans eat less often is no problem, the fact that obese rats also eat less often is awkward, for it is a bit difficult to see how food stimulus intensity can vary for a caged rat on an ad-lib schedule. This may seem farfetched, but there is some experimental evidence that this may be due to the staleness of the food. Brooks, Lockwood, and Wiggins,[2] using mash for food, demonstrated that lesioned rats do not outeat normals when the food is even slightly stale. Only when the food was absolutely fresh and newly placed in the cage did lesioned rats eat conspicuously more than normal rats. It seems doubtful, however, that this could be the explanation for results obtained with pellets.

4. As with food, one should expect from this formulation that the animal's water intake would increase following the lesion. There does not appear to have been much systematic study of the problem, but what data exist are inconsistent from one study to the next. Several studies indicate decreased water intake; at least one study[13] indicates no change following the operation; and there are even rare occasional case reports of polydipsia. Possibly my interactional hypothesis can cope with this chaos, and systematically varying the salience of the water cue will systematically affect the water intake of the ventromedial animal. It is also possible that under any circumstance, water, smell-less and tasteless, is a remote cue.

There are, then, difficulties with this formulation. These may be the kinds of difficulties that will ultimately damn the theory, or at least establish its limits. Alternatively, these may mostly be apparent difficulties, and this view of matters may help us clarify inconsistent sets of data, for I suspect that by systematically varying cue prominence we can systematically vary the lesioned animal's reactivity on many dimensions. We shall see. Granting the difficulties, for the moment this view of matters does manage to subsume a surprisingly diverse set of facts about animals and men under one quite simple theoretical scheme.

Since I have presented this chapter as a more or less personal history of the development of a set of ideas, I would like to conclude by taking a more formal look at this body of data, theory, and speculation, by examining what I believe we now know, what seems to be good guesswork, and what is still out-and-out speculation.

With some confidence, we can say that obese humans are externally controlled or stimulus-bound. There is little question that this is true of their eating behavior, and evidence is rapidly accumulating that eating is a special case of the more general state.

I have suggested that stimulus prominence and reactivity are key variables in understanding the realms of behavior with which I have been concerned. The specific shapes of the curves are, of course, pure guesswork, and the only absolute requirement that I believe the data impose on the theory is that there be an interaction such that at low levels of stimulus prominence, the obese are less reactive, and at high levels of prominence more reactive, than normals.

With considerably less confidence, I believe we can say that this same set of hypotheses may explain many of the differences between the ventromedial lesioned rat and his intact counterpart. This conclusion is based on the fact that so much of the existing data either fit or can be plausibly reinterpreted to fit these ideas. Obviously, the crucial experiments have yet to be done.

Finally, and most tentatively, one may guess that the obesity of rats and men has a common physiological locus in the ventromedial hypothalamus. I must emphasize that this guess is based *entirely* on the persistent and tantalizing analogies between lesioned rats and obese humans. There is absolutely no relevant independent evidence. However, should future work support this speculation, I suspect, in light of the evidence already supporting the stimulus-binding hypotheses, we are in for a radical revision of our notions about the hypothalamus.

REFERENCES

1. Brooks, C. McC. and Lambert, E. F.: A study of the effect of limitation of food intake and the method of feeding on the rate of weight gain during hypothalamic obesity in the albino rat. *Am J Physiol,* 147:695-707, 1946.
2. Brooks, C. McC., Lockwood, R. A. and Wiggins, M. L.: A study of the effect of hypothalamic lesions on the eating habits of the albino rat. *Am J Physiol,* 147: 735-741, 1946.
3. Bullen, B. A., Reed, R. B. and Mayer, J.: Physical activity of obese and nonobese

adolescent girls appraised by motion picture sampling. *Am J Clin Nutr,* 14: 211-223, 1964.

4. Cannon, W. B.: *Bodily Changes in Pain, Hunger, Fear and Rage.* (2nd ed.) New York, Appleton, 1915.

5. Carlson, A. J.: *The Control of Hunger in Health and Disease.* Chicago, University of Chicago Press, 1916.

6. Decke, E.: Effects of taste on the eating behavior of obese and normal persons. Cited in S. Schachter, *Emotion, Obesity, and Crime.* New York, Academic Press, 1971.

7. Gladfelter, W. E. and Brobeck, J. R.: Decreased spontaneous locomotor activity in the rat induced by hypothalamic lesions. *Am J Physiol,* 203:811-817, 1962.

8. Goldman, R., Jaffa, M. and Schachter, S.: Yom Kippur, Air France, dormitory food, and the eating behavior of obese and normal persons. *J Pers Soc Psychol,* 10: 117-123, 1968.

9. Grossman, S. P.: The VMH: A center for affective reactions, satiety, or both? *Int J Physiol Behav,* 1:1-10, 1966.

10. Grossman, S. P.: *A Textbook of Physiological Psychology.* New York, Wiley, 1967.

11. Hetherington, A. W. and Ranson, S. W.: Hypothalamic lesions and adiposity in the rat. *Anat Rec,* 78:149-172, 1940.

12. Johnson, W. G.: The effect of prior-taste and food visibility on the food-directed instrumental performance of obese individuals. Unpublished doctoral dissertation, Catholic University of America, 1970.

13. Krasne, F. B.: Unpublished study cited in N. E. Miller, Some psycho-physiological studies of motivation and of the behavioural effects of illness. *Bull Brit Psychol Soc,* 17:1-20, 1964.

14. Maren, T. H.: Cited in J. L. Fuller and G. A. Jacoby, Central and sensory control of food intake in genetically obese mice. *Am J Physiol,* 183:279-283, 1955.

15. Miller, N. E.: Some psycho-physiological studies of motivation and of the behavioural effects of illness. *Bull Brit Psychol Soc,* 17:1-20, 1964.

16. Miller, N. E., Bailey, C. J. and Stevenson, J. A. F.: Decreased "hunger" but increased food intake resulting from hypothalamic lesions. *Science,* 112:256-259, 1950.

17. Mrosovsky, N.: *Hibernation and the Hypothalamus.* New York, Appleton-Century-Crofts, 1971.

18. Nisbett, R. E.: Determinants of food intake in human obesity. *Science,* 159: 1254-1255, 1968a.

19. Nisbett, R. E.: Taste, deprivation, and weight determinants of eating behavior. *J Pers Soc Psychol,* 10:107-116, 1968b.

20. Nisbett, R. E.: Eating and obesity in men and animals. In press, 1971.

21. Pliner, P.: Effects of liquid and solid preloads on the eating behavior of obese and normal persons. Unpublished doctoral dissertation, Columbia University, 1970.

22. Rabin, B. M. and Smith, C. J.: Behavioral comparison of the effectiveness of irritative and non-irritative lesions in producing hypothalamic hyperphagia. *Physiol Behav,* 3:417-420, 1968.

23. Reeves, A. G. and Plum, F.: Hyperphagia, rage, and dementia accompanying a ventromedial hypothalamic neoplasm. *Arch Neurol,* 20:616-624, 1969.

24. Reynolds, R. W.: Ventromedial hypothalamic lesions with hyperphagia. *Am J Physiol,* 204:60-62, 1963.

25. Rodin, J.: Effects of distraction on performance of obese and normal subjects. Unpublished doctoral dissertation, Columbia University, 1970.

26. Ross, L. D.: Cue- and cognition-controlled eating among obese and normal sub-jects. Unpublished doctoral dissertation, Columbia University, 1969.
27. Schachter, S.: The interaction of cognitive and physiological determinants of emotional state. In L. Berkowitz (Ed.), *Advances in Experimental Social Psychology*. Vol. 1, New York, Academic Press, 1964.
28. Schachter, S.: Cognitive effects on bodily functioning: Studies of obesity and eating. In D. C. Glass (Ed.), *Neurophysiology and Emotion*. New York, Rocke-feller University Press and Russell Sage Foundation, 1967.
29. Schachter, S.: Obesity and eating. *Science*, 161:751-756, 1968.
30. Schachter, S.: *Emotion, Obesity, and Crime*. New York, Academic Press, 1971.
31. Schachter, S., Goldman, R. and Gordon, A.: Effects of fear, food deprivation, and obesity on eating. *J Pers Soc Psychol*, 10:91-97, 1968.
32. Singh, D.: Comparison of hyperemotionality caused by lesions in the septal and ventromedial hypothalamic areas in the rat. *Psychonom Sci*, 16:3-4, 1969.
33. Stellar, E.: The physiology of motivation. *Psychol Rev*, 61:5-22, 1954.
34. Stunkard, A. and Koch, C.: The interpretation of gastric motility: I. Apparent bias in the reports of hunger by obese persons. *Arch Gen Psychiat*, 11:74-82, 1964.
35. Teitelbaum, P.: Sensory control of hypothalamic hyperphagia. *J Comp Physiol Psychol*, 48:156-163, 1955.
36. Teitelbaum, P.: Random and food-directed activity in hyperphagic and normal rats. *J Comp Physiol Psychol*, 50:486-490, 1957.
37. Teitelbaum, P. and Campbell, B. A.: Ingestion patterns in hyperphagic and nor-mal rats. *J Comp Physiol Psychol*, 51:135-141, 1958.
38. Turner, S. G., Sechzer, J. A. and Liebelt, R. A.: Sensitivity to electric shock after ventromedial hypothalamic lesions. *Exp Neurol*, 19:236-244, 1967.

II
BODY IMAGE

3

Obesity and the Body Image

Albert J. Stunkard

and

Myer Mendelson

O F the many behavioral disturbances to which obese persons are subject, only two seem specifically related to their obesity. The first is overeating, the second is a disturbance in body image. This paper attempts to characterize these disturbances in body image, to describe their determinants, and to discuss their implications for theory and therapy. It is based upon one-hour interviews with seventy-four randomly selected obese persons in the general medical and psychiatric clinics of the Hospital of the University of Pennsylvania, plus a background obtained by psychotherapy of about twenty obese persons for periods of from one to ten years.

The median age of the sample was forty-three, with a range from eighteen to seventy. It was about equally divided between men and women, with medical clinic patients generally of lower class and psychiatric clinic patients of lower middle class. Although the psychotherapy patients had not been selected for this purpose, their demographic characteristics were similar to those of the psychiatric clinic patients.

The term "body image" refers to "the picture that the person has of the physical appearance of his body."[17] Disturbances in body image may range from "gross depersonalization . . . through distorted thoughts and feelings about the body, to distorted perceptions. . . ."[10] The disturbances to be described are primarily in the area of feelings. One might expect that derogatory feelings about one's body occurred in all obese persons and that they were a central feature of the neurosis of all emotionally disturbed obese persons. Such is not the case. Body image disturbances do not occur in emotionally healthy obese persons, and we have found them in only a minority of neurotic obese persons.

NATURE OF THE DISTURBANCE

We have divided the manifestations of body image disturbances rather arbitrarily into three areas: views of the self, self-consciousness in general, and self-consciousness in relation to the opposite sex. A disturbance in one area usually meant also a disturbance in the other two.

Views of the Self

A simple and revealing method of assessing a person's body image is to ask him how he views himself in a mirror.[3] We have systematically col-

41

lected data on this topic. An obese woman reported, "I call myself a slob and a pig—I look in the mirror and I say 'you're nothing but a big fat pig.' "

The experience of looking at oneself in a mirror can become so disturbing to obese persons that it can even interfere with such activities as shopping, which requires looking into store windows. One obese man reported,

> Just looking at myself in a store window makes me feel terrible. It's gotten so I am very careful not to look by accident. It's a feeling that people have the right to hate me and hate anyone who looks as fat as me. As soon as I see myself, I feel an uncontrollable burst of hatred. I just look at myself and say "I hate you, you're loathesome!"

As we have indicated, a disturbance in body image is not present in all obese persons, and many view their obesity in a thoroughly realistic manner. As one obese man put it, "You know, I caught a glimpse of myself in the mirror this morning, and I was surprised at how fat I have become. It made me feel that it's time to get some of this weight off."

Self-consciousness in General

The private views which some obese persons hold about their bodies are frequently paralleled by an intense self-consciousness and even misperception of how others view them. It sometimes seems as if they feel that nothing ever happens to them except in some kind of (usually derogatory) relationship to their weight. One young man said, "Weight was always a problem. If I missed a note in my music class and someone said, 'You always mess it up, man,' then I would think, 'Maybe it's because of my weight.' " A sixty-one-year-old housewife said, "I've always been self-conscious—I was always fat. It made me shyer than most people, I was withdrawn and kind of backward. I was never pleased with myself at all, never, never. . . ."

That obesity is not a sufficient cause for such self-consciousness is indicated by the remarks of a man who was at the time 46 per cent overweight: "The cosmetic point of view really bothers me only indirectly—through my wife. She objects to it; I think that she thinks a lot about it."

Self-consciousness in Relation to the Opposite Sex

Almost all of the subjects with body-image disturbances had serious difficulties in relationships with the opposite sex. These difficulties seemed both to arise from, and to reflect, self-consciousness about how others viewed their obesity. One of the most common complaints dealt with humiliations at parties. As one woman put it, "Nobody wants to go out with a tub, which was my nickname. By going to a dance all I did was stand against the wall listening to music. Nobody ever asked me to dance. I made believe I didn't care. But I just thought I was a big nothing." An attractive young woman who, in other days, would have been considered pleasingly plump, put in even more succinct terms the despair with which recurrent disappointments had brought her to consider the possibility of marriage, "Who would want to marry an elephant?"

These disturbances ranged from avoidance and inhibitions to hateful devaluation of the opposite sex. For example, a forty-five-year-old man reported,

> Physical appearances seemed to exclude me from social activities and I resented it. I felt I was not physically attractive to women. Now I consider being short and heavy an advantage. I don't have anything to do with women. I hate their guts. I get such a revulsion when I see how women act that I can't bring myself to go after sex.

An obese woman said that her body made her feel embarrassed with men she thought were "normal." "So I pick up abnormal men. I'll tend to hang out with fairies. That way I don't feel that I have to compete with real women."

The obese persons who escaped a disturbance in the body image had far fewer difficulties in their relations with the opposite sex. One such man boasted, "I can get a woman any time I want. I'm a good-looking guy, and if you know anything about how women are, you know that I can get one without any trouble."

FACTORS INFLUENCING THE DISTURBANCE

The intensity of the body image disturbances fluctuates widely even over short periods of time. When things are going well and a person with a body image disturbance is in good spirits, he may be troubled little or not at all by his disability, although it is rarely far from awareness. Let things go badly, however, let a depressive mood ensue, and at once all of the derogatory and unpleasant things in his life become focused upon his obesity, and his body becomes the explanation and the symbol of his unhappiness. A kind of circular relationship obtains between body image disturbances which predispose to esteem-lowering experiences and depressive moods which in their turn reinforce the disturbed body image.

Despite these short-term fluctuations in intensity, body image disturbances persist with remarkably little change over long periods of time and in the face of considerable variation in life circumstances. Weight reduction, for example, appears to have little effect upon them, a finding which has been made by a number of obese persons to their surprise and dismay. Neither the extent of the weight reduction, as illustrated by persons suffering from anorexia nervosa, nor its duration, as exemplified by the subjects described in the second paper of this series,[15] seems able to correct the disturbance in body image. And we have not heard reports of spontaneous remission of the disorder.

The relatively intractable nature of the disturbance in body image highlights the one form of treatment which has ameliorated it. In each of five persons suffering from the disturbance who were significantly benefited by long-term psychotherapy there was a concomitant improvement in the body image disturbance, which has persisted as long as six years. It is of interest that this improvement occurred prior to the control of the obesity and has appeared to be a favorable prognostic sign. As one young man said shortly before embarking on a weight loss of 140 pounds, which he has maintained for five years, "It's strange to see myself in the mirror looking so fat, because I feel so differently about it now. I *feel* thin."

ORIGINS OF THE DISTURBANCE

Three factors predisposed an obese person to the development of a disturbed body image: age of onset of the obesity, presence of emotional disturbance, and negative evaluation of the obesity by others during the formative years. Three other factors did not seem of importance. They were: gender, extent of overweight, and intelligence.

Age of Onset

The most surprising aspect of the body image disturbances was the great importance of age of onset. Disturbances occurred almost exclusively among persons who became obese during childhood or adolescence. Table 3-I shows that not one of forty subjects with adult-onset obesity showed a severe body image disturbance, while such disturbances were found in half of those with onset of obesity in childhood or adolescence, the so-called "juvenile obesity."

Our interviews suggested that adolescence was the period during which the disturbed body image was most likely to begin. Again and again subjects reported bitter adolescent experiences which had colored their whole later evaluation of their obesity. By contrast, childhood seemed to have been a time of relative indifference for the elaboration of this disorder. The second paper of this series describes further studies concerning the period of onset.[15]

Presence of Emotional Disturbance

The relatively short interviews of this study frequently uncovered evidence of emotional disturbance. Among subjects with adult-onset obesity

TABLE 3-I

DEGREE OF BODY IMAGE DISTURBANCE ACCORDING TO AGE
OF ONSET OF OBESITY IN SEVENTY-FOUR PERSONS

Onset Category	Severe	Mild	None
Juvenile	17	8	9
Adult	0	10	30

$\chi^2 = 19.44$, df = 2, p < .001.

a wide variety of diagnostic pictures was observed, few if any of which seemed related to their obesity. Among subjects with juvenile obesity, on the other hand, a disturbance in body image was usually a central feature of any emotional disorder. Nine juvenile obese subjects showed no disturbance in body image. No emotional disturbance was detected in six of them, while three manifested well-defined neurotic patterns not involving body image disturbance. Emotional disturbance apparently constitutes a necessary but not sufficient cause of a disturbance in body image.

Negative Evaluation of Obesity by Significant Others

The almost universal devaluation of obesity in our society today might make it appear redundant to mention this factor as significant in the development of a disturbed body image. The occasional instance in which an obese youth did not face such censure, however, reminds us of the force of these attitudes. Two obese men in this series, both with onset of obesity in childhood and both from disturbed early family environments, escaped body image disturbances. The families in which both men were raised valued large size and looked upon overweight as a sign of strength and health. This favorable family evaluation was shared by their peers, and both men were much in demand as football players. Despite the fact that they showed clearly defined neurotic patterns at the time of their examinations, neither showed any evidence of a disturbance in body image.

DISCUSSION

The disturbances in body image of obese persons are different from those which occur in brain-damaged and schizophrenic persons and in normal persons under the influence of drugs, hypnosis, and fatigue.[1, 2, 4, 6, 7, 11, 12, 16] In the greater emphasis on affective than on cognitive disorder they resemble instead the disturbances reported among persons suffering from deformities of the face, breasts, and genitals.[8, 9, 13] The main feature is a preoccupation with obesity, often to the exclusion of any other personal characteristic. It may make no difference whether the person be talented, wealthy, or intelligent; his weight is his overriding concern and he sees the world in terms of body weight. He may divide society into persons of differing weights, and his orientation toward others may be largely in terms of this division. He envies persons thinner than he and feels contempt for those who are fatter. At the center of this attitude is the appraisal of his own body as grotesque and even loathesome, and the feeling that others view it only with horror and contempt.

The more we have learned about obesity, the more we have been impressed with the need for specificity in linking neurosis and obesity. Many obese persons have severe neurotic problems. From this observation it has often been inferred that the neurosis is a cause of the obesity. On methodologic grounds alone this is a shaky inference, and the results of recent population surveys emphasize its weakness. In one sample, for instance, some degree of emotional disturbance was found in 80 per cent of the population and obesity in 20 per cent.[5, 14] In this population, chance alone could ensure a high concordance of neurosis and obesity.

Furthermore, it is our clinical impression that the presence of neurosis in an obese person does not explain his obesity, nor is it even necessarily relevant to it. Understanding the relationship of neurosis to obesity requires careful description of which neurotic features are and which are not specific to obesity. The disturbance in body image constitutes one such specific feature.

This concern with specificity is particularly important in assessing the role of psychotherapy in the treatment of obesity. The results of psychotherapy have been disappointing, particularly when it has been used without careful selection of patients and when weight reduction has served as the only criterion of improvement. This disappointment does not deny the frequent usefulness of psychotherapy to obese persons suffering from emotional disturbances; it does emphasize the ineffectiveness of treatment of their obesity. In such a situation the delineation of specific indications for psychotherapy should permit our limited psychotherapeutic resources to be invested where they have the greatest prospects of success. The favorable results of long-term psychotherapy with persons suffering from body image disturbances, and the ineffectuality of other treatment, including prolonged weight reduction, suggests that this disorder constitutes a specific indication for psychotherapy.

SUMMARY

Of the many behavioral disturbances to which obese persons are subject, only two seem specifically related to their obesity. One is overeating, the other is a disturbance in body image. The disturbance in body image is characterized by a feeling that one's body is grotesque and loathesome and that others view it with hostility and contempt. This feeling is associated with self-consciousness and with impaired social functioning. It arises among emotionally disturbed persons whose obesity began prior to adult life, in families which did not value their obesity. The disturbance is not affected by weight reduction but has been favorably altered by long-term psychotherapy.

REFERENCES

1. Bruch, H.: *The Importance of Overweight*. New York, W. W. Norton & Co., 1957, pp. 182-187.
2. Federn, P.: Some variations in ego feeling, *Int J Psychoanal*, 7:434-444, 1926.
3. Fisher, S. and Cleveland, S. E.: *Body Image and Personality*. Princeton, N. J., D. Van Nostrand Co., 1958.

4. Gerstmann, J.: Psychological and phenomenological aspects of disorders of body image, *J Nerv Ment Dis,* 26:499-512, 1958.
5. Goldblatt, P. B., Moore, M. E. and Stunkard, A. J.: Social factors in obesity, *JAMA,* 192:1039-1044, 1965.
6. Klemperer, E.: Changes of body image in hypnoanalysis, *J Clin Exp Hypnosis,* 2:157-162, 1954.
7. Kolb, L. C.: Disturbances of body-image, in Arieti, S. (Ed.): *American Handbook of Psychiatry.* Vol. I. New York: Basic Books, 1959.
8. MacGregor, F. C., Abel, T. M., Bryt, A., Lauer, E. and Weissman, S.: *Facial Deformities and Plastic Surgery: A Psychosocial Study.* Springfield, Ill., Charles C Thomas, 1953.
9. Money, J. and Hampson, J. G.: The evidence of human hermaphroditism, *Bull Hopkins Hosp,* 97:301-319, 1955.
10. Orbach, J., Traub, A. C. and Olson, R.: Psychophysical studies of body image, *Arch Gen Psychiat,* 12:41-47, 1966.
11. Savage, C.: Variations in ego feeling induced by D-lysergic acid diethylamide (LSD3), *Psychoanal Rev,* 42:1-16, 1955.
12. Schilder, P.: *Image and Appearance of the Human Body.* London, Kegan Paul, Trench, Trubner & Co., 1935.
13. Schonfeld, W. A.: Gynecomastia in adolescence: Effect on body image and personality adaptation, *Psychosom Med,* 24:379-389, 1962.
14. Srole, L., Langner, T. S., Michael, S. T., Opher, M. K. and Rennie, T. A. C.: *Mental Health in the Metropolis: The Midtown Manhattan Study,* vol.. 1, New York, McGraw-Hill Book Co., 1962.
15. Stunkard, A. J. and Burt, V.: Obesity and the body image: II. Age of onset of disturbance in the body image. *Am J. Psychiat,* 123:1433, 1967.
16. Stunkard, A. and Mendelson, M.: Disturbances in body image of some obese persons. *J Am Diet Assoc,* 38:328-331, 1961.
17. Traub, A. C. and Orbach, J.: Psychodynamical studies of body image. *Arch Gen Psychiat,* 11:53-66, 1964.

4

The Perception of Body Size

MYRON L. GLUCKSMAN
AND
JULES HIRSCH

THE RESPONSE OF OBESE PATIENTS TO WEIGHT REDUCTION

DISTURBANCES of body image are often observed in obese patients.[1-6] These disturbances range from feelings of self-consciousness and contempt toward one-self to denial or distortion of one's appearance. Stunkard and Mendelson[3] suggested that three factors predisposed an obese individual to the development of a disturbed body image: the onset of obesity prior to adult life, the presence of a neurotic behavior pattern, and censure by significant family members.

The evaluation of body image has been traditionally obtained through interviews, questionnaires, and projective tests. Recently, an objective estimation of body image was developed by Traub and Orbach[7] using a body-distorting mirror. They concluded that it was a useful instrument for the quantitative measurement of body image. Studies of obese patients in this laboratory[5, 6] have indicated that body size is an important component of body image. Our definition of body size is the subjective estimation of total body girth or area. Previous data[5, 6] suggested that body size perception plays an important role in both the obese and reduced state. Some patients reported persistent feelings of obesity following weight loss. Moreover, their human figure drawings, following weight loss, contained larger waist diameters and total body areas, in contrast to their figure drawings before weight loss.

In this study, a body-sizing apparatus was utilized for the measurement of body size perception in obese patients before, during, and following weight loss.

MATERIALS AND METHODS

Six severely obese adult patients seeking weight reduction were hospitalized during the same period of time on the behavioral-metabolic unit of the University hospital. They included three males and three females, aged from twenty to thirty-six years. The mean admission weight of the group was 334 lb. All the patients had been obese since childhood and unsuccessful with previous attempts at weight reduction.

The experimental program consisted of an initial six-week period of weight maintenance (Period I), followed by a fifteen-week period of weight loss (Periods II and III), and a final six-week period of weight maintenance (Period IV). The mean length of hospitalization for the group was eight months, and the mean weight loss was 86.7 lb. Caloric intake during each of the four periods of hospitalization has been described elsewhere.[5]

A contrast group was utilized in the study, consisting of four adult, non-obese, hypercholesterolemic patients. Included in this group were three males and 1 female, aged from thirty-nine to fifty-seven years. These patients were in the same hospital, lived under similar conditions, and were fed the identical diet as the obese patients.[8] However, instead of losing weight, they were maintained at their admission weights throughout hospitalization. The mean admission weight of the contrast group was 132 lb, and the mean length of hospitalization was seven months.

The body-sizing apparatus used in this study consisted of a Hilux 102 variable anamorphic lens with a magnification of 1.0 to 2.0 times and with a regular, fixed-distance, corrector lens.* Attached to the lens was a 16 mm Agfa Diamator slide projector. The anamorphic lens was motorized, allowing both subject and experimenter to control it by means of manual devices. A dial, consisting of ten equal units, was attached to the anamorphic lens, enabling the experimenter to measure the amount of distortion in two directions—obese or thin. The midpoint on this dial corresponded to an undistorted image. Thus, with the dial set at midpoint, a slide placed in the slide projector and projected through the anamorphic lens onto a screen resulted in an undistorted image. With the dial at other settings, an obese or thin image resulted. The subject was not allowed to observe the dial.

Three different images of a female subject, when projected through the anamorphic lens (thin, undistorted, and obese), would be illustrated.

Subjects were tested once weekly, on the same day, and at the same hour. Each week, a few days prior to testing, a photograph was taken of each subject and converted into a 2-inch by 2-inch slide. Testing consisted of the following steps:

1. A slide of the subject was projected on a screen in front of the seated subject. Prior to projection on the screen, the slide was distorted in either the direction of obesity or thinness at a predetermined dial setting. The subject was requested to make the distorted screen image correspond to his or her body size, as it was perceived by the subject at that moment. The subject accomplished this by manipulating the manual device which controlled the motorized, anamorphic lens. The subject was given four trials at this task, consisting of two trials in which the screen image was initially distorted in the direction of obesity, and

* Projection Optics Co., Inc., Rochester, N. Y.

two trials in which the screen image was initially distorted in the direction of thinness.

2. A slide of a symmetrical vase was presented to the subject in a manner similar to that for the previous slide. However, the subject was initially shown an undistorted image of the vase for 10 seconds instead of a distorted image. Following this, the screen image was distorted in the directions of obesity (two trials) and thinness (two trials). During these presentations, the subject was requested to make the screen image correspond to the initial, undistorted one.

3. A slide of an anonymous average-weight male was presented in the same manner as the symmetrical vase slide.

4. A slide of an anonymous average-weight female was presented to the subject in the same manner as the two previous slides.

5. All slides and all trials were presented in a randomized fashion throughout the study.

The contrast or nonobese subjects were each tested only weekly for six successive weeks. Since they were not all hospitalized simultaneously, it was not technically possible to test each of them for twenty-seven successive weeks, as were the obese subjects. However, the six-week period of testing was not performed during the same phase of hospitalization for each subject. Therefore, the effects of the initial, middle, and terminal phases of hospitalization were taken into account for the nonobese group.

RESULTS

The basic unit of data was the "size estimation score." This consisted of a subject's total score for a particular stimulus in a given test during four trials. A trial score was simply the numerical value of the dial setting arrived at by the subject.

Table 4-I presents the results of an analysis of variance of the periods of weight reduction and of the size estimation of stimuli by the obese subjects. Table 4-I indicates that the "self" body size estimations of the obese

TABLE 4-I

ANALYSIS OF VARIANCE OF PERIODS OF WEIGHT REDUCTION AND SIZE ESTIMATION OF "SELF," "VASE," "MALE," AND "FEMALE" STIMULI FOR OBESE SUBJECTS

Source of Variation	df	Self Mean sq.	F	Vase Mean sq.	F	Male Mean sq.	F	Female Mean sq.	F
Periods	3	58.44	5.52*	6.19	0.95	2.30	0.40	0.35	0.06
Subjects	5	427.37	4.04*	50.07	7.68*	62.59	10.89*	68.31	13.30*
Interaction	15	40.71	5.78*	5.64	0.86	6.34	1.10	8.67	1.85*
Residual	120	6.82		6.51		5.75		4.68	
Total	143								

* $p \leqq 0.05$,

TABLE 4-II

ANALYSIS OF VARIANCE OF NONOBESE SUBJECTS AND SIZE ESTIMATION
OF "SELF," "VASE," "MALE," AND "FEMALE" STIMULI

Source of Variation	df	Mean sq.	F
Subjects	3	59.76	5.01*
Stimuli	3	60.57	5.08*
Interaction	9	30.83	3.15*
Residual	80	9.79	
Total	95		

* $p \lesssim 0.05$.

subjects differed significantly between periods. This difference consisted of an increasing overestimation of their own body size from Period I to Period IV. By contrast, their size estimations of the other three stimuli ("vase," "male," and "female") did not differ significantly between periods. There were significant differences in size estimation scores between subjects for all stimuli. Interaction between obese subjects and the periods was significant for the "self" and "female" stimuli.

Table 4-II presents the results of an analysis of variance of the nonobese subjects and their size estimation of the stimuli. There was a significant difference between subjects in their size estimations of all stimuli. Moreover, each stimulus differed significantly from the other for all subjects. Interaction between nonobese subjects and the stimuli was significant.

Obese and nonobese subjects differed, although not significantly, in their estimations of "self." The nonobese subjects underestimated their own body sizes, in comparison to the obese subjects. The obese subjects overestimated and the nonobese subjects underestimated the "vase" size, although this difference was not significant. Both groups overestimated the "male" and "female" body sizes, but without a significant difference.

DISCUSSION

The results of this study suggest that it is possible to evaluate quantitatively the perception of body size. The anamorphic-lens technique is especially advantageous for the quantification of body size perception, because it distorts only body girth.

The most striking observation was that the obese subjects increasingly overestimated their own body size during and following weight loss. Prior to weight loss (Period I), the obese group slightly underestimated their actual body size. During weight loss (Periods II and III), they overestimated their actual body size. The amount of overestimation was significantly larger than their slight underestimation of themselves during Period I. Following weight loss (Period IV), they continued to overestimate their actual body size. The amount of overestimation during Period IV was significantly larger than the amount of overestimation during Periods II and III. By measuring the screen body size (waist diameter) which the obese subjects estimated of themselves, it was possible to determine the difference between their screen body sizes from one period to the next. It was apparent that those subjects who increasingly overestimated their body size during Periods II, III, and IV were actually perceiving themselves as they had during Period I. In effect, despite their weight loss, they perceived themselves as if they had lost almost no weight. This "phantom body size" phenomenon was accompanied by supportive clinical and figure-drawing data.[6] For example, these same subjects drew progressively larger isosexual figure drawings during hospitalization. They also reported that they continued to feel obese, following weight loss.

In contrast to their progressive overestimation of "self" during and following weight loss, the obese subjects did not make the same perceptual error with regard to the "vase," "male," and "female" stimuli.

Although they consistently overestimated the size of the "vase," "male," and "female" stimuli during each period of hospitalization, the amount of overestimation was not significantly different from one period to the next.

There are several possible explanations for their increasing overestimation of "self" and their rather consistent overestimation of the other stimuli from one period to the next. First, they were never shown their own actual body size but were shown the actual size of the other stimuli during testing. Thus, they never had a reference point for their own body size, in contrast to the other stimuli. Second, there may have been a significant difference in the way they perceived their own body size and the way they perceived stimuli external to themselves. This difference became more marked with weight loss because of the "phantom body size" phenomenon—that is, continued maintenance of their before-weight-loss "body size image" necessitated an increasing overestimation of their actual body size, because of their increasing weight loss. This mechanism was not necessary for the external stimuli, since the actual sizes of these were never changed during the study. One reason for the "phantom body size" phenomenon may be that, in subjects obese since childhood, the "body size image" before weight loss is relatively fixed, and cannot be altered as rapidly as the actual change in body configuration. Moreover, there may be psychodynamic determinants for the maintenance of a before-weight-loss "body size image." Of interest is the subsequent finding that three of the obese subjects in this study, who were retested after an additional year of weight loss, continued to overestimate their actual body size.

The greatest difference between the obese and nonobese subjects was in their perception of "self." The nonobese subjects underestimated their body size, in comparison to the obese subjects. In view of their cardiovascular pathology, the importance of remaining thin may have been an important determinant for their underestimation of body size. Entirely normal nonobese subjects might not have responded in this manner. Shipman and Sohlkhah[9] observed that normal nonobese women were accurate in their body size estimates, in contrast to obese women who estimated themselves as substantially broader than they actually were. As a group, the nonobese subjects in this study underestimated the "vase," but overestimated the "male" and "female" stimuli. It is of interest that they did not perceive stimuli external to themselves in as uniform a manner as the obese subjects. Except for their before-weight-loss "self" body size estimation, the obese subjects overestimated all other stimuli before, during, and following weight loss. In view of the small number of subjects used in this study, further exploration of the perceptual differences between obese and nonobese subjects is indicated, especially now that an apparatus is available for the quantitative measurement of body size perception.

SUMMARY

An apparatus was constructed and utilized for the measurement of body size. Six obese and four nonobese (contrast) subjects were studied under similar hospital conditions. The obese subjects were studied prior to, during, and following weight loss, while the nonobese subjects were studied only during weight maintenance.

Once weekly, the subjects estimated the real size of distorted photographs projected on a screen of a) themselves, b) a symmetrical vase, c) an average-weight male, and d) an average-weight female. The results indicated that the obese subjects increasingly overestimated their own body size during and following weight loss. They also overestimated the size of the other stimuli, but the amount of overestimation did not differ significantly before, during, and following weight loss. Those obese subjects who overestimated their own body size during and following weight loss were perceiving themselves, in fact, as if they had lost almost no weight. A delay in the appropriate correction of the before-weight-loss "body size image," as well as psychodynamic factors, may contribute to this "phantom body size" phenomenon.

The nonobese subjects underestimated their own body size, in comparison to the obese subjects. They did not perceive the other stimuli uniformly, in contrast to the obese subjects who consistently overestimated all the stimuli external to themselves.

REFERENCES

1. Bruch, H.: *The Importance of Overweight*. New York, Norton, 1957.
2. Stunkard, A. and Mendelson, M.: Disturbances in body image of some obese persons. *J Am Diet Assoc*, 38:328, 1961.
3. Stunkard, A. and Mendelson, M.: Obesity and the body image: I. Characteristics of

disturbances in the body image of some obese persons. *Am J Psychiat,* 123: 1296, 1967.

4. Stunkard, A. and Burt, V.: Obesity and the body image: II. Age at onset of disturbances in the body image. *Am J Psychiat,* 123:1433, 1967.

5. Glucksman, M. L. and Hirsch, J.: The response of obese patients to weight reduction: A clinical evaluation of behavior. *Psychosom Med,* 30:1, 1968.

6. Glucksman, M. L., Hirsch, J., McCully, R. S., Barron, B. A. and Knittle, J. L.: The response of obese patients to weight reduction: II. A quantitative evaluation of behavior. *Psychosom Med,* 30:359, 1968.

7. Traub, A. C. and Orbach, J.: Psychophysical studies of body image: I. The adjustable body-distorting mirror. *Arch Gen Psychiat (Chicago),* 11:53, 1964.

8. Ahrens, E. H., Jr., Dole, V. P. and Blankenhorn, D. H.: The use of orally fed liquid formulas in metabolic studies. *Am J Clin Nutr,* 2:336, 1954.

9. Shipman, W. G. and Sohlkhah, N.: Body image distortion in obese women. (abst.) *Psychosom Med,* 29:540, 1967.

III
PSYCHOSOCIAL FACTORS

5

Social Factors in Obesity

Phillip B. Goldblatt
Mary E. Moore
and
Albert J. Stunkard

THIS report is an extension of our previous finding that social factors play an important role in human obesity.[1] Current theories as to the etiology of obesity, whether behavioral, biochemical, or physiological, have directed their attention to the individual. We were, therefore, very much interested in a finding incidental to our earlier study, which was undertaken to assess the relationship of mental health to obesity in a large, representative, urban population.[1] Parental social class, introduced as a controlling variable, showed a high correlation with the prevelance of obesity and was a more powerful predictor of overweight than a number of psychological measures. The present study, undertaken to investigate this relationship further, showed obesity to be related to each of the following additional social variables: the respondent's own socioeconomic status, social mobility, and generation in the United States.

METHODS AND MATERIALS

The data reported here were collected as part of the Midtown Manhattan Study, a comprehensive survey of the epidemiology of mental illness. The details of the sample and the data collection techniques have been fully described elsewhere.[2,3] The data in the present analysis were obtained from the Midtown Home Survey of 1,660 adults, consisting of 690 males and 970 females between the ages of twenty and fifty-nine. One female in the Home Survey was omitted from our study because she was under four feet (122 cm) in height. The population was divided into three weight categories: "obese," "normal," and "thin," based upon the self-reported heights and weights as described in our previous paper. The validity of such reports has been attested to by an independent survey.[4]

The relationships of these categories to the widely accepted standards for "desirable" weight of the Metropolitan Life Insurance Company[5] is shown in Table 5-I. The "desirable" weights are those for which the mortality rates are lowest, so that even the group which we have designated "normal" exceeds their "desirable" weight by about 10 per cent. The means for our "obese" groups were 34 per cent and 44 per cent above the

TABLE 5-I

RELATIONSHIP OF MIDTOWN HOME SURVEY WEIGHT
CATEGORIES TO STANDARDS OF "DESIRABLE" WEIGHT*

Midtown Weight Category	Average % Over (+) or Under (–) Desirable Weight	
	Females	Males
Thin	–13	–16
Normal	+11	+ 9
Obese	+44	+34

* Standards of Metropolitan Life Insurance Company for desirable weight.

"desirable" weight, indicating a significant degree of overweight. The corresponding means for the "thin" groups were 13 per cent and 16 per cent below the "desirable" weight.

The respondent's own socioeconomic status (SES) at the time of the interview was rated by a simple score devised by Srole et al.[2] based upon the respondent's occupation, education, weekly income, and monthly rent. Each of these four variables was subdivided into six categories. In the scoring, each variable was given equal weight. Thus, an individual in the lowest category of each variable (unskilled labor, no schooling, income less than 49 dollars per week, and monthly rent less than 30 dollars) received a score of four. Conversely, an individual in all of the highest categories (high white collar, graduate school education, income over 300 dollars per week, and monthly rent greater than 200 dollars) received a score of 24. (Unmarried working women were rated on the basis of their own occupation. Unmarried nonworking women were classified by their fathers' occupation. Married women, whether working or not, were rated on the basis of their husbands' occupation.) In order to obtain subgroups of sufficient size to permit control by variables which the analysis showed to be relevant, the population was divided into three socioeconomic groups as nearly equal in number as feasible. Individuals with scores of 4 to 10 were designated low status; those with scores of 11 to 16 were middle status; and those with 17 to 24 points were high status.

In our first paper we used the respondent's social class of origin as a controlling variable. This measure was employed so as to avoid any reciprocal relationship that might exist between a respondent's present SES and his obesity. Obesity may in part depend on social status but, at the same time, social status may in part depend on obesity. The SES of origin is a measure of important social influences on a respondent which are in no sense a product of his obesity. The social class of origin was based on the education and occupation of the respondent's father when the respondent was eight years old.

The scores for SES of origin were divided into "low," "medium," and "high" socioeconomic categories in a manner analogous to that used for the respondent's own SES. These two sets of scores permitted us to study the relationship of obesity to social mobility by comparing the socioeconomic status of the respondent at the age of eight with that at the time of the interview.

RESULTS

The present analysis extended in a most dramatic way our previous finding of the importance in the understanding of human obesity of one socioeconomic variable—socioeconomic status of origin. Every one of the three additional social factors investigated was also strongly related to obesity. Furthermore, each was more strongly related to obesity among women than among men. The analysis of the data for women will be presented first.

Obesity Among Women

Own Socioeconomic Status

There was a marked inverse relationship between the prevalence of obesity and the respondent's own SES. The prevalence of obesity among lower SES women was 30 per cent, falling to 16 per cent among the middle SES, and to only 5 per cent in the upper SES. A chi-square test of the relationship between socioeconomic status and the three weight categories was significant at the 0.001 level ($x^2 = 120.7$).

Socioeconomic Status of Origin

Just as the respondent's own socioeconomic status was inversely related to her obesity, so also was her socioeconomic status of origin ($x^2 = 66.5$, $P < 0.001$). Note that the relationship between this factor and obesity was nearly as strong as that between the respondent's own socioeconomic status and her weight category.

Social Mobility

The close correspondence between the results for the respondent's own SES and SES of origin suggested the possibility that these two variables were measuring the same underlying dimension. This would be the case in a society in which the vast majority of people lived out their entire lives in the same social class into which they were born. Such was not the case, however, in Midtown Manhattan which showed a high degree of social mobility. Indeed, 44 per cent of the women belonged to a different social class from that of their parents. In other words, many people were classified differently by our two indices of social status, and these two variables did not measure the same underlying dimension. A measure of this discrepancy be-

The Psychology of Obesity

tween the respondent's own SES and the SES of her origin is given by our index of social mobility.

Of women who remained in the socioeconomic status into which they were born 17 per cent were obese, whereas among women who moved down in social status there was a higher prevalence of obesity (22%), while among those who moved upwards there was a lower prevalence (12%) ($\chi^2 = 20.5$, $P < 0.001$). Thus, movement *among* the social classes as well as membership *in* a social class was predictive of obesity.

Generation in the United States

The fourth variable, generation in the United States, was also strongly linked to obesity. To assess this variable, respondents were divided into one of four groups on the basis of the number of generations their families had been in this country. Generation I consisted of foreign-born immigrants; generation II, of all those native-born respondents with at lease one foreign-born parent; generation III, of all those who were native-born of native born parents but had at least one foreign-born grandparent; and generation IV, of all those who had no foreign-born grandparents and who otherwise met the qualifications for generation III.

The longer a woman's family had been in this country, the less likely she was to be obese. Of first generation respondents 24 per cent were overweight, in contrast to only 5 per cent in the fourth generation ($\chi^2 = 56.5$, $P < 0.001$).

It seemed probable that generation in the United States was closely related to socioeconomic status, and that the longer a family had been in this country, the higher its status was likely to be. The data in Table 5-II show that this is indeed the case. Thus, in the first generation, 194 out of 365 respondents were of low SES, while in the fourth generation, 102 out of 140 were of high SES ($\chi^2 = 235.6$, $P < 0.001$).

To determine whether this phenomenon accounted for the finding that

TABLE 5-II

PERCENTAGE OF OBESE FEMALES BY GENERATION IN UNITED STATES—
CONTROLLING THE FACTOR OF SOCIOECONOMIC STATUS (SES)

	Generation											
	I			*II*			*III*			*IV*		
	Own SES Low	*Own SES Med*	*Own SES High*	*Own SES Low*	*Own SES Med*	*Own SES High*	*Own SES Low*	*Own SES Med*	*Own SES High*	*Own SES Low*	*Own SES Med*	*Own SES High*
Obese, %	30	21	7	34	19	6	22	6	2	13	4	4
N (100%)*	194	113	58	96	126	78	23	52	87	15	23	102

* N = Number in sample falling into particular category, e.g., 30% of 194 first generation low SES females are obese. Excludes two females about whom no information on generation is available.

obesity was less common the longer a respondent's family had been in the country, we examined the prevalence of obesity for each SES within each generation. Table 5-II clearly demonstrates that the inverse relation between obesity and generation was independent of socioeconomic status. Of the generation I respondents who were of low status 30 per cent were obese, but only 13 per cent of generation IV low-status females were overweight. This trend obtained in all the social classes (χ^2 for low SES = 21.5, $P < 0.01$; χ^2 for middle SES = 18.1, $P < 0.01$; χ^2 for high SES = 21.5, $P < 0.01$).

Obesity Among Men

The relationship between social factors and the prevalence of obesity among males paralleled that among the women, but in each instance was less marked.

Own Socioeconomic Status

There was an inverse relationship between his own SES and obesity. The effect was far weaker than in the case of females ($\chi^2 = 17.4$, $P < 0.01$). Whereas obesity was six times more common among women of lower socioeconomic status than among those of high status, the corresponding ratio among men was only 2:1.

Socioeconomic Status of Origin

Socioeconomic status of origin had an effect upon the prevalence of overweight among men, although, as was true for women, the effect was weaker than that of the respondent's own SES. Furthermore, the influence of SES of origin was far weaker among men than among women. Whereas obesity was four times more common among women of lower socioeconomic status of origin than among those of high status, the corresponding ratio among males was less than 2:1.

Social Mobility

Social mobility was even more common among the men in our sample than among the women, with 47 per cent of the males belonging to a different social class than their parents.

In regard to obesity among men who moved downward, stayed in the same class, or moved upward, once again the same trend obtained as for females. In this instance, however, the chi-square did not reach a level of statistical significance.

Generation in the United States

Among the men as among the women the percentage of obese respondents decreased as the number of generations in the United States increased. Obesity was three times more common among the males in the first generation as compared to those in the fourth generation ($\chi^2 = 18.7$, $P < 0.001$). There was, however, no sharp drop in the percentage of obese between generation II and III, as was the case among females. As among women, these findings resulted even when socioeconomic status was held constant.

The Thin Category

At the beginning of the analysis of the weight categories, we expected that "thinness" would behave as though it were the opposite of obesity. We found, however, a striking difference in this regard between men and women. With increasing status, women moved from the "obese" to the "thin" category, whereas men moved from the "obese" to the "normal." Thus, thinness did operate as the opposite of obesity for women, but not for men. Table 5-III shows that there were four times as many thin respondents among women of high status as there were among those of low status. Among men, however, about 10 per cent were thin in all classes, and it was the percentage of normal-weight respondents that increased with increasing status.

COMMENT

The most important finding of this study was the remarkable consistency with which social factors correlated with body weight. Such a strong correlation, appearing in all the factors investigated, is highly significant. The only other attempt to study obesity as a social phenomenon, that by Pflanz[6] in Germany, has reported similar findings. It is now apparent that obesity can no longer be viewed as simply an abnormal characteristic of the individual. It must also be viewed as one of the possible, and not to infrequent, normal responses of persons in certain subgroups of society to the perceived expectations of their social milieu.

Although not being obese, indeed, being thin, seems culturally desirable for the women of Midtown, almost one out of three lower class females was obese. Such a high percentage implies that in this subgroup of Midtown society, overweight is common enough that it need not be viewed as abnormal.

TABLE 5-III

WEIGHT CATEGORIES BY RESPONDENT'S OWN SOCIOECONOMIC STATUS (SES)

| Weight Categories | *Per Cent of Each Weight Category in Each SES* | | | | | |
| | *Low SES* | | *Middle SES* | | *High SES* | |
	Males	*Females*	*Males*	*Females*	*Males*	*Females*
Thin	10	9	9	19	12	37
Normal	59	61	64	65	73	58
Obese	31	30	27	16	15	5
N (100%)*	215	329	240	315	235	325

* Number of individuals in sample falling into particular category.

In the Midtown society we do not have to look far to see the image of the slim, attractive female as portrayed throughout the popular culture. Motion picture stars, television personalities, women in advertisements, fashion models, and, indeed, the fashionable clothes themselves, all reflect the definition of the beautiful female as the one who is thin. How does such an ideal of beauty exert its impact on the body weight of persons in the different elements of society? At least two mechanisms seem plausible.

First, a selection process may operate so that in any status-conferring situation, such as a promotion at work or marriage to a higher status male, thinner women may be preferentially selected over their competitors.

Second, an acculturation phenomenon may be operating. For example, an individual's adult weight can be seen to be partly a product of social influences operating in his childhood. That this occurred in Midtown is demonstrated by our finding of a marked relationship between obesity and the SES of one's origin. A similar process may also be operating throughout life. Thus a female who acquires upper socioeconomic status for desirable attributes other than thinness will perceive that among her new peers more emphasis is placed upon being slim than was true in her old environment. She is likely, therefore, to make a greater effort to lose weight than she might previously have done.

The lesser importance of social factors as related to body weight among men, as contrasted to women, may arise from a lesser importance that society attaches to the physical appearance of men, as well as from a different definition of culturally desirable weight for them. In advertisements, for example, men are as likely to be exhorted to avoid being "ninety-seven-lb weaklings," as to avoid being obese. It is, perhaps, not surprising that the normal weight category correlates so highly with upper socioeconomic status.

The extent to which a respondent has adopted the Midtown values about body weight apparently depends upon at least two factors: first, on the length of his family's exposure to these values (as measured by number of generations in the United States) and second, the amount of pressure to conform to these values, which is a function of his proximity to the upper classes where the values are most strongly exemplified.

Although generation and socioeconomic status are related to each other, it has been shown in this study that each makes an independent contribution to the prevalence of obesity. It is unfortunate that the size of the sample precluded more precise estimates of their relative contributions.

It is obvious that there were important differences among our respondents besides those of class and generation. The Midtown sample included nine ethnic groups (British, Russian-Polish-Lithuanian, German-Austrian, Irish, Puerto Rican, Italian, Hungarian, Czech, and fourth generation

American) as well as many religions and sects. We discovered several relationships between ethnic and religious backgrounds and obesity. These were so intertwined with each other and with other social factors such as generation and socioeconomic status that we were unable to control all of the relevant factors simultaneously. Nevertheless, some of the data are worth describing briefly.

For example, only 9 per cent of female respondents of British descent were obese, whereas 27 per cent of those of Italian extraction were in this weight category. These differences diminished when social class was the control. Thus, for example, when only the upper classes of both ethnic groups were contrasted, the prevalence of obesity was 10 per cent for the British and 20 per cent for the Italian. Such differences can be related to what is known about the traditional diets and social implications of eating of these two ethnic groups. Joffe,[7] for example, has reported that first generation Italian mothers regard obesity in their children as protection against tuberculosis. Childs[8] found the basic diet of Italian-Americans to have a high fat content. Finally, a recent study in a small Pennsylvania town inhabited almost entirely by Italian-Americans revealed that the diet had a greater proportion of fat than that of the average American diet and that the prevalence of obesity was also significantly above average.[9]

Another example of such a phenomenon may be found among our data for Americans of eastern European extraction. Joffe notes that the Czechs love food and are less Americanized than the Poles as far as cooking habits are concerned. Among the Czechs, there is a great deal of visiting on Sundays during which time large quantities of food are consumed. Refusing a second or even a third helping of food is considered impolite. Our data reflect the results of these customs. Of the lower-class Czechs 41 per cent were obese as compared with only 18 per cent of the lower-class Polish-Russian-Lithuanians that were obese.

We also found differences among respondents of different religions. Lutherans, for example, were more often obese (24%) than Episcopalians (3%), but any statement made about the Lutherans and Episcopalians reflects also the difference between respondents of German and of British extraction. Unfortunately, we did not have enough cases to sift out the effects of religion *per se.*

What has been reported in this study about obesity in Midtown in 1954 is not necessarily applicable *in toto* to any other country, or any other urban area, or even to the Midtown of today. Indeed, Pflanz found an increased incidence of obesity among upwardly mobile German men and a decreased incidence among German women; in contrast, a decreased incidence among the upwardly mobile of both sexes was found in the present study. It thus appears that the same social mechanisms which discourage obesity among the socially mobile in this country may encourage it among

German men. Even though Pflanz's specific findings differed from ours, his conclusion was the same: human obesity must be understood in part as a social phenomenon.

Many of the present theories about human obesity were formulated by psychiatrists on the basis of their treatment of middle and of upper class women, for whom obesity was a severe social liability. In other segments of society, however, obesity appears to be by no means such a handicap. Future researchers will have to explore the ways in which some respondents in all classes develop the attitude that a slim appearance is very important. Studies will be needed to determine the reasons why certain subgroups have a higher incidence of this belief than others, the mechanisms by which this belief is inculcated, and the ages at which it appears with differing frequencies in differing social classes. Future theories will have to take into account the differing implications of overweight for the different social classes.

It seems quite possible that the lack of success in the control and treatment of obesity stems from the fact that until now physicians have thought of obesity as always being abnormal. This is certainly not true for persons in the lower socioeconomic population. Obesity may always be unhealthy, but it is not always abnormal.

Unfortunately, our weight control programs have directed their appeals in a nonspecific way to rich and poor alike. The present study reveals an unexpected opportunity for increasing the selectivity of public health measures for the control of obesity. Would it not be more effective to initiate programs tailored specifically for subgroups of society where obesity is most common? The success of a similar approach has been demonstrated by Johnson et al.,[10] who studied the epidemiology of polio vaccine acceptance in Dade County, Fla. They pointed up the importance of ethnic background and social class as an index of commonly held beliefs, shared feelings, group values and attitudes, and social participation. Utilizing such information in work with a high-risk population (lower-class, Spanish-speaking residents of Dade County), they significantly increased the percentage of respondents who took polio vaccine over the percentage who had done so in previous campaigns.

The present study shows the feasibility of identifying obese populations at high risk. Such identification has generally been a prerequisite for effective public health programs. Recognition of the significance of social factors in obesity may lay the foundation for our first effective public health program for the control of obesity.

REFERENCES

1. Moore, M. E., Stunkard, A., and Srole, L.: Obesity, social class, and mental illness, *JAMA,* 181:962-966 (Sept 15) 1962.

 2. Srole, L., *et al.: Mental Health in the Metropolis: Midtown Manhattan Study.*
    New York, McGraw-Hill Book Co., Inc., vol 1, 1962.
 3. Langner, T. S. and Michael, S. T.: *Life Stress and Mental Health: Midtown
    Manhattan Study.* New York, The Free Press of Glencoe, Inc., vol 2, 1963.
 4. Perry, L. and Learnard, B.: Obesity and mental health. *JAMA,* 183:807-808
    (March 2) 1963.
 5. New weight standards for men and women. *Statist Bull Metrop Life Insur Co,*
    40:2-3 (Nov-Dec) 1959.
 6. Pflanz, M.: Medizinische-soziologische Aspekte der Fettsucht. *Psyche,* 16:575-591,
    1962-1963.
 7. Joffe, N. F.: Food habits of selected subcultures in United States. *Bull Nat Res
    Council,* 108:97-103 (Oct) 1943.
 8. Childs, A.: Some dietary studies of Poles, Mexicans, Italians, and Negroes. *Child
    Health Bull,* 9:84-91, 1933.
 9. Stout, C., *et al.:* Unusually low incidence of death from myocardial infarction:
    Study of Italian-American community in Pennsylvania. *JAMA,* 188:845-849
    (June 8) 1964.
10. Johnson, A. L., *et al.: Epidemiology of Polio Vaccine Acceptance—Social and
    Psychological Analysis.* Monograph No. 3, Florida State Board of Health, 1962.

6

Psychosocial Aspects of Obesity

J. Trevor Silverstone

IN spite of a multitude of publications on the subject of obesity very little is known for certain about its etiology. It is, of course, generally accepted that in order for weight gain to take place calorie intake must exceed calorie expenditure, but the relative importance of factors which might influence calorie intake and expenditure, such as age, social class, and psychiatric state, have been relatively little studied. There are several possible criteria by which to define obesity and the most widely used is based on the concept of "ideal" weight. This is the weight, for each height, which was found to be associated with the greatest longevity in an actuarial study of insured persons.[11] As these "ideal" weights do not vary with age and are not likely to alter much from culture to culture, they are more useful for comparative purposes than average weights. Significant obesity is considered to be present when a subject is 30 per cent or more above his ideal weight. For a woman of 5 ft 4 in (1.63m) the ideal weight (clothed) is 123 lb (56 kg), for a man of 5 ft 6 in it is 140 lb (64 kg).

Age: In all published height and weight surveys the average weight of the population tends to increase with age.[6] In keeping with this observation it was found, in a sample of New Yorkers, that the prevalence of significant obesity also increased with age.[7]

Social class: Examining the data obtained during a study in "Midtown" New York, Goldblatt *et al.*[3] discovered that the prevalence of obesity was greater in the lower socioeconomic categories than the higher, particularly in women.

Psychiatric factors: Although a number of authors have suggested that obesity is largely the consequence of neurotically-induced eating behavior, there is little controlled evidence to support this suggestion. In fact, what evidence there is appears contrary to it.

Little major difference in psychiatric status between obese and nonobese subjects in New York could be found after analysis of the data obtained at a large number of standardized interviews.[7] Using a symptom check-list, the Cornell Medical Index (CMI), to detect neuroticism, McCance[5] could find no evidence of increased neuroticism among a group of obese patients attending the dietetic department of a London teaching hospital when compared to a group of nonobese patients attending the medical clinic of the same hospital. In a small general practice study employing the CMI, we

67

could find no greater prevalence of neuroticism in a group of thirty-two obese women[10] than might be expected to occur in London women generally.[8] The present investigation was planned to compare a group of normal-weight subjects to a group of obese subjects with respect to certain psychological factors, both groups being relatively unselected.

INVESTIGATION

The investigation was conducted in two stages. During the first stage a random sample was taken from two general practices selected to cover between them a wide range of social class. One was situated in the northwest suburbs of London and contained a high proportion of social classes I and II, while the other was in the "East End" of London, and contained a higher proportion of social classes IV and V.

In each practice every fifth patient whose medical notes were in the files was selected. Of these patients, all those who were aged between twenty and sixty on January 1, 1966 were included in the sample, there were 563 in all. Each patient in the sample was then requested to attend by appointment at his general practitioner's surgery to be weighed and measured. Enclosed with the letter asking him to come was a CMI form. The patient was asked to complete it at home and to bring it with him when he attended.

When the patients attended, their height and weight was measured with shoes and jacket off. In addition, skin thickness measurements were made over the left triceps and just below the angle of the left scapula. Three readings were taken at each site and the mean of these recorded. The instrument used was a Harpenden skinfold calliper.[12] On the basis of his occupation (or her husband's occupation in the case of a married woman) each subject was allocated to one of the five social classes specified by the General Register Office.[2]

If a patient failed to attend he was given a further appointment, and if he again failed he was written to a third time and given yet another ap-

TABLE 6-I

AGE AND SOCIAL CLASS DISTRIBUTION OF MEN IN THE SAMPLE

Social Class	Age				Total
	20-29	30-39	40-49	50-59	
I	2	5	5	2	14 ⎫ (28%)
II	4	9	11	8	32 ⎭
III	26	23	19	30	98 (60%)
IV	1	6	1	2	10 ⎫ (12%)
V	2	3	1	3	9 ⎭
Total	35 (21.5%)	46 (28.2%)	37 (22.7%)	45 (27.6%)	163

TABLE 6-II

AGE AND SOCIAL CLASS DISTRIBUTION OF WOMEN IN THE SAMPLE

Social Class	Age 20-29	30-39	40-49	50-59	Total
I	4	4	4	3	15 ⎱ (34%)
II	7	11	15	13	46 ⎰
III	14	21	27	33	95 (52%)
IV	3	2	4	9	18 ⎱ (14%)
V	1	3	0	3	7 ⎰
Total	29 (16%)	41 (22.6%)	50 (27.6%)	61 (33.8%)	181

pointment. Of those who had been originally included in the sample, 115 (20%) were no longer available for the study as they had either moved (113) or died (2). Of the remaining 448, 344 (77%) attended, while 17 (4%) expressed reluctance to participate. Even after three requests a fifth of the available subjects failed to attend.

The results presented are from the 344 subjects on whom adequate information was collected. The age and social class distribution of this sample of 344 is given in Tables 6-I and 6-II. In the case of the male subjects the age distribution is reasonably close to that for London as a whole, but in the sample of women there were fewer young women aged 20 to 29 and more older women aged 50 to 59 (General Register Office 1963-6). Although a wide spectrum of social classes was represented, there was a relative underrepresentation of social classes IV and V and an overrepresentation of social classes I and II compared to London as a whole.

Prevalence of Obesity in the Sample

Each patient's actual weight was compared to his ideal weight. If the patient was less than 15 per cent above his ideal weight he was classified as normal, if he weighed 15 to 29 per cent above his ideal weight he was classified as being "moderately" obese. If he weighed 30 to 45 per cent above his ideal weight he was placed in the "marked" obesity group, and if he was more than 45 per cent above his ideal weight he was classified as "massively" obese. In Table 6-III the distribution of these grades of obesity in the sample is shown; 18 per cent of the men and 25 per cent of the women were at least 30 per cent above their ideal weight.

The measurements of skin thickness showed that these overweight subjects were suffering from true adiposity, not increased muscularity. Almost all the men who were in the "normal" group had a combined triceps and subscapular skin thickness of under 30 mm, while almost all those who were 30 per cent overweight and more had a combined skin thickness of

TABLE 6-III

DISTRIBUTION OF SAMPLE IN TERMS OF OVERWEIGHT

	Normal (< 15% Overweight)	Moderate Obesity (15-29% Overweight)	Marked Obesity (30-45% Overweight)	Massive Obesity (> 45% Overweight)	Total
Men	78 (48%)	56 (34%)	23 (14%)	6 (4%)	163
Women	79 (44%)	57 (31%)	28 (16%)	17 (9%)	181
Total	157	113	51	23	344

over 30 mm. For the women the "normals" had a combined skin thickness of below 40 mm and the "marked" and "massively" obese had a combined skin thickness of 40 mm or more.

The prevalence of obesity in the sample increased with age for both men and women. This was particularly striking in the case of women. Very few women under thirty were obese; a considerable proportion of those over forty were.

The proportion of those who were "markedly" or "massively" obese was increased in social classes IV and V as compared with social classes I to III. Again this uneven pattern of distribution was particularly noticeable among the women in the sample. Taking the age and social class distribution together, obesity was proportionately more prevalent among older women of social classes IV and V than in any other subgroup.

Obesity and Neuroticism

A score of 10 or more positive responses in the M-R sections of the CMI was taken to indicate a tendency to neuroticism. The distribution of such scores obtained in the sample is given in Table 6-IV (in two cases the rele-

TABLE 6-IV

CMI-M-R SCORES AND DEGREE OF OVERWEIGHT

	M-R Score			
	0-4	5-9	10+	Total
Men				
Normal	57	13	8	78
Moderately obese	36	9	11	56
Markedly obese	15	6	1	22
Massively obese	3	3	0	6
Total	111	31	20	162
Women				
Normal	28	19	32	79
Moderately obese	27	16	14	57
Markedly obese	8	13	6	27
Massively obese	5	3	9	17
Total	68	51	61	180

vant data were not available). Considering the figures for the "markedly" and "massively" obese together and comparing them to the combined figures for the "normals" and "moderately" obese it was found that proportionally fewer of the men in the "marked" and "massively" obese groups had scores in the neurotic range than of those in the "normal" and "moderately" obese groups. Of the latter, 14 per cent could be classified as neurotic. This compares closely to the figure of 15.6 per cent obtained by Shepherd *et al.*,[8] using the same criterion of neuroticism in a sample of fourteen general practices in the London area.

The significantly obese women (30% or more above their ideal weight) tended to have similar M-R scores to the "normals" and "moderately" obese. In both groups 34 per cent had scores indicating neuroticism (in Shepherd *et al.*'s sample 35.2% of women had M-R scores above 10). Thus, by the criterion adopted, the majority of obese subjects could *not* be classified as neurotic.

Stage II of the study was designed to detect any differences between the obese and nonobese regarding their attitudes to body weight, eating and dieting, and to determine whether the obese were more prone to psychiatric disturbance than the nonobese. In order to obtain a suitable control group I matched each obese patient, who was at least 30 per cent above his ideal weight, as closely as possible with respect to sex, age, and social class to a member of the normal-weight group described above. As there was a prevalence of social class IV and V women in the obese group it was not possible to match five of these, and they will be considered separately where necessary.

The 138 members of the sixty-nine selected pairs (plus the five unpaired obese women) were all requested to attend at a specified time at their practitioner's surgery for a standard interview to be conducted by the investigator. Of those requested to attend fifty-eight obese (80%) and fifty-two nonobese (76%) did so. Three patients had died since the first stage of the survey and six had moved away. Four patients, all men, said they could not spare the time to attend; nineteen (12%) failed to reply. Interviews were obtained with both partners in fifty of the matched pairs, twenty male pairs and thirty female pairs.

Attitude to Weight

Each partner was asked whether he considered himself very thin, thin, normal weight, overweight, or very overweight; he was also asked if weight was a problem for him and whether or not he wished to lose weight. The replies are summarized in Table 6-V. It is apparent that by no means all of those who were 30 per cent above their ideal weight considered themselves to be overweight. Almost a third of the obese men and a fifth of the obese women denied being overweight. An even greater number of obese

TABLE 6-V

ATTITUDE TO WEIGHT

	Men Normal (n = 20)	Obese (n = 20)	Women Normal (n = 30)	Obese (n = 30)
Number who consider themselves overweight	2	14	4	24
Number for whom their weight is a problem	0	7	6	20
Number who want to lose weight	2	15	10	25

patients did not consider their weight to be a problem, yet a proportion of these did admit to a desire to lose weight. A number of women in the normal weight range considered themselves as overweight, yet none of them were more than 12 lb (5.4 kg) above their ideal weight. An even greater number of the normal women (a third of the total) wanted to lose weight.

Attitude to Eating

Each person interviewed was asked if he thought he overate, ate a normal amount of food, or underate. In addition each was asked whether he ate more when he was anxious, and whether or not food was "very," "moderately," or only "slightly" important to him. The results are presented in Table 6-VI. Although more obese subjects than normal subjects considered that they overate, the majority of obese subjects denied overeating.

With regard to the importance of food there was no difference between the obese and nonobese men, whereas obese women regarded food as "very important" more frequently than their nonobese counterparts. There was a similar difference between the sexes concerning eating and anxiety. Almost none of the men in either the obese and nonobese groups had noticed any association between anxiety and increased food intake. In contrast, almost a quarter of the nonobese women and over half of the obese women remarked on the association between feeling anxious and eating more.

TABLE 6-VI

ATTITUDE TO EATING

	Men Normal (n = 20)	Obese (n = 20)	Women Normal (n = 30)	Obese (n = 30)
Number who think they overeat	1	5	0	4
Number who consider food to be "very" important to them	6	6	6	11
Number who say they eat more when anxious	1	1	7	17

Neuroticism and Previous Psychiatric Symptoms

None of the men in either group had a CMI score in the neurotic range. Eight of the normal-weight women and eleven obese women had scores in this range, but this difference was not statistically significant. Two men in each group gave a past history of psychiatric symptoms (three anxiety, one depression). Six normal-weight women had a history of previous psychiatric disturbance (five anxiety, one depression) compared to three obese (two depression, one anxiety). These findings would suggest that the obese were no more likely to develop psychiatric symptoms than those of normal weight.

CONCLUSIONS

It is apparent from the present study, as from others, that obesity becomes more prevalent with increasing age. This probably results more from a reduction in calorie output associated with advancing years than from a change in calorie intake. We all tend, as we get older, to ride where we used to walk, to take the elevator where we used to climb the stairs, and so on. Our eating habits do not change correspondingly and we therefore tend to gain weight. Such weight gain occurring in middle age is rarely the consequence of any psychological disturbance.

This association between age and obesity was more marked among women, and was particularly striking among those women in social classes IV and V. It might be that all women tend to put on weight as they grow older, but the women in the upper social classes care more, and are subject to greater social pressures to be slim. Therefore they take appropriate dietary action to correct any weight gain which might occur.

The prevalence of neuroticism and psychiatric disturbance among obese patients was found to be no greater than among normals, even when any possible influence of age and social class had been allowed for. It has been suggested that obesity is often a psychological defense against depression. If this were so, loss of weight might be expected to be associated with the onset of depressive symptoms, but in a previous study[9] we could find no evidence that dieting and weight loss resulted in any increase whatsoever in such symptoms.

The only finding which did point to an association of psychological factors to obesity was the number of women, particularly among the obese group, who stated that they ate more when they were anxious. They tend to spend more of their time at home, where there is likely to be a supply of readily-available food, and in times of stress they may turn to this food for comfort and relief. The figures obtained in the present study suggest that obese women are more likely to act in such a manner than those of normal weight.

The majority of obese subjects of both sexes denied overeating. While such denials may be regarded as somewhat suspect, they are in keeping with the finding, obtained in many dietary surveys, that most obese people do not eat significantly more than the majority of normal-weight people.[13]

In conclusion, I would suggest, on the basis of the information outlined above, that psychiatric factors are unlikely to be of primary etiological significance in the majority of cases of obesity, although they may well play a secondary part.

REFERENCES

1. General Register Office: *Classification of Occupations.* London, Her Majesty's Stationer Office, 1966.
2. General Register Office: *Census 1961, County Reports.* London, Her Majesty's Stationer Office, 1963-66.
3. Goldblatt, P. B., Moore, M. E. and Stunkard, A. J.: Social factors in obesity. *JAMA,* 192:1039-1044, 1965.
4. Kemsley, W. F. F.: *Ann Eugen,* 16:316, 1952.
5. McCance, C.: *Psychiatric Factors in Obesity.* Dissertation for Diploma in Psychological Medicine, University of London, 1961.
6. Metropolitan Life Insurance Company. *Statistical Bull,* 40:2, 1959.
7. Moore, M. E., Stunkard, A. J. and Srole, L.: Obesity, social class, and mental illness. *JAMA,* 181:962-966, 1962.
8. Shepherd, M., Cooper, B., Brown, A. C. and Kalton, G. W.: *Psychiatric Illness in General Practice.* London, 1966.
9. Silverstone, J. T. and Lascelles, B. D.: *Brit J Psychiat,* 112:513, 1966.
10. Silverstone, J. T. and Solomon, T.: Psychiatric and somatic factors in the treatment of obesity. *J Psychosom Res,* 9:249-255, 1965.
11. Society of Actuaries: *Build and Blood Pressure Study.* Chicago, 1959.
12. Tanner, J. M. and Whitehouse, R. H.: *Brit Med J,* i:446, 1962.
13. Thomson, A. M., Billewicz, W. Z. and Passmore, R.: *Lancet,* i:1027, 1961.

7

An Anthropological Approach
to the Problem of Obesity

HORTENSE POWDERMAKER

MY role as an anthropologist is to attempt to set the problem of obesity in the context of the culture. In this day of specialists we cultural anthropologists are the specialists in a holistic approach. In our studies of primitive or preliterate tribal societies, we have asked questions concerning relationships between different elements of culture. How are the functioning of the family, the economic and class organization, the political system, the religious and magical beliefs, the values that men live by, related to each other and integrated in that abstraction we call culture? In this chapter I shall give a cultural approach to the problem of obesity, raise questions, and, quite tentatively, offer some hypotheses. These will provide some understanding of the complexities of the problem and a basis for future research.

In setting the problem of obesity in the frame of the culture of contemporary society, my focus will be on the roles of food and of physical activity in our value systems. Incidentally, I wonder why so much of the education designed to reduce the incidence of obesity is centered on food rather than on activity. Is it assumed that food habits may be modified more easily than those of physical activity?

My basic questions are concerned with the symbolism of fatness and thinness in our society and the relationship of each to other symbols and to our values. I would be interested in differences in the symbols and in the relative strength of the same symbols in class, ethnic, religious, sex, and age groups, and among individuals. I would assume that there might be conflicting values concerning fatness and thinness, about eating and physical activity, as there are in many other areas of our life, and that some of this conflict might stem from the fact that we live in a rapidly changing society, where traditional values linger beside new ones. I would also be interested in the cultural study of people who are not obese as well as those who are, i.e. some kind of control group in which variables are limited. As an anthropologist, I am naturally interested in a comparative approach, i.e. the symbolism of obesity and thinness in other cultures and the many-sided role of food and eating in them, assuming that this comparative knowledge would illuminate the problem in our society.

Beginning with the last point, let me summarize briefly some relevant facts from pre-literate, tribal societies. In a large number of these societies the economy was a subsistence one, whether characterized by food gathering, hunting, fishing, agriculture, raising cattle, or some combination of these activities. A major part of all activity was concerned with the production of food. Tools were crude—a wooden hoe and a stone axe. The only means of transportation was by foot or canoe. Food-growing plots were often several miles from the village; the clearing of the dense bush in tropical and semi-tropical parts of the world by the men was a strenuous job, as was also the planting and weeding by the women. Strenuous physical activity was the norm for men and for women, whatever the type of economy. But although everyone worked hard and long in the production of food, hunger was a common experience. Famines and periods of scarcity were not unusual. Seasonal changes, plagues, pests, and many other natural causes tended to produce alternate periods of shortage and relative plenty. It is, therefore, not difficult to understand that gluttony, one of the original sins in our society, was an accepted and valued practice for these tribal peoples whenever it was possible. In anticipating a feast a Trobriand Islander in the Southwest Pacific says, "We shall be glad, we shall eat until we vomit."[1] A South African tribal expression is, "We shall eat until our bellies swell out and we can no longer stand."[2]

The function of food and eating was, and still is, not restricted to the biological aspects. Food is the center of a complex value system and an elaborate ideology centers about it. Religious beliefs, rituals, prestige systems, etiquette, social organization, and group unity are related to food. Throughout the Pacific, in Africa, and in most other parts of the tribal world, kinship groups work together in the production of food. Distribution of food is part of traditional obligations between people related biologically and through marriage ties, between clans, and between chiefs and their subjects. The accumulation of food, particularly for ritual occasions, is a major way of obtaining prestige. At all significant events in the individual's life history—birth, puberty, marriage, death—there must be a feast, and the amount of food reflects the prestige of those giving it. Less formal but of equal significance, is the relationship of food-giving to hospitality, valued even more among tribal peoples than among ourselves.

The importance of food is not limited to relations among the living. It plays a significant role in relationships with dead ancestors and gods. Offerings of food are made to them, so that they will grant the requests of the living and protect them from sickness and other misfortunes. The spirits of the dead and the ancestral gods presumably have to eat and, among some tribes, observe the same eating etiquette as do the living. In Haiti the gods are very demanding, and providing their food becomes a means of controlling and manipulating them, for the gods depend on men for their strength. In the same country death is symbolized in many instances as being "eaten" by evil gods and, in a modern context of a railroad accident, the locomotive is said to be a machine that eats people. This oral aggression of evil gods (and, presumably, the locomotive, too) is regarded as being motivated by the desire to acquire strength through being fed.[3] The function of food in magical and religious practices throughout the world is well known, and food taboos are part of many religious rituals in both tribal and modern societies. We could go on almost indefinitely describing the social role of food.[4, 5]

But we turn now to the more personal role of food for the individual. The infant's first relationship with his mother is a nutritive one. In primitive societies it is fairly common for a child to be nursed at his mother's breast for several years. For the infant in all societies, suckling and eating appear to be among the earliest sensory experiences and pleasures. The psychoanalysts call it the oral stage. We tend to agree with them that early infantile experiences have lasting effects. In some tribal societies such as the one I studied in the Southwest Pacific, the stomach is the seat of the emotions. "Bel belong me hot" is the pidgin English way of expressing deep feeling, whether occasioned by anger, sexual desire, or eating well.[6] The same concept appears in Africa and other parts of the world.

Given the scarcity of food and the ever-present fear of famine in many tribal societies, the significant social role of food, and the lasting impact of the infant's first sensory satisfactions, it is not surprising to find that stoutness or some degree of obesity is often regarded with favor. This is particularly true for the concept of female attractiveness. Among the Banyankole, a pastoral people in East Africa, when a girl began to prepare for marriage at the age of eight, she was not permitted to play and run about, but kept in the house and made to drink large quantities of milk daily so that she would grow fat. By the end of a year she could only waddle. "The fatter she grew the more beautiful she was considered and her condition was a marked contrast to that of the men, who were athletic and well-developed." The royal women, the king's mother and his wives, vied with each other as to who should be the stoutest. They took no exercise, but were carried in litters when going from place to place.[7]

Among the Bushmen of South Africa, the new moon is spoken of as a man because of its slenderness, and the full moon is a woman because of its roundness. Masculine and feminine endings are given to the same roots to denote sex: male endings for strong, tall, slender things and female for weak, small, round ones.[8] Today in a mining community on the Copperbelt of Northern Rhodesia where I have done fieldwork, in one popular song a young man sings,

> Hullo, Mama,* the beautiful one, let us go to town;
> You will be very fat, you girl, if you stay with me.

---

* "Mamma" is a term of address for a woman.

The standard of beauty for a woman here was not the fatness which we mentioned earlier, but rather a moderate plumpness.

Summarizing briefly for tribal pre-literate societies, we note that hunger was common and that a high proportion of men's and women's energy was spent in producing enough food to stay alive; that food was not only a biological necessity, but that its social and psychological functions were also very significant. The giving of food was a prominent part of all relationships: between kindred, between clans, with dead ancestors, and with gods. Food played a role in ritual, magic and witchcraft, and in hospitality. The accumulation of food was a mark of great prestige. Fatness was a mark of beauty and desirability in women.

We turn now to our contemporary society. It is characterized by an economy of plenty as compared to the economy of scarcity in tribal societies. We eat too much. We have too much of many things. According to the population experts, there are too many people in the world, due to the decline in mortality rates. A key theme in this age of plenty—people, food, things—is consumption. We are urged to buy more and more things and new things such as food, cars, refrigerators, television sets, and clothes. We are constantly advised that prosperity can be maintained only by ever-increasing consumption. This is in sharp contrast to our own not too distant past, when saving and thrift were among the prized virtues and emphasis was on production rather than consumption.

Another important change in our modern industrial society is that physical activity is almost nonexistent in most occupations, particularly those in the middle and upper classes. We think of the ever-increasing white-collar jobs, the managerial and professional groups, and even the unskilled and skilled laborers in machine and factory production. For some people there are active games in leisure time, probably more for males than females. But, in general, leisure time activities tend to become increasingly passive. We travel in automobiles, we sit in movies, we stay at home and watch television. Most people live too far away to walk to their place of work. Walking for pleasure is very rare. Former President Truman's daily walk is regarded as one of his peculiarities. The trend for those who are advised to take exercise and who also have the necessary wealth is a passive form—massage, the electric table which vibrates the body, and other electrical devices.

But while people may exercise less and live in an economy of plenty, they are becoming increasingly aware of the problem of obesity. There is a continuing enlargement of our knowledge of nutrition, of the relationship between obesity and certain diseases, and to health and longevity in general, and a wide popularization of this knowledge. This past month we had a "Nutrition Week," and every day our mass media—newspapers, radio and television—carried information about food and its relationship to health, disease, and physical attractiveness.

Our standards of beauty, particularly for the female, have undergone a great change from tribal societies and from our own past. The slender, youthful-looking figure is now desired by women of all ages. The term "matronly," with its connotation of plumpness, is decidedly not flattering. Although the female body is predisposed to proportionately more fat and the male to more muscle,[9] the plump or stout woman's body is considered neither beautiful nor sexually attractive. Our guess is that a hundred years ago the term "matronly" was not unflattering. The role of a wife to-day as an active sex mate, as compared to her role in our more Puritanical past with its emphasis on motherhood rather than on the pleasures of sexual experiences, may be significant in this context. For this and for other reasons the contemporary cult of youthfulness appears to be stronger among women than among men. At almost any middle and upper class gathering of middle-aged men and women, a large proportion of the latter will have dyed their hair, while most of the men will have the symbolic grey hair of aging. It is generally assumed that physical attractiveness is more important for the female than for the male in their respective search for a mate. Success, wealth, and vigor are significant eligibility criteria for potential husbands and fathers. Of course, sex appeal is important for men, too, but it seems not to be so much associated with seeming youth-fulness as it is for women.

However, the cult of youthfulness is not confined to women. As science enables us all to live longer and longer, men and women want to remain young longer and longer. This is not a new desire. The quest for the foun-tain of youth is one of the well-known themes in mythology. The desire to remain healthy and "fit" as long as possible seems quite normal to us. Yet our excessive need to *look* young may also be related to other trends in our culture. Middle-aged people often find it difficult to get jobs, and they are faced with enforced, and sometimes unwanted, retirement at a fixed age. The cult of youthfulness may also have some connection with our apparent concern about sexual potency and sexual pleasure. Many books and articles discuss these as a difficult problem, and their large sale presumably indi-cates considerable anxiety about sexuality in our culture. Do people with this kind of anxiety have more, or less, difficulty in dieting and keeping their bodies young-looking?

We have indicated a number of strong trends in our culture which run counter to obesity. The desire for health, for longevity, for youthfulness, for sexual attractiveness is indeed a powerful motivation. Yet obesity is a problem. We ask, then, what cultural and psychological factors might be counteracting the effective work of nutritionists, physicians, beauty specialists, and advertisements in the mass media? We have a number of hypotheses. We think there may be considerable ambivalence for many people in regard to being fat or thin, to overeating or to dieting. This ambivalence could, in turn, come from conflicting patterns in our culture.

I have a hypothesis that, consciously or unconsciously, our symbolism for a maternal woman is on the plump or obese side. There is the figure of a pregnant woman and, as already indicated, the infantile satisfactions gained from food given by a mother or mother-surrogate. The image for mother and for mate may be in conflict.

Then, too, food is a very significant symbol in our prestige system. The kind of food, the quantity, and the manner in which it is served are among the important criteria of social class. In most tribal societies, even those with a highly stratified social system, everyone—royalty and commoners—ate the same kind of food, and if there was famine everyone was hungry. In our society there are sharp distinctions. Although there are probably relatively few people today who know sustained hunger because of poverty, poor people eat differently from rich people. Fattening, starchy foods are common among the former, and in certain ethnic groups, particularly those from southern Europe, women tend to be fat. Obesity for women is therefore somewhat symbolic for lower class. In our socially mobile society this is a powerful deterrent. The symbolism of obesity in men has been different. The image of a successful middle-aged man in the middle and upper classes has been with a "pouch," or "bay-window," as it was called a generation ago. We are all familiar with pictures of this type, resplendent with gold watch chain across the large stomach. Today this particular male class-symbolism is changing, probably because of the increased knowledge of the relationship of obesity to heart-malfunctioning and to other diseases.

Although slenderness becomes increasingly a symbol of social status, the food of the wealthy is still rich and plentiful, and their dinner parties are often, quite literally, a sign of conspicuous consumption. With the ever-increasing diversity of foods, food has become not only a matter of social status, but also a mark of one's personality and taste. More and more people are becoming gourmets, and with the declining number of servants, the hostess—and often the host, too—display their individual style and taste in cooking.[10] We become more personally interested in food as we become more aware of the problems connected with overeating.

The giving of food to people who are in trouble is a still widely prevailing folk custom and is reflected in our radio "soap operas." When someone is having marital or financial problems, or when there is illness in the family, a good neighbor brings in food and says, "You must eat to keep up your strength." The same correlation of eating with strength runs through many food advertisements, particularly those designed to reach young, growing children in the television audience. It would be interesting to do an analysis of the mass media advertisements of food which are directed toward children. It would be equally desirable to analyze the advertisements concerning reducing foods, pills, and other products, directed toward adults.

Our symbols for fatness or thinness are not clear-cut, as old and new patterns mingle. We have the beliefs that fat people are good-natured, contented, likable, funny, and also that they are foolish, "greasy," and greedy. There is the well-known image from Shakespeare's *Julius Caesar,* in which Caesar prefers his followers to be fat, and fears those who are lean and hungry.* A study of heroes and heroines and villains in our mass media, in terms of their fatness and thinness, might be revealing. I cannot offhand remember any fat movie villains, male or female. But this would be interesting to check.

While the family in our society is no longer an economic unit for the production of food, as it was in primitive society, the family meal remains one of the few times when the family is united and drawn together. Parents still are the givers of food, and most of us are aware of the intense interest with which young siblings watch mother cut a pie and their anxiety over whether the slices are even. This is true in homes where food is plentiful, and obviously food is a symbol for the mother's favoring or not favoring one child more than another.

Eating well, a full stomach, is still one of our main ways of achieving a state of euphoria. A really good dinner sets all of us up. This is probably connected with the fact that one of the earliest forms of security and of sensory pleasure is connected with the intake of food, and that about it are centered the first human relations. The eating of food and the giving of it thus remains a symbol of love, affection, and friendliness, as well as a source of pleasure in itself.

It is often stated and rather commonly believed that indulgence in overeating is a conscious or unconscious compensation for frustration or neurotic problems. We ask a further question: why do some people seek this form of compensation rather than another form? Is there, for instance, one type of person who tends to be alcoholic and another to overeat? A number of studies have indicated a comparatively low rate of alcoholism among Jews.[11, 12] They show that sobriety is a strong moral virtue among orthodox and pious Jews, and that drunkenness is associated with the outgroup, the Gentiles. The Jewish norms of moderate drinking and sobriety are

---

* "Let me have men about me that are fat,
  Sleek-headed men, and such as sleep o'nights:
  Yond Cassius has a lean and hungry look;
  He thinks too much; such men are dangerous."
    Shakespeare, William. *Julius Caesar,* Act I, Scene 2.

bound up with the ceremonial and ritual observances, with their religious beliefs, and with the value of remaining separate from Christians. It is assumed that Jews have the same proportion of neurotic and other problems that could lead to alcoholism as do Christians. The norms favored by any group for meeting problems are part of its culture and are internalized in childhood. It would be interesting to find out whether overeating and obesity are more common among orthodox Jews than among reformed Jews and Christians of the same class. We think, too, that there could be regional as well as religious differences in attitudes toward obesity. One suspects that there would be considerable difference between the South and New England.

We have a number of other questions concerning possible correlations of cultural and psychological factors with obesity. Is the ability to diet, and to diet consistently, related to belief in a measure of control over one's fate? Is it related to the strength of the belief in science? Is obesity correlated with orientations toward asceticism versus sensory pleasures? Has there been any study of obesity among monks and nuns? Do people who value sensory pleasures in general, such as those derived from perfumes, from physical contacts, from sexual experience, demonstrate an ability to diet more, or less, successfully than others? The degree of emphasis on sensory pleasure may be culturally determined, may vary from one historical period to another in the same culture, and from one class and ethnic group. And within each group there can be variations due to genetic idiosyncratic factors in the life history of individuals.

There are time limits to the number of questions we can raise. We have tried to indicate some of the cultural factors underlying the problem of obesity. Our society, with its economy of plenty and lack of physical activity, as compared to the economy of scarcity and the hard physical work in tribal societies, provides increasing opportunities for people to eat more food and to become obese. At the same time, other cultural factors, such as the knowledge of nutrition and of the relationship of obesity to disease and longevity and the popularization of the knowledge, our cult of youthfulness and the emphasis on the beauty of the slender body, particularly for the female, our class stereotypes, all tend to keep people from taking advantage of the opportunities to gorge on food. Yet there are many who overeat. We have hypotheses that this may be related to our deeply imbedded desire for the euphoria which comes from a full stomach, with other sensory indulgences or a lack of them, with conflicting imagery about a motherly woman versus a sex mate, with the use of food as a status symbol and as an expression of personality tastes, and with cultural norms about food and standards of beauty in different religious, class, ethnic, and regional groups. We have asked a number of questions relating to possible cultural correlations, for which there is no data. Mainly we have tried to show some of the intricate and complex ramifications of eating and of obesity in the tribal societies of the past characterized by too little food, and in our contemporary culture characterized by too much food.

REFERENCES

1. Malinowski, B.: *Argonauts of the Western Pacific.* New York, E. P. Dutton and Co., 1922, p. 171.
2. Kropf, A.: *Das Volk der Xosa-Kaffern.* Berlin, 1889, p. 88.
3. Bourguignon, E.: Persistence of folk belief: Some notes on cannibalism and zombis in Haiti. *J Am Folklore,* 72:42, 1959.
4. Richards, A. I.: *Hunger and Work in a Savage Tribe.* Glencoe, Ill., The Free Press, 1948.
5. Radcliffe-Brown, A. B.: *The Andaman Islanders.* Cambridge Univ. Pr., 1922.
6. Powdermaker, H.: *Life in Lesu. The Study of a Melanesian Society in New Ireland.* New York, W. W. Norton and Co., 1933, pp. 232-34.
7. Roscoe, J.: *The Northern Bantu.* Cambridge Univ. Pr., 1915, p. 38. Ibid., *The Banyankole,* 1923, pp. 116-17, 120.
8. Schapera, I.: *The Khoisan Peoples of South Africa; Bushmen and Hottentots.* London, Routledge and Keegan Paul, 1930, p. 427.
9. Scheinfeld, A.: *Women and Men.* New York, Harcourt, Brace and Co., 1943, p. 147.
10. Riesman, D., Glazer, N. and Denney, R.: *The Lonely Crowd.* New York, Doubleday and Co., 1953, pp. 168-69.
11. Bales, R. F.: The "Fixation Factor" in Alcohol Addiction: An Hypothesis Derived from a Comparative Study of Irish and Jewish Social Norms. Doctoral dissertation. *Arch Widener Libr,* Harvard Univ., 1944.
12. Snyder, C. R.: Culture and Jewish Sobriety: The Ingroup-Outgroup Factor. In *The Jews, Social Patterns of an American Group,* M. Sklare, ed. Glencoe, Ill., The Free Press, 1958.

8

Overweight as a Social Disability with Medical Implications

GEORGE L. MADDOX

AND

VERONICA LIEDERMAN

A PURPORTED relationship between leanness and longevity is frequently reported in the scientific literature. The deleterious consequences of fatness are widely publicized by insurance companies and are a factor in their determination of insurance rates. An undetermined number of physicians also treat overweight more or less seriously as an undesirable condition and thus contribute at least tacitly to the concern Americans have about being overweight.

The leanness-longevity relationship has been severely criticized on at least two counts. The supporting evidence is less than convincing to some. Moreover, the physician's reaction to overweight is said to be colored substantially by his evaluation of the fat person as unaesthetic and morally weak. Thus, the social transaction between physicians and overweight patients appears to reflect a complex mixture of medical fact and sociocultural values. That is, whatever medical implications overweight may have, fatness is first and foremost a social disability. This state of affairs makes the medical facts about overweight difficult to assess and even more difficult to apply in the management of patients.[1]

In an earlier study the authors investigated the medical management of overweight patients in a public outpatient clinic and some of the factors associated with physicians' identification of patients as overweight, their entry of their observations in the charts, and any proposal they made to manage the overweight patients.[1] The purpose of the study was to assess whether and how selected physicians managed patients who were, by a commonly used measure of body size, significantly overweight. To this end two stratified random samples (total N = 491) were drawn from new patients in the clinic in such a way as to insure their adequate distribution by body build, race, and sex. These samples were supplemented by a special panel of severely overweight individuals whose course was followed in detail over a period of months. A commonly used height-weight table was employed to identify moderately and severely overweight patients, that is, those who exceeded by 10 per cent and by 20 per cent their "best weight" as determined by actuarial standards. A study of clinic charts indicated that

84

entries about weight were almost never made for the moderately over-weight patients and proposals for weight management were never offered in such cases. For severely overweight patients the chances were one in two that an entry about weight would be made and one in four that weight management would be proposed. And even when weight management was proposed, actual follow-up was infrequent except in instances in which the patient presented cardiovascular or diabetic symptoms.

The apparent medical irrelevance of overweight suggested by these find-ings seemed to be explained, at least in part, by a complex interaction of information, experiences, and attitudes of both physicians and patients. The salience of overweight as a condition to be managed medically was demonstrably low for both groups and deviations from actuarially derived standards of "best weight" appeared to be meaningless to both. This was the central finding. There were indications, however, that overweight, while rarely addressed consciously or directly by physicians or patients, did color their relationship. Physicians, for example, indicated in informal conversa-tions that the overweight patients were difficult to manage, that attempt-ed management more often than not was unsuccessful, and that the over-weight individual was for other reasons not a preferred patient. The physi-cians did not appear to have at their disposal authoritative information about overweight and its management.

These observations led the authors to study in detail the training, ex-perience, and attitudes of physicians in the clinic with regard to over-weight. As in the earlier study, the intent was not to be pejorative. We do not presume to know what perspective the physicians ought to have toward overweight, what they ought to be taught about this condition and its management, or the attitudes they ought to have toward overweight pa-tients. Rather, the authors wished to ascertain what physicians remembered being taught, and what they felt they learned, and how they felt about the problem of overweight.

SELECTION OF PHYSICIANS

The senior physicians, house officers, and student clerks ($N = 197$) work-ing in the public out-patient medical clinic in the spring of 1965 were asked to complete a self-administered questionnaire. The purpose of the inquiry was initially discussed at a regular staff meeting of the Department of Med-icine, and questions regarding the investigators (one of whom was a senior member of the Department) and the investigation were answered. A num-ber of senior staff physicians were eventually consulted about the question-naire and their recommendations were, for the most part, incorporated in the final instrument. In spite of the fact that a covering letter from the De-partment chairman encouraged full participation in the research, only 51 per cent of the questionnaires were returned: 41 of 57 (72%) from senior physicians; 44 of 87 (52%) from house officers; and 15 of 53 (28%) from student clerks. An even 100 respondents constituted the final sample.

The biases which follow from this selective return cannot be assessed with any degree of certainty. However, conversations between the investigators and a number of nonrespondents indicated that the latters' hostility was directed toward any demand to assume additional responsibility for making unnecessary reports and not toward the research per se. Although hostility to behavioral research cannot be discounted as a source of nonresponse, the inverse relationship between status in the system, and, presumptively, freedom from a great deal of paper work, and response rate lends support to this interpretation. Moreover, it seems reasonable to presume that those most favorable to behaviorial research in medicine and those most interested in overweight would be most likely to respond.

METHODS

The self-administered questionnaire required about one-half hour to complete. The physicians and student clerks were asked to list the sources of information about overweight in their medical education, with particular attention being given to the medical literature they would recommend to colleagues interested in overweight and its management. They were also asked to indicate how they concluded that a patient was significantly overweight, the factors associated with deciding to manage perceived overweight, and their estimated success in such management. Finally, a semantic differential procedure[2] was used to explore descriptions of themselves, a competent physician, patients in general, and an obese patient. Twenty-one 7-point scales were selected equally from lists of words known to tap evaluative, power, and activity dimensions which Osgood and his associates[2] have identified in their work. From specific responses to the various stimulus phrases it is possible to construct descriptions of the respondents, and of their conceptions of a competent physician, patients in general, and significantly overweight (obese) patients. It is also possible to calculate difference scores, that is, the distance or semantic space between a given respondent and his response to the persons indicated in the stimulus phrases such as "myself as I really am" or "a competent physician."* A respondent may indicate that any particular scale does not apply to the stimulus phrase or that the scale is neutral. Moreover, the extremity and direction of characterizations in response to the various stimulus phrases can be determined. For the purposes of the present study a response was considered extreme when a polar value (1, 2 or 6, 7) was chosen on a par-

---

* Difference scores are calculated as follows: Differences in a subject's responses to 2 stimulus phrases are compared for the 21 scales. Differences on each pair of scales are squared and summed. The square root of this sum constitutes the difference score.

ticular scale and negative when it was in the direction of the description which, in our society, would be considered less desirable. In the typical case the socially desirable description was that given "a competent physician."

RESULTS

Among those physicians studied, personal experience rather than formal training was reported to be the primary source of information about over-weight and its management: 93 per cent stressed experience; 66 per cent indicated that personal research contributed to their knowledge; and 50 per cent mentioned rounding. In contrast, 22 per cent considered lectures in medical school to have been important; and only 20 per cent were able to report an article or textbook that they would recommend to a colleague interested in overweight and its management.

What had experience taught the respondents about overweight patients? Most importantly, only 10 per cent reported that successful management of overweight was characteristically his experience; more than half (56%) admitted that they were usually unsuccessful. Forty per cent indicated "careful management" as preferred management of severe overweight in spite of this modest success rate. This proportion, incidentally, is twice the observed proportion of management proposals actually recorded on the charts of severely overweight patients who were treated in the clinic served by the physicians in the sample; the proportion of proposed programs actually carried out was even smaller. Among the minority reporting a preference for careful management, personal experience and rounds were imputed to be important sources of information in contrast to formal lectures, professional literature, and research.

Almost all of the respondents (96%) estimated that social and emotional factors are important in the etiology of overweight. There is some evidence that physicians ordinarily prefer patients who do not present with conditions presumed to have substantial social and emotional components.[3]

There are surely other factors which contribute to the observed non-management of severe overweight in this clinic[1] in addition to the experience of failure and an apparent lack of support for management of overweight in the prevailing clinic culture. The overweight patient also clearly evoked a strong negative affect in these respondents.

AFFECTIVE RESPONSES TO OVERWEIGHT

The evidence that Americans generally disvalue fatness is extensive and convincing.[4] Keys[5] speculated that physicians, typically subscribers to middle-class American values, would view fatness as unaesthetic and an indication of lack of personal control. The authors' evidence supports Keys' impression. The image which the respondents had of overweight patients

The Psychology of Obesity

TABLE 8-I

SELECTED CHARACTERIZATIONS OF SEVERELY OVERWEIGHT PERSONS,
BY PERCENTAGES OF SAMPLES OF PHYSICIANS AND STUDENTS AND
OVERWEIGHT PATIENTS

| | Description of Severely Overweight Person | | |
Characteristics	By Physicians and Students	Self-Description by Overweight Patients *	Description of Other Overweight Persons by Overweight Patients *
Fast	3	31	40
Sharp	8	57	58
Successful	10	45	50
Strong	10	39	66
Active	14	37	52
Nice	31	82	92
Happy	35	48	68

* Responses from patients in the clinic served by the physicians described in this article; for a description of the research on patients see Maddox, Anderson, and Bogdonoff.[1]

is clearly much more negative than the self-descriptions of overweight patients themselves (Table 8-I).

The response of the study subjects to the semantic differential itself warrants a brief comment. In the instructions to respondents regarding this procedure, it was stressed that any one of the twenty-one scales could be perceived as not relevant to a given stimulus phrase and that the respondent could leave the item blank to distinguish this response from one in which a neutral evaluation was intended, in which case the midpoint of the scale was to be marked. Twenty-three of the one hundred respondents did not mark any of the semantic differential items. Some of the respondents were quite frank in specifying their reasons for not completing this portion of the questionnaire; occasionally notes were written on the questionnaires and systematic inquiry supplemented these notes.

Most of those who refused to deal with the semantic differential objected to "playing a game in which important variations in people, whether physicians, competent physicians, patients, or obese patients, are submerged in a single impression." In this sense they reacted as clinicians impressed with the importance of emphasizing the particularity of the individual. A few also hinted darkly that such information might be used for invidious comparisons of physicians and patients as their reason for nonresponse. Nonetheless, seventy-seven study subjects were willing to characterize themselves and a "competent physician" in terms of the twenty-one scales.

In contrast, fewer of those questioned were willing to characterize patients. Only forty-four described patients in general, although sixty-eight characterized the obese patient. Thus, the image of an obese patient was more likely to overcome the study subjects' reluctance to categorize people than was the image of the patient in general.

The strong negative reaction to the obese patient is reflected by a measure of extremity of response. The seventy-seven respondents who characterized themselves and a "competent physician" in terms of the twenty-one scale items made cumulatively 1,617 judgments in each instance. Of these judgments fifteen (less than 1%) were extremely negative when a "competent physician" was being described; and only fifty-three (3.3%) were extremely negative when they were describing themselves.

With regard to the evaluation of patients, on the other hand, 157 of the 924 judgments (17%) made about patients in general were intensely negative as were 271 of the 1,428 judgments (19%) made about the obese patient. One fifth of these intense negative judgments about the obese patient are accounted for by two scales, strong-willed/weak-willed and handsome/ugly as Keys' observation about physicians would have led one to suspect. This unflattering assessment is also suggested by the data in Table 8-II in which "awkward" is added to "weak-willed" and "ugly" as characterizations of obese patients.

Although a more detailed analysis of factors associated with variations in the tendency to extreme negative responses within this small sample of physicians is unwarranted, several general observations are in order. In the study by Martin[3] noted previously, the tendency to express preference for one or another type of patient was in part a function of the felt competence of student physicians. Insofar as years of practice after receiving one's medical degree can be taken as a rough indicator of perceived competence, the patient study data suggest that perceived competence is associated with the avoidance of extreme responses on the semantic differential scales. For example, physicians who received their medical degree after 1950, including a few advanced medical students yet to be graduated, were twice as likely to respond extremely and in a negative direction as those graduated prior to 1950. Moreover, difference scores derived from descriptions of self, a competent physician, and an obese patient were compared. Difference scores of self as compared with a competent physician were, as expected, also positively associated with having been graduated prior to 1950. In turn, the greater the perceived discrepancy between physicians' self-de-

TABLE 8-II

SELECTED CHARACTERIZATIONS OF COMPETENT PHYSICIANS, SELF,
PATIENTS, AND OBESE PATIENTS, BY PERCENTAGES OF A
SAMPLE OF PHYSICIANS AND STUDENTS

	Description			
Characteristics	*Competent Physician*	*Self*	*Patients*	*Obese Patients*
Weak-willed	1	5	24	60
Ugly	0	3	11	54
Awkward	0	19	39	55

scriptions and their descriptions of a competent physician, the greater were the differences between their self-descriptions and their characterizations of both patients in general and obese patients.

The post-1950 graduate was significantly more likely than those graduated earlier, however, to report a preference for detailed management of the severely overweight patient. This is interesting in view of his tendency to be extremely negative in his descriptions of such patients. The apparent contradictions may shed some light on the observation with which this report began. The medical student, as a product of his culture, disvalues fatness. He learns informally about the medical relevance or irrelevance of overweight in an environment in which basic science information is at best ambiguous and clinic experience suggests a poor prognosis for attempted management. This prognosis, which may be in part self-fulfilling, is nonetheless rather quickly confirmed in his experience. Medical school lectures and research on significant overweight and its management, both apparently rare, do not counteract the negative thrust of clinical experience. Counterbalancing professional literature remains unknown.

SUMMARY AND CONCLUSIONS

In this study of one-hundred physicians and student clerks in a Department of Medicine the investigators found that informal experience rather than formal medical training is the imputed source of information about significant overweight, its etiology, and its management. Typically, the study subjects preferred not to manage the overweight patient and other evidence indicates that they did not in fact do so. They are, by their own report, more often than not unsuccessful when they try. The imputed etiology of overweight stresses social and emotional factors. The presence of such factors is not preferred by physicians generally and the respondents are apparently no exception. Their characterization of the severely overweight patient is extremely negative. Although there is some indication that this negative evaluation of fatness is ameliorated somewhat by the physician's confidence that he is competent, clinical experience appears to reinforce his tendency not to attempt the management of overweight and not to expect success when he does so. If the management of overweight is as important to health as is sometimes claimed, this message has made little impact on what the study subjects appear to believe or actually do.

Although it is possible that the present findings are unique to a particular department of medicine or that they reflect the experience of the respondents with a type of clinic patient for whom the various costs of weight management overbalance any possible benefits, one implication of the findings definitely warrants additional investigation. All physicians would probably agree that weight management is called for in particular instances and yet the culture of this medical outpatient clinic, reinforced by the disvalue of fatness and the experience of failure in weight management, provides a poor context for learning how to manage the overweight patient when such management is indicated.

REFERENCES

1. Maddox, G. L., Anderson, C. F. and Bogdonoff, M.: Overweight as a problem of medical management in a public outpatient clinic. *Am J Med Sci*, 252:395-402, 1966.
2. Osgood, C., Suci, S. and Tannenbaum, R.: *The Measurement of Meaning*. Urbana, University of Illinois Press, 1957.
3. Martin, W.: Preferences for Types of Patients. In *The Student-Physician*. Merton, R. K., Reader, G. G. and Kendall, P. L. (Eds.): Cambridge, Massachusetts, Harvard University Press, 1957.
4. Maddox, G. L., Back, K. and Liederman, V.: Overweight as social deviance and disability. *J Health Soc Behav*, 9:287-298, 1968.
5. Keys, A.: Editorial. *J Chronic Dis*, 1:456, 1955.

9

Social Correlates of Weight in an Aging Population

ROBERT G. BURNIGHT

AND

PARKER G. MARDEN

E VIDENCE is accumulating which shows an association between health problems and overweight.[1] Accordingly, warnings against obesity have become an important part of the physician's practice of preventive medicine. Despite the general acceptance of such cautions, however, the amount of social and epidemiological research concerning weight differences has been limited.[2] The purpose of the present study is to explore certain dimensions of this problem within an urban population that is approaching old age.

The data are drawn from a longitudinal study of a probability sample of 605 white, married couples living in Providence, Rhode Island, on May 1, 1962, in which the husband was sixty to sixty-four years of age.[3] A goal of this study is the investigation of the important changes in health which occur during the seventh decade of life. The probability of developing a chronic disease, of encountering a disability that requires confinement, or of dying increases throughout this period. As a consequence, the study of the implications of weight differences for health takes on new meaning, since being overweight and the possibility of becoming ill come into closer juxtaposition. Although a weight condition may interfere with good health at any age, it grows in importance as the body ages and becomes increasingly relevant to many of the types of diseases in older age groups.

A necessary prerequisite for the full understanding of such a relationship between health and weight in this, or any other age group is the investigation of the social correlates of weight differences. Such an epidemiological investigation is reported here.[*] This investigation seeks to discover whether obesity and other weight conditions are randomly distributed throughout the study population or whether they are more frequently found in certain groups within that population.

Few other analyses have been undertaken concerning this question. In 1965, findings were published of an investigation of the relationship between obesity and several social factors within the sample population in

---

[*] Analysis of the relationship between weight and a variety of indices of health condition (e.g. presence of chronic disease, evaluation of health and medical expenditures) is being carried out for future publication.

the Midtown Manhattan Study.[4] The authors could report only one other study which examined weight condition as a social phenomenon rather than as a random and individual occurrence.[5] Therefore, the examination of weight differences should be extended to another study population and the results compared with the findings already reported.

DEVELOPMENT OF THE WEIGHT VARIABLE

A person's weight relative to that of others can be measured in many ways. Perhaps the soundest procedures are clinical in nature. Among these are the estimation of body fat from specific gravity[6] or the measurement of folds of skin and subcutaneous fat.[7] But measures that involve determining the weight of the body in air and under water or applying calipers to various parts of the body—and even the comparatively innocuous procedure of directly weighing and measuring people—are generally inappropriate to household interview studies. Thus, a measure must be developed from the objective information which an individual can provide: his height and weight.* Such information was obtained from all but four of the 1,210 respondents (605 couples) in the Providence study population at the time of interview (1962).

Given the need to use self-reported figures, the soundest procedure would be to compare the person's height and weight with the "desirable" height-weight tables developed in medico-actuarial studies for the various age groups.[8] Unfortunately, such figures take into consideration another factor that is unobtainable in large surveys—body build. An alternative procedure, however, represents a reasonable compromise. In the absence of detailed information on desirable weight by height and age that does not include body build, the general recommendation of physicians and others concerned with this problem is for persons to maintain their weight at the level of ages twenty to twenty-four.[9] Therefore, the present weight condition of the respondents in the Providence survey will be measured relative to the average weights of persons of their height and sex between the ages of twenty and twenty-four.† These figures are presented in Table 9-I (columns 1 and 3).

---

* Such self-reporting imposes certain limitations on the study. But, as the Midtown Manhattan Study authors indicated in their report, the errors of respondents in reporting their weight is in the direction of the mean. Thus, some persons who are either overweight or underweight may be mistakenly included in the "normal" weight grouping, thereby understating relationships that are present. *See* Moore, Stunkard and Srole, *op. cit.,* p. 963.

† Use of the average weights at age 20 to 24 as a standard presents one problem. A person for whom a desirable weight would be 160 pounds at age 20 might well be obese some 40 years later without gaining a pound, since "maintenance" of constant weight with advancing years obscures the critical change in the muscle-fat ratio relative to the progressive reduction in lean body mass. *See* Pomeranze, Julius, Obesity as a Health Factor in Geriatric Patients, *Geriatrics,* 12:481, August, 1957. Fortunately, this fact can lead to greater confidence in whatever definite results are obtained since it will cause some of the existing relationships to be hidden or understated.

This procedure can be challenged by contending that the comparisons between the height-weight figures for the aging population being studied and persons who are twenty to twenty-four years old at the same time fails to take into account the fact that members of the study population were actually in their twenties four decades ago. This challenge can be answered in several ways. In the first place, comparison of the height-weight tables presently in use with one for the early 1920's, when members of the study population were themselves twenty years old, shows a remarkable agreement, as seen in Table 9-I (columns 2 and 4). Secondly, the respondents' weights at age twenty were also recorded in the 1962 interview and the correlation could be computed between: a) the deviation of the individual's present weight from his desirable weight—the measure of weight condition used in this study and b) the actual weight change that he has undergone over the forty-year period. The correlation coefficients were .712 for males and .797 for females, indicating that the statistical measure being employed is a good reflection of actual trends over time. Both sets of comparisons demonstrate that the use of weight at age twenty to twenty-four as a

TABLE 9-I

COMPARISON OF "DESIRABLE" WEIGHT USED AS A MEASURE OF
WEIGHT CONDITION WITH AVERAGE WEIGHT IN EARLY 1920'S,
PERSONS 20 TO 24 YEARS OLD, BY HEIGHT AND SEX

Height (inches)	Men "Desirable" Weight*	Average Weight in 1920's†	Height (inches)	Women "Desirable" Weight	Average Weight in 1920's†
62	128	124	58	102	108
63	132	128	59	105	109
64	136	132	60	108	113
65	139	136	61	112	116
66	142	141	62	115	119
67	145	144	63	118	122
68	149	149	64	121	125
69	153	154	65	125	128
70	157	157	66	129	132
71	161	161	67	132	135
72	166	165	68	136	139
73	170	169	69	140	142
74	174	174	70	144	145
75	178	178	71	149	149
76	181	183	72	154	154

* "Desirable" weight is the average weight of persons 20 to 24 as given in the Society of Actuaries Study; see Metropolitan Life Insurance Company, op. cit., p. 2.[9]

† The average weights given for the 1920's (when most of the Providence respondents were in their twenties) are from Wood, T. D.: *Personal Health Standard and Scale.* New York, Columbia University Teacher's College, 1923; data were published *in* Hathaway, Millicent L. and Foard, Elsie D.: *Heights and Weights of Adults in the United States.* Home Economics Research Report No. 10, Washington, United States Department of Agriculture, 1960, p. 48. Data presented are for age group 21 to 22.

TABLE 9-II

WEIGHT CONDITION IN AN AGING POPULATION, BY SEX

	Males		Females		Total	
	N	%	N	%	N	%
Thin	30	5.0	6	1.0	36	3.0
Normal	262	43.3	183	30.4	445	36.9
Overweight	200	33.0	197	32.8	397	32.9
Obese	113	18.7	215	35.8	328	27.2
Total	605	100.0	601	100.0	1,206	100.0

$x^2 = 61.8$ p $< .05$.

standard for desirable weight is a fair measure and appropriate for the purposes of this research.*

For the purposes of this analysis, four categories of weight condition are employed: a) those individuals who were within fifteen pounds of their desirable weight (i.e. average weight of twenty to twenty-four-year-olds for their sex and height group) were classified as *normal*,[†] b) those who were more than fifteen pounds below their desirable weight were classified as *thin;* c) those who were between sixteen and thirty-five pounds over their desirable weight were categorized as *overweight;* and d) those who were more than thirty-five pounds in excess of their desirable weight were identified as *obese.*

The use of these four categories distributes the respondents in the manner shown in Table 9-II, reflecting a high prevalence of obesity and overweight among both males and females. Indeed, 60 per cent of all respondents were above normal weight and more than one of every four could be identified as obese. Because of the extent to which these conditions are found, the discussion which follows will focus upon those individuals who are overweight or obese.[‡]

SOCIAL FACTORS ASSOCIATED WITH WEIGHT DIFFERENCES

Sex

The data presented in Table 9-II indicate important sex differentials when weight condition is considered in the Providence study population. More

---

* Although weight at age 20 was available, it could not be used as a substitute for the "desirable weight" standard because ascertaining the persons who were obese at that earlier age was impossible in summary calculations.

† The figure of 15 lb represents an average of 10 to 12 per cent gain in weight for this study population between age 20 and the 1962 interview.

‡ This decision must be made to render the discussion as clear as possible. Since very few persons are clasified as thin, normality in weight can generally be considered as the reciprocal of overweight and obese.

than twice as many women as men could be classified as obese while the proportion of each group that was overweight is nearly identical. Furthermore, this four-category presentation conceals the magnitude of the amount of obesity in the study population and the differences between males and females in this regard. Considering, for example, only the 215 women who were categorized as obese, 18, or 8.4 per cent, were 100 pounds or more over their desirable weights and one woman was 164 pounds overweight. In contrast, only three of the 113 obese males or 2.7 per cent were 100 pounds or more in excess of the desirable weight for persons of their height. Conversely, at the lower end of the range in this obese category, 57.5 per cent of the men and only 39.1 per cent of the women were between 36 and 50 pounds over their desirable weight. These figures reinforce the findings concerning the sex differentials in Table 9-II. Not only is obesity more prevalent among women, but the males so categorized are generally closer to their desirable weight than are their female counterparts.

Table 9-II suggests another aspect of the sex differentials in weight condition. Although interpretation must be qualified by the small number of cases,* five times as many males as females could be classified as thin—fifteen or more pounds below desirable weight. Since analyses such as the Framingham Study have shown that weight loss (crudely reflected here as thinness) is closely associated with ill-health,[10] it is revealing to discover that 26 per cent of all males in the Providence study had one or more serious chronic illnesses,† as compared with only 17 per cent of the females. This aspect of the weight differences by sex, therefore, may be intertwined with the greater morbidity among males. The longitudinal design of the larger study of which this analysis is a part will permit elaboration on this point.

Socioeconomic Status

Differentials in weight by sex is emphasized when other social characteristics are examined. Variables which have great meaning for one sex group may not be as important for the other. Analysis of the relationship between socioeconomic status‡ and weight condition is especially illustrative. The data presented in Table 9-III show that differences do exist in the frequency of obesity for males by socioeconomic status, with the greatest prevalence

---

* Because of the small number of cases when spread into an additional variable, analysis of those who are thin is limited to prevent misinterpretation.

† Serious chronic illnesses are those which are considered life-threatening. These are, as reported in the interview, malignant neoplasms, cerebrovascular accidents, heart disease, vascular disease, and cirrhosis of the liver.

‡ The measure used to determine socioeconomic status is an index based upon occupation, education, and income as developed and employed by the United States Bureau of the Census. For a full discussion *see Methodology and Sources of Socioeconomic Status,* Working Paper No. 15, Technical Paper Series, United States Bureau of the Census, Washington, 1962. Women are categorized according to the socioeconomic status of their husbands.

TABLE 9-III

WEIGHT CONDITION IN AN AGING POPULATION, BY
SOCIOECONOMIC STATUS

| | Socioeconomic Status* | | | | | | Total | |
| | Low | | Medium | | High | | | |
	N	%	N	%	N	%	N	%
Males								
Thin	12	5.9	17	6.1	1	0.8	30	5.0
Normal	80	39.6	113	40.5	69	55.7	262	43.3
Overweight	64	31.7	99	35.5	37	29.8	200	33.0
Obese	46	22.8	50	17.9	17	13.7	113	18.7
Total	202	100.0	279	100.0	124	100.0	605	100.0
$x^2 = 15.5\ p < .05.$								
Females								
Thin	1	0.5	3	1.1	2	1.6	6	1.0
Normal	47	23.4	79	28.5	57	46.4	183	30.4
Overweight	61	30.3	87	31.4	49	39.8	197	32.8
Obese	92	45.8	108	39.0	15	12.2	215	35.8
Total	201	100.0	277	100.0	123	100.0	601	100.0
$x^2 = 42.8\ p < .05.$								

* Categories of socioeconomic status are based upon the following ranges of socioeconomic-status scores: low, 1-33; medium, 34-66; high, 67-99. Scores developed by the method set forth in *Methodology and Sources of Socioeconomic Status, op. cit.*

of this condition being found among those in the low category. These differences pale into insignificance, however, when compared with the differences for females. Women of high socioeconomic status are infrequently found to be obese (12.2% as compared to 35.8% of all females studied), while those who fall into the low grouping are much more likely to be classified in this manner (45.8%).

Table 9-III shows the merits of identifying an extreme group within those who are above normal weight. Although the terms "overweight" and "obese" are admittedly arbitrary, those respondents who fall into the obese category are a distinctive group. This is demonstrated by the fact that, although women in the higher socioeconomic status are seldom obese, they are frequently found to be overweight. This tendency reflects a general departure from normality in weight that is less pronounced in the case of males and shows that substantial excesses over desirable weight among women are positively associated with socioeconomic status, but that obesity is inversely related.

Nativity

Examination of the relationship between weight condition and nativity produces some additional insights into the problem under study. As Table 9-IV indicates, prevalence of obesity and overweight appears to be related to generation in the United States. In general, an increasing prevalence of these two weight conditions accompanies decreases in the length of time that respondents and their families have been in this country. Again, differences are found between males and females in this regard. Not only is the relationship found to be stronger (and statistically significant) for women, but the point at which the differences appear also varies. In the case of the males, the major difference was between the native-born of native parents and the other two groupings, while the difference for females was most noticeable between those who were foreign-born and the two native-born categories.

With socioeconomic status and generation in the United States perhaps being closely related, it is important to determine whether the inverse relationship between obesity and nativity is independent of socioeconomic positon. Accordingly, the association between socioeconomic status and weight condition was examined for each of the nativity categories. The results of this analysis are shown in Table 9-V. In general, differences by nativity disappear when socioeconomic status is held constant. In the case of women in the middle status, for example, 42 per cent of the foreign-born, 36 per cent of the native-born of foreign parents, and 43 per cent of the native-born of native parents can be classified as obese. The percentages for overweight in the same category were 34, 29, and 34 per cent, respectively.

Only in a few instances does a relationship between nativity and weight condition remain in the presence of controls for socioeconomic status, but these are worthy of note. The proportion of women in the upper socioeconomic status who could be identified as obese or overweight drops sharply as length of residence in the United States (as measured by generation)

TABLE 9-IV

WEIGHT CONDITION IN AN AGING POPULATION, BY NATIVITY

	Native-Born Native Parents		Native-Born Foreign Parents		Foreign-Born		Total	
	N	%	N	%	N	%	N	%
Males								
Thin	9	7.8	12	4.9	8	3.3	29	4.8
Normal	55	47.8	100	41.1	106	43.3	261	43.3
Overweight	33	28.7	83	34.2	84	34.3	200	33.2
Obese	18	15.7	48	19.8	47	19.1	113	18.7
Total	115	100.0	243	100.0	245	100.0	603	100.0

$x^2 = 5.8$ not significant.

Females								
Thin	3	2.3	2	0.7	1	0.6	6	1.0
Normal	48	37.2	100	32.6	35	21.2	183	30.4
Overweight	35	27.2	99	32.2	63	38.2	197	32.8
Obese	43	33.3	106	34.5	66	40.0	215	35.8
Total	129	100.0	307	100.0	165	100.0	601	100.0

$x^2 = 13.8$ p $<$ .05.

TABLE 9-V

WEIGHT CONDITION IN AN AGING POPULATION, BY NATIVITY AND
SOCIOECONOMIC STATUS

	Native-Born, Native Parents Socioeconomic Status			Native-Born, Foreign Parents Socioeconomic Status			Foreign-Born Socioeconomic Status		
	Low	*Medium*	*High*	*Low*	*Medium*	*High*	*Low*	*Medium*	*High*
Males									
Thin	10.7	12.0	0.0	1.8	8.3	0.0	5.9	0.0	3.2
Normal	42.9	42.0	59.5	38.2	36.8	54.5	39.8	44.2	53.1
Overweight	25.0	28.0	32.4	36.4	35.3	29.1	31.4	40.0	28.1
Obese	21.4	18.0	8.1	23.6	19.6	16.4	22.9	15.8	15.6
Total	100.0	100.0	100.0	100.0	100.0	100.0	100.0	100.0	100.0
N	28	50	37	55	133	55	118	95	32
Females									
Thin	3.5	1.8	2.3	0.0	1.3	0.0	0.0	0.0	5.6
Normal	31.0	21.4	61.4	25.0	33.1	42.6	18.8	23.9	22.2
Overweight	13.8	33.9	27.3	28.3	29.2	45.9	38.7	34.3	50.0
Obese	51.7	42.9	9.0	46.7	36.4	11.5	42.5	41.8	22.2
Total	100.0	100.0	100.0	100.0	100.0	100.0	100.0	100.0	100.0
N	29	56	44	92	154	61	80	67	18

increases. Among the males in the upper category, approximately the same pattern of prevalence of obesity is observed. Although the difference is slight between those who are native-born of foreign parents (16.4%) and those who are foreign-born (15.6%), a sharp drop occurs in the case of those who are native-born of native parents (8.1%). Unlike the women, however, the decline in prevalence of obesity among these males is not paralleled by similar changes in the amount of overweight as the proportion who are classified in this fashion remains generally constant by nativity group.

Religion-Ethnicity

Two other social variables, religion and ethnicity, were also considered. Because consideration of religion in many industrial communities lacks meaning without a sensitivity to ethnic factors, and because the number of cases was insufficient to make a detailed analysis of ethnicity, these two variables were combined into a set of five categories: Italian Catholic, Irish Catholic, other Catholic, Protestant and Jewish. Careful reading of the results presented in Table 9-VI, however, can lead to solid inferences about the importance of each of these variables.

The weight condition of the respondents, as reflected in Table 9-VI, shows important differentials by religion and ethnicity for both males and females. Again, the differences are less pronounced in the case of the males than females. The prevalence of obesity is much higher among Italian Catholics, men and women alike, than among any of the other groups.

The Psychology of Obesity

TABLE 9-VI

WEIGHT CONDITION IN AN AGING POPULATION, BY RELIGION-ETHNICITY

	Italian Catholic		Irish Catholic		Other Catholic		Protestant		Jewish		Total	
	N	%	N	%	N	%	N	%	N	%	N	%
Males												
Thin	3	1.5	7	6.5	12	11.9	6	5.6	2	2.5	30	5.0
Normal	72	35.8	49	45.8	45	44.5	54	50.4	39	48.1	259	43.4
Overweight ...	78	38.8	35	32.7	29	28.7	31	29.0	25	30.9	198	33.2
Obese	48	23.9	16	15.0	15	14.9	16	15.0	15	18.5	110	18.4
Total	201	100.0	107	100.0	101	100.0	107	100.0	81	100.0	597	100.0

$x^2 = 29.1$ p $<$ .05.

	Italian Catholic		Irish Catholic		Other Catholic		Protestant		Jewish		Total	
Females												
Thin	0	0.0	3	3.3	1	0.8	2	1.8	0	0.0	6	1.0
Normal	32	17.8	31	33.7	44	33.8	44	38.9	32	40.5	183	30.8
Overweight ...	56	31.1	23	25.0	43	33.1	39	34.5	35	44.3	196	33.0
Obese	92	51.1	35	38.0	42	32.3	28	24.8	12	15.2	209	35.2
Total	180	100.0	92	100.0	130	100.0	113	100.0	79	100.0	594	100.0

$x^2 = 54.4$ p $<$ .05.

In addition, Catholic women in general are disproportionately represented in the obese category in comparison to Protestant and Jewish women, but no such clear pattern could be found for males. Although the differences were somewhat offset by a higher proportion of their numbers being classified as overweight, the Jewish women were found to be much less frequently obese than women in the other groups.

Because religion-ethnicity and socioeconomic status may be closely related, the combined effects of these factors are assessed in relation to weight condition. This more complex analysis, presented in Table 9-VII, reveals some interesting patterns. In the case of females, the relationship between obesity and religion-ethnicity nearly vanishes among women of low socioeconomic status. The prevalence of obesity in each of the three Catholic groupings in this category is nearly identical and only the Jewish women deviate sharply from that figure. (The number of cases in this last group, however, is very small.) But as above, the low proportion of obesity among the Jewish women is offset by a very high prevalence (71.4%) of overweight. In the middle and high socioeconomic categories, the relationship between religion-ethnicity and weight returns as Italian women are found to be relatively more obese than women in the other groups, although this pattern was less pronounced in the upper socioeconomic grouping.

Among the males of low socioeconomic status, the greatest prevalence of obesity is found among the Italians and the Jews (although the small number of cases in the latter group makes interpretation difficult). The highest prevalence of obesity among the men in the middle group is also found among the Italians, and, as with the women, the relationship between re-

TABLE 9-VII

WEIGHT CONDITION IN AN AGING POPULATION, BY RELIGION-ETHNICITY AND SOCIOECONOMIC STATUS

	Italian Catholic			Irish Catholic			Other Catholic			Protestant			Jewish		
	Low	Medium	High	Low	Medium	High	Low	Medium	High	Low	Medium	High	Low	Medium	High
Males															
Thin	2.8	0.0	0.0	4.3	9.4	0.0	8.5	16.0	0.0	15.4	2.4	2.5	14.3	2.7	0.0
Normal	34.6	33.3	56.3	56.5	40.6	50.0	42.9	41.1	70.0	34.6	48.8	62.5	57.1	45.9	48.6
Overweight	35.5	44.9	31.3	26.1	32.8	40.0	34.3	28.6	10.0	30.8	31.7	25.0	0.0	35.2	32.5
Obese	27.1	21.8	12.4	13.1	17.2	10.0	14.3	14.3	20.0	19.2	17.1	10.0	28.6	16.2	18.9
Total	100.0	100.0	100.0	100.0	100.0	100.0	100.0	100.0	100.0	100.0	100.0	100.0	100.0	100.0	100.0
N	107	78	16	23	64	20	35	56	10	26	41	40	7	37	37
Females															
Thin	0.0	0.0	0.0	5.9	1.7	5.9	0.0	1.4	0.0	0.0	2.1	2.6	0.0	0.0	0.0
Normal	22.1	6.8	29.4	29.4	31.0	47.1	25.6	37.0	42.9	26.9	27.1	61.5	14.3	45.9	40.0
Overweight	29.8	28.8	47.1	17.6	25.9	29.4	25.6	34.2	50.0	38.5	35.4	30.8	71.4	35.2	48.6
Obese	48.1	64.4	23.5	47.1	41.4	17.6	48.8	27.4	7.1	34.6	35.4	5.1	14.3	18.9	11.4
Total	100.0	100.0	100.0	100.0	100.0	100.0	100.0	100.0	100.0	100.0	100.0	100.0	100.0	100.0	100.0
N	104	59	17	17	58	17	43	73	14	26	48	39	7	37	35

ligion-ethnicity and weight largely disappears among those of high socio-economic status.

SUMMARY AND INTERPRETATIONS

Two important conclusions can be reached immediately concerning the data which have been presented. First, a very high amount of obesity and overweight was discovered in the aging population under study. Whenever statistics are found which reveal that more than 50 per cent of the men and 60 per cent of the women are above normal weight for their age, they deserve attention. In a study population composed of individuals who are at an age when the possibility of becoming ill is rapidly increasing, the magnitude of these figures cannot be ignored.

Secondly, the data clearly show that differences in weight are not randomly distributed throughout the population. High proportions of obesity, for example, are found to be concentrated in certain segments of that population. This finding agrees with the few other studies that have also examined weight condition as a social phenomenon rather than an individual occurrence. As the Midtown Manhattan Study's authors observed, obesity may always be unhealthy, but it may not always be viewed as abnormal in various population subgroups such as persons of low socioeconomic status or those of Italian backgrounds.[11] With most discussions of the etiology of obesity having focused upon the individual, this conclusion should not be treated lightly.

With respect to more specific findings, the following general observations can be made: a) Substantial differences exist in weight condition by sex. Although more males than females could be classified as thin, possibly reflecting differences in health, the most significant departure from normality occurs in the direction of obesity where more than twice as many women as men could be identified in this manner. b) Important socioeconomic differences in the prevalence of overweight and obesity were also found. Although 54 per cent of the men and 76 per cent of the women in the low-socioeconomic groupings were either overweight or obese, the comparable percentages for men and women of high socioeconomic status were 44 and 53 per cent, respectively. These socioeconomic differences were more marked for females than for males. c) When socioeconomic status was controlled, relationships between weight condition and a third variable, nativity, generally disappear. Only among those persons of high socioeconomic status did this relationship remain when the controls were applied. Here, the proportion of those individuals who were obese drops with increasing generation in the United States. d) The same controls for socioeconomic status also produced some very interesting patterns when the relationship between weight and religion-ethnicity was examined. For women, overweight and obesity were highly prevalent in the low socioeconomic grouping regardless of religion-ethnicity, but the Italian males in this grouping were much more frequently found to be above normal weight. In the case of both males and females, the highest prevalence of obesity and overweight in the middle grouping is also found among Italians, and the relationship between religion-ethnicity and weight disappears among those of high socioeconomic status.

These results are similar to those presented in the Midtown Manhattan Study despite differences in study population and research design. Weight differentials by socioeconomic status were found in both studies as were such differences by ethnicity, although the Midtown researchers were not able to treat this variable as completely. Both analyses discovered differences in the prevalence of obesity and other weight conditions by sex, but the direction of this relationship differed between the two studies. In the present analysis the prevalence of obesity among females was much more pronounced than among males, although the opposite pattern was found in the Midtown Manhattan Study. Comparisons are marred by the different methods used to identify weight condition,* but part of the variation may be influenced by the age composition of the respective study populations. The Providence Study involved an "aging" group while the respondents in the Midtown Manhattan Study ranged from twenty to fifty-nine years of age. This raises the question as to whether obesity among females is a condition that occurs later in life, at which time it becomes more prevalent among this sex than among males. Additional research is needed to investigate the differences in results obtained in these two studies. The similarity of many of the findings, however, is worthy of careful note.

As an explanation for the weight differences discovered in their study population, the Midtown Manhatten researchers developed a social-psychological interpretation. In a nation where the popular culture emphasizes slimness as a desirable attribute among females, they suggested that this value will influence weight condition in several ways. Pressure to conform to this value will be felt and will increase with proximity to the upper class where the value is most strongly held, and increasing exposure to these values with length of generation in the United States will lead to its adoption.[12] In this fashion, the Midtown researchers were able to explain the patterns they found.

---

* The height-weight index employed by the Midtown Manhattan Study uses broad categories for both height and weight and is uniformly applied to both males and females, thus creating great differences in the identification of obesity. For example, if the Midtown Manhattan Study's height-weight index had been applied to the Providence Study population, obesity could range from 14 to 30 per cent over desirable weight depending upon an individual's height. Measuring the deviation of an individual's present weight from the "desirable" weight for persons of the same sex and his exact height eliminates that problem in the present analysis.

In the present analysis, this "value-orientation" approach requires some modification. The prevalence of obesity among Italian Catholics, even when social class is controlled, suggests that dietary factors are important as well. Studies have shown, for example, that the Italian-American's diet has a high caloric and fat content[13] and that some members of this ethnic group still hold to the belief that obesity provides protection from certain diseases.[14] Apparently, both dietary considerations and orientation to the popular culture's value of "slimness" affect the weight condition of Italians in the study population, although the latter may be sufficient to explain the patterns found for other religious-ethnic groups. For example, tendencies toward a diet that is inappropriate to maintain normal weight may disappear with improvements in socioeconomic status, thereby explaining why Italian Catholics of high socioeconomic status were not noticeably more obese than other religious-ethnic groups of the same status. On the other hand, the very high prevalence of obesity among all women in the low socioeconomic group may mask any ethnic factor that might be operative.

Additional investigation on these two alternative explanations and extension of the research to other subgroups of the population and additional social variables are needed. The message of the present study centers upon the word "epidemiological" in the announced form of the analysis. McMahon, Pugh, and Ipsen make a distinction between descriptive and analytic epidemiology:[15]

> Epidemiology is the study of the distribution and determinants of disease prevalence in man. Two main areas are indicated in the definition. These are the study of the *distribution* of disease (descriptive epidemiology) and the search for the *determinants* of the noted distribution (analytic epidemiology).

This study is an example of the former and has discharged its responsibility by a) emphasizing the prevalence of obesity in an aging population, b) noting that weight differences do not occur randomly throughout the population, and c) pointing to some of the differentials in weight which exist between subgroups of the population. Some interpretation was undertaken and points of comparison and contrast with the Midtown Manhattan Study were noted. With this information, the work of analytic epidemiology should begin by asking persons of different ages about their value orientations concerning weight, making assessments of their diet, and analyzing weight changes and the ages at which they occurred. The present study has pointed to the need for such information and with the importance of weight condition for health, these are appropriate questions for further study.

REFERENCES

1. United States Public Health Service: *Obesity and Health.* Washington, United States Government Printing Office, 1966.

2. Goldner, Martin: Obesity and its relationship to disease. *New York State J Med,* 56:2064, July 1, 1956.
3. Burnight, Robert G.: Chronic morbidity and the socio-economic characteristics of older urban males. *Milbank Memorial Fund Quart,* 43:312-314, July, 1965.
4. Goldblatt, Phillip B., Moore, Mary E. and Stunkard, Albert J.: Social factors in obesity. *JAMA,* 192:1039-1044, June 21, 1965; and Moore, Mary E., Stunkard, Albert and Srole, Lee: Obesity, social class and mental illness. *JAMA,* 81: 962-966, September, 1962.
5. Pflanz, M.: Medizinische-soziologische Aspekte der Fettsucht. *Psyche,* 16:575-591, 1962-1963; cf. Goldblatt, Moore and Stunkard, *op. cit.,* p. 1042.
6. Brozek, Joseph and Keys, Ancel: Relative body weight, age and fatness. *Geriatrics,* 8:70-74, 1953.
7. Edwards, K. D. G. and Whyte, H. M.: The simple measurement of obesity. *Clin Sci,* 22:347-352, 1962.
8. Society of Actuaries: *Build and Blood Pressure Study.* Washington, 1959.
9. Metropolitan Life Insurance Company: *Statistical Bull,* 40:4, November-December, 1959.
10. Kannel, William B.: Director of the Framingham Heart Study, Personal communication.
11. Goldblatt, Phillip B., Moore, Mary E. and Stunkard, Albert J.: Social factors in obesity. *JAMA,* 192:1040, June 21, 1965.
12. Goldblatt, Phillip B., Moore, Mary E. and Stunkard, Albert J.: Social factors in obesity. *JAMA,* 192:1042-1043, June 21, 1965.
13. Joffe, Natalie: Food habits of selected subcultures in the United States. *Bull Nat Res Council,* 108:98, October, 1943; and Stout, Clarke, *et al.:* Unusually low incidence of death from myocardial infarction: Study of an Italian-American community in Pennsylvania. *JAMA,* 188:848, June 8, 1964.
14. Joffe, Natalie: Food habits of selected subcultures in the United States. *Bull Nat Res Council,* 108:98-99, October, 1943.
15. McMahon, Brian, Pugh, Thomas F. and Ipsen, Johannes: *Epidemiologic Methods.* Boston, Little, Brown and Company, 1960, p. 3.

IV
CHILDHOOD AND ADOLESCENT OBESITY

10

Obesity in Children

ERIC J. KAHN

RECENT interest in preventive approaches to childhood obesity[1,2] can be attributed to the poor response of this condition to present treatment methods. In discussing preventive measures, stress is usually laid on screening programs which detect early cases. Ideally, however, individuals at risk should be identified and given surveillance before the onset of rapid weight gain, because obesity tends to become self-perpetuating and treatment resistant at some unpredictable stage of development. Unfortunately, knowledge of the factors which predispose young children to obesity is still fragmentary. Thus Bruch[3] showed that the obese were frequently the youngest or the only child in the family or that they were the products of unwanted pregnancies; she also described psychological trauma as an etiologic factor, including that associated with hospitalization. Predisposition to obesity is also indicated by the presence of this condition in parents or siblings,[4] by a somatotype characterized by endomorphism, mesomorphism, and ectopenia,[5] by physical handicaps which limit mobility,[6] or a family setup in which the father is subordinate to the mother.[7]

This paper reports an additional predisposing factor, namely separation of children from their mothers. Working in an obesity clinic which serves a ghetto population, the author was impressed by the high percentage of children living with mother surrogates. This observation was investigated in the present study by comparing relevant data of the clinic population with those of a control group from the same environment.

MATERIAL AND METHODS

The report is based on the records of seventy-two obese children, twenty-seven boys and forty-five girls under the age of twelve years, and seventy-two control children matched for age and sex. Seven of the obese children and four of the control children were Puerto Rican; all others were Negro.

The obese group comprised all referrals to the pediatric obesity clinic at Harlem Hospital Center made during the period from December, 1967 to March, 1969, by physicians, nurses, and social workers at hospitals, health stations, and schools in the district, usually on the basis of the child's appearance and occasionally because there had been a recent, rapid weight gain. No referrals were rejected, but six patients were eliminated from the study because their records were incomplete. One girl was slightly mentally

109

retarded; no children had any severe physical handicaps or diseases. Compared with the "Physical growth standards for children from birth to eighteen,"[8] the weights of all obese children were above the ninety-fifth percentile; the height was above the ninety-fifth percentile in thirty, between the fiftieth and ninety-fifth percentiles in thirty, and between the twenty-fifth and fiftieth percentiles in twelve children. The age at onset of obesity could be ascertained in fifty-six children; in fifteen (27.3%) it started during the first year of life and in an additional twenty-one (37.8%), during the subsequent two years. Only six patients had become obese after six years of age. Twenty-one of the children had no siblings, and only five had three or more. A reliable assessment of family stability, or even the *de facto* marital status of the mother, was not possible.

The control subjects were chosen at random from children attending the pediatric walk-in and general surgical follow-up clinics, which serve the same district and socioeconomic segment of the population as the obesity clinic. Excluded were five children whose weights were above the ninety-fifth percentile, but their data are shown as *eliminated controls.* Matching for age was correct to within the same year but not the same month. Children in the control group were of shorter stature than the obese children. Only one was above the ninety-fifth percentile in height, thirty-four were between the fiftieth and ninety-fifth percentiles, twenty-eight were between the fifth and fiftieth percentiles, and seven were below the fifth percentile. They also tended to be members of larger families, only thirteen having no siblings and seventeen having three or more.

Separation was defined as placement of a child in the home of a person other than the mother. In both groups the shortest period of such separation happened to be about six months. In most instances there was no contact with the mother during this time, but in some instances the mother visited the child at intervals or the child returned to the mother on weekends.

RESULTS

A history of separation from the mother was obtained in twenty-three (31.9%) of the obese children (seven boys and sixteen girls) and in six (8.3%) of the seventy-two control subjects (two boys and four girls). The difference between the two groups is statistically significant ($p < 0.001$). Only one of the twenty-three children had been legally adopted; the others were living with relatives or friends of the mother. The reasons for the inability of the mothers to take care of their children were resumption of employment in six instances, death in two, heroin addiction in two, mental illness in two, and desertion in two. In the remaining nine, the child's guardian was reluctant to discuss the whereabouts of the mother. The age at the onset of obesity could be ascertained in eighteen of the twenty-three children. In fourteen of these a rapid weight gain commenced shortly after a separation episode; the other four were already obese prior to separation. However, the families of two of these four children had long-standing histories of periodic turmoil, caused by mental illness of one of the parents, and this situation almost certainly precluded a normal mother-child relationship.

In four additional children, the obesity was said to have started after a brief episode of hospitalization; however, documentary proof for this time relationship could be obtained for only one patient.

As previously stated, five children were excluded from the control group because they were obese. Even in this small sample, two children gave a history of separation from their mothers; one spent the first four years of her life with the maternal grandmother and was obese when she rejoined her mother, and the other began to gain weight rapidly after her mother had been admitted to an institution for mental illness.

Though forty-nine obese children and sixty-six control children had remained in daily contact with their mothers, twenty-six (53.0%) of the former and thirty-nine (59.0%) of the latter had been left for several hours of the day with baby sitters or at day-care centers while the mother was working outside the home. In 46.1 per cent of the obese children and 41.0 per cent of the corresponding control subjects, the mother entered employment before the child was one year of age.

DISCUSSION

It is unlikely that the composition of the group of obese children was significantly influenced by considerations other than body weight or appearance, because the decisions for the referrals were made by medical and nonmedical personnel at a variety of institutions. Indeed, these children conformed to the well-described pattern of childhood obesity in the United States in respect of family size, age at onset of the obesity, acceleration of longitudinal growth, and absence of certain diseases which may cause obesity, although the numerical preponderance of females over males was somewhat more marked than usual.

However, in this group of obese children a history of separation from the mother was nearly four times more frequent than among control children, even after excluding patients whose weight gains were said to have been precipitated by hospitalization. In contrast, absence of the mother from the home for part of the day was recorded with equal frequency in patients and control subjects.

Mother-child separation has long been recognized as a precipitating factor of "failure to thrive";[9] it has not previously been directly implicated as a factor in the pathogenesis of childhood obesity, although Bruch[3] observed that rapid weight gain sometimes followed discharge of patients from a hospital.

The pathogenesis of obesity in children who are separated from their mothers is uncertain. It is suspected that some of our patients had been, at least initially, overfed by anxious mother surrogates who were intent on proving their competence in child rearing. Separation anxiety in children is another possible cause of obesity; Schachter[10] showed that some adults react to a stressful situation with overeating and others with a reduced food intake. It is not known whether this mechanism explains the paradox of separation causing wasting in some children and obesity in others.

Regardless of these uncertainties, excessive weight gain could probably have been prevented in some of our patients without imposing diet restrictions, had children of working mothers been placed in day-care centers or with baby sitters rather than in the homes of mother surrogates. The effectiveness of such measures, the relative predictive value of known predisposing factors, and their potential for reinforcing each other need to be tested in prospective studies.

REFERENCES

1. Committee on Nutrition: Obesity in childhood, *Pediatrics,* 40:455, 1967.
2. Mayer, J.: Some aspects of the problem of regulation of food intake and obesity. *New Engl J Med,* 274:722, 1962.
3. Bruch, H.: Obesity in childhood. *Am J Dis Child,* 59:739, 1940.
4. Ellis, R. W. B. and Tallerman, K. H.: Obesity in childhood: Study of 50 cases. *Lancet,* 2:615, 1934.
5. Seltzer, C. C. and Mayer, J.: Body build and obesity—who are the obese? *JAMA,* 189:677, 1964.
6. Greene, J. A.: Clinical study of the etiology of obesity. *Ann Intern Med,* 12:1797, 1939.
7. Bruch, H.: *The Importance of Overweight.* New York, W. W. Norton Co., Inc., 1957, p. 198.
8. United States Department of Health, Education, and Welfare: *Obesity and Health,* Pub. No. 1485, p. 11.
9. Bakwin, H.: Loneliness in infants. *Am J Dis Child,* 63:30, 1942.
10. Schachter, S.: Obesity and eating. *Science,* 161:751, 1968.

11

Obesity in Adolescence

Frank Carrera III

THE demand for psychiatric, diagnostic, and therapeutic services for adolescents has increased markedly over the past few years and projective studies indicate that these clinical demands will continue to increase. It becomes imperative, then, as recommended by the APA Committee on Psychiatry of Childhood and Adolescence, for child psychiatrists and general psychiatrists to enhance their effectiveness in dealing with the emotional problems of adolescents. How to best approach the evaluation of that group of adolescents who present with obesity is the purpose of this chapter.

Obesity among adolescents seems to be a significant clinical problem. Garell's[15] survey of fifty-five hospitals in the United States and Canada revealed that sixteen of these hospitals had special adolescent clinics. He reported that the majority of adolescents who were seen in these adolescent specialty clinics were seen because of obesity and that in ten of these clinics obesity was listed as the most frequent diagnosis. That obesity in teenagers often interferes with healthy personality development is agreed upon by anyone who has even had a casual relationship with an obese adolescent. Yet it seems that child psychiatry clinics see relatively few of these patients. If they are referred, they frequently get lost in clinic waiting lists. This is probably due to two main factors: the pressures for child psychiatrists to focus on other more urgent and dramatic psychiatric problems, and general clinical experience that obese adolescents are "poor therapy" candidates.

This lack of exposure to obese adolescents on the part of psychiatrists seems to result too often in a stilted "classical" view of the problem—namely, that all obese adolescents are "fixated in the oral stage of psychosexual development." It seems relevant, then, in view of the prevalence of the problem, to review the recent literature on obesity which seems pertinent to a more up-to-date understanding of obesity in adolescence, and which seems to define the role of the clinical psychiatrist in his work with obese adolescents.

The old basic physiological mechanism in obesity of a positive energy balance still remains basic today in our physiologic understanding of how obesity begins and how it is maintained, i.e. obesity results when a person takes in more calories than he uses. But Bruch[6] noted that this basic phys-

113

iological mechanism is part of the symptomatology and *not* an explanation of the underlying factors.

Over the past twenty-five years the scientific view of childhood and adolescent obesity has changed from one of "it's all soma" or "it's all psyche" to the more reasonable present view that there are multiple etiological factors and probably a variety of obesities. Factors reported in the literature which influence food intake and energy output include social, economic, somatic, emotional, and genetic elements. Relevant to the focus of this paper is that this present view of obesity points to the necessity for the psychiatric clinician to focus on the individuality of each obese adolescent he sees and that any tendency to lump all obese adolescents in one formulation frame would put him at least ten years behind the times.

Although some of the literature on the natural history of obesity in children and adolescents points to this imperative to individualize our diagnostics with obese teen-agers, the literature in most other instances still reflects the old view of lumping all obesity together. This fact seems to define for the present the primary role of the clinical psychiatrist with obese adolescents as one of researcher, data-gatherer, or "fact-finder." I would propose, then, the following checklist to be used during the history taking and physical examination of every obese adolescent. The data obtained would serve as either an important bit of information for a differential diagnosis of obesity based on our present knowledge, or would provide more research data to clarify certain issues which are still unresolved.

BIRTH WEIGHT

Heald[20] recently reported conflicting evidences regarding whether obese children or adolescents are obese at birth or tend to have higher birth weights. It is likely that this contradictory evidence reflects the heterogeneity of the obese adolescent population. The importance of obtaining birth weight information on each obese adolescent becomes clearer when we consider the next bit of data on our checklist.

AGE OF ONSET

The age of onset of the obesity would seem to be a particularly valuable factor in differential diagnosis. Unfortunately, very few studies have focused on the age of onset specifically. However, Forbes,[29] studying body compositional changes in adolescents, was able to identify two types of obesity when the lean body mass was determined by the whole body potassium counter. Interestingly, and of great significance, is the fact that each of these two types of obesity had *different* ages of onset. Forbes' work suggested the following *two* types: Type I, characterized by an increase in lean body mass, a tendency to tallness, advanced bone age, and a history of overweight since infancy; Type II, showing no increase in lean body mass, normal growth characteristics, with obesity developing during the childhood years. This data suggests that a number of subgroups exist among obese youngsters and that they are obese for different reasons. In view of this, the necessity for intensive and detailed history-taking concerning life events and the general family milieu during the time of age of onset becomes critical. It would help differentiate between a Type I juvenile obesity as Forbes suggests in which psychological factors may play a relatively minor role, and a Type II juvenile obesity whose ages of onset may be largely determined by psychological and social factors.

RATES OF GROWTH AND MATURATION

Wolff,[30] in reviewing the literature on the relationship between obesity and height in children, reported that obese children tended to be above average height during childhood but Lloyd, *et al.*,[31] reported that the ultimate height of these same youngsters after puberty was significantly below the standard height. They then concluded that what appeared to be accelerated growth during childhood seemed to be really accelerated maturation. These cases would seem to correspond to Forbes' Type I of childhood obesity characterized in part by a tendency to tallness and advanced bone age.

It would appear that the heterogeneity of obese children again explains the contradictory reports in the literature concerning the age of menarche in obese girls. This should be part of the checklist in adolescent girls' evaluations in order to provide more data concerning this event's relationship to obesity and particularly to possibly differentiate subtypes of obesity. It would seem reasonable to assume that for this Forbes I type of accelerated maturer, the psychological effects of menarche may play a lesser role in obesity than in Forbes Type II where the psychological factors centering around the menarche may play a more prominent role.

BODY TYPES

A study[23] by Seltzer and Mayer, of the somatotypes and anthropomorphic measurements of obese adolescent girls and nonobese teen-age girls, demonstrated that obesity did not occur in all the varieties of physical types but occurred in greater frequency in some physical types than in others. Their findings suggest that a prime prerequisite for the development of obesity in the group of adolescent girls they studied is a physique with at least a moderate degree of endomorphy under normal conditions, the endomorphy predisposing to the laying on of additional quantities of fat *unless* excessive activity, disease, or voluntary weight control supervened.[22] The theoretical implication of this last statement which makes detailed history-taking important is that the phenotypic expression of a somatotypic genotype may be altered by environmental factors such as the eating patterns in the family, by psychological factors or even by other constitutional factors such as differences in temperament as Stella Chess proposes, particularly the individual child's characteristic activity level which she has reported persists from infancy into childhood. This study of the role of somatotype on the subsequent development of obesity in adolescent girls may best be considered as another evidence of the significance of constitutional and genetic factors in the predisposition to obesity.

FAMILY OCCURRENCE

It has been reported many times that a high incidence of obesity in one or both parents is associated with the development of obesity in the child. Familial occurrence of obesity in some of these studies ranges from 69 per cent to 80 per cent of obese children having had one or both parents obese. In the diagnostic evaluation of obese adolescents it would be important to inquire not only into the incidence of obesity in the family but also to obtain a detailed history of family life in order to better evaluate the relative weight of genetic factors versus other factors such as family eating patterns and family attitudes toward food which are operating, interacting, and possibly modifying the genetic components.

ACTIVITY VERSUS INACTIVITY

Evaluation of the obese adolescent's usual activity level pattern is of major importance in the differentiation of obesity at the very basic physiological level as regards the concept of positive energy balance. Two broad types of obesity in childhood and adolescence appear in relation to this physiological factor: a) the hyperphagic type of obesity in which the imbalance seems primarily due to excesses at the intake end of this equation, and b) the low activity type in which the imbalance in the equation seems to be on the output side of the equation.

It is difficult to estimate from the literature the relative frequency of the hyperphagic type in childhood and adolescence since these are reported primarily in the form of clinical case studies. A recent survey however, conducted by the Department of Agriculture of adolescents in Iowa, reported that only 4 per cent of the obese teen-agers they studied ate excessively. By comparison, the low activity type of obesity in children and adolescents has been reported many times. Bruch[1] had called attention to the relative inactivity of many obese children back in 1940. More recently Johnson, *et al.*,[32] compared twenty-eight obese high school girls with twenty-eight average weight controls and reported that the obese girls ate *less* than the controls but that they spent two-thirds less time than the controls in active pursuits. Stefanik, *et al.*,[33] also called attention to this phenomenon in fourteen obese adolescent males as compared to fourteen nonobese controls. Bullen,[10] using photographic time-motion studies, also noted that the average obese adolescent girl expends far less energy than the average nonobese adolescent girl during scheduled exercise periods. This inactivity which seems to be most characteristic of obese adolescents may be the result of physiological factors, constitutional factors, or psychological factors. A possible physiological explanation for the inactivity comes from the study of Wenzel *et al.*, in which he noted that among an out-patient clinic adolescent population the obese youngsters had a significantly lower serum iron (with normal serum hemoglobin) than did nonanemic, nonobese controls. Whether this lower serum iron represents a physiological basis for the inactivity or whether it is a concomitant effect of the inactivity is yet to be determined.

For another possible interpretation of this relative inactivity we could refer again to Chess' work concerning individual differences in temperament, particularly activity level present at birth and stable through early childhood. Since these subjects in Chess' follow-up study have not yet reached adolescence no definite connection between these two factors can yet be made. The psychodynamic factors in personality formation which may tend to result in a child's "passive" solution to stresses and which may also directly affect activity level is another factor which must be investigated.

It appears important from these studies that urging these obese teen-agers to increase their activity level seems imperative in treatment. How to best promote this change from their usual low activity level will depend to a large extent on the specific etiology and/or attached meanings of this behavioral manifestation in the individual, pointing to the need for individualized, focused interviewing.

HUNGER AND SATIETY SENSATIONS

In evaluating obese teen-age patients, we can no longer fall back comfortably on old and familiar formulations derived from classical drive theories—formulations which assumed that all obesity was the result of an increased drive to eat and in which the concept of orality was used across the board in understanding obesity and the obese individual.

Research data does not support this exclusive reliance on these classical drive theory assumptions.

Brobeck[34] demonstrated in his animal studies that there were two anatomically and behaviorally distinct centers in the hypothalamus, the one regulating feeding and the other regulating satiety. Since then it has been repeatedly demonstrated in animals that experimental obesity due to overeating may result from either increased activity of the feeding centers with an apparent increase in the "hunger drive" *or* from decreased activity of the satiety centers with a resultant disorder in satiety mechanisms. The point to be emphasized is that the one behavior, overeating, may result from two quite different mechanisms at hypothalamic cellular level. Stunkard[35] and others have reported many instances in obese adult humans in which the associated overeating seemed to be due to disturbances in satiety mechanisms. Monello[18] recently reported that in adolescent obesity, satiety abnormalities also occur and, in fact, suggested that they were more prevalent than differences in hunger among the obese adolescent girls he studied. In comparing hunger and satiety sensation differences between obese teenage girls and nonobese controls, his preliminary findings indicate that at the end of the meal, obese subjects require more conscious willpower to stop eating even though they report more frequently than controls that they experience sensations of discomfort at the end of the meal, particularly distention and nausea. Increased hunger and disturbed satiety appear to be two different mechanisms leading to overeating and obesity. As clinicians we should identify the type of overeating in the individual patient.

PSYCHOLOGICAL FACTORS

That we cannot approach an obese adolescent with preconceived fixed psychodynamic notions is reflected in Gluckman's recent statement that "all we do know is that obese patients do not have a common personality structure and their obesity does not have a common meaning." However, the necessity of a close look at psychological-emotional factors is evident from common clinical knowledge that among obese adolescents there seems to be a clear connection between heightened emotional tension, eating behavior, and weight gain.

Bullen, *et al.*[10] reported that in the 115 obese adolescent girls he studied, the majority stated they went on eating sprees when they felt bad, tense, nervous, depressed, bored, worried, etc. However, the underlying mechanisms mediating this relationship of psychic tension to increased eating have not been elucidated although it is likely that learned patterning in reaction to stress plays a part.

Along these lines, Bruch[36] reformulated her thinking about the etiology of certain cases of obesity in terms of learning theory when she noted that these patients seemed to suffer from an inability to identify their bodily sensations correctly, in particular, hunger and satiation. Her hypothesis is that the deficit occurred as the result of disturbed early mother-child interactions in which the mother would repeatedly feed the child inappropriately when he was *not* hungry—so that the child never learned the significance of the stimuli arising from his own stomach.

Bruch describes other psychological characteristics of this type of "I can't feel when I'm hungry" obese adolescent which indicate a more general lack of a sense of basic trust in their own feelings and in their ability to identify their own feelings. Her patients in this group frequently made statements like "Mother always knew how I felt when I myself did not know it." She concluded that a prerequisite for psychotherapy with any lasting success with obese adolescents of this type must focus on this conceptual disturbance —the therapy directed to helping the patient express how he feels right now rather than an approach that suggests in any way how he *should* feel.

It would seem then, that on the basis of our present information, among certain obese adolescents psychological factors leading to overeating may form distinct subgroups which are themselves distinct from those where psychological factors lead to inactivity, and distinct from those where psychological factors lead to disturbances in satiety mechanisms.

A quantity of research showing the interplay between emotions and obesity has been done. When we look to the literature for the prevalance of significant emotional illness occurring in obese adolescents we find a broad range reported. Tolstrup[4] reported evidence of significant psychological disturbances in 45 per cent of forty obese children and adolescents studied. Bruch[37] reported that 40 per cent of her obese child patients who were seen in twenty-year follow-up remained obese *and* significantly emotionally maladjusted. Ostergaard[5] reports an even higher prevalence of 81 per cent emotional disorders among fifty-eight obese children. These studies underscore the danger of underestimating the significant psychological disorders associated with obesity in children and adolescents. A recent study by Monello and Mayer[38] of one-hundred adolescent obese girls compared to sixty-five nonobese controls focuses our attention on how serious the psychological maladjustments tend to be in the adolescent obese female group specifically. The results of three projective tests administered to these girls revealed that the obese teen-age girls showed personality characteristics strikingly similar to the traits of ethnic and racial minorities: a) "obsessive concern" with heightened sensitivity and preoccupation with status, b) "passivity," withdrawal, sense of isolation, and feeling of rejection by their peers; c) "acceptance of dominant values" and considered obesity, and therefore their own bodies, as undesirable and somewhat harmful.

Stunkard and Mendelson[9] had reported similar minority group personality characteristics in a small percentage of obese adult female subjects who also demonstrated distorted body images.

The three prerequisites for the development of a distorted body image in his study were as follows: the person developed obesity in childhood or adolescence; the person suffers from an emotional disturbance; the obesity was the focus of derogatory parental concern.

Since these serious psychological problems all carried into adulthood, it appears that prolonged intensive psychotherapy is indicated for those obese adolescents who demonstrate these particular characteristics.

Bruch[6] reported on her more than twenty-year study on obese children whose onset occurred before puberty. She found a high correlation between a congenial family environment and a favorable outcome, i.e. with normal weight (15%) or a stable condition of overweight (20%) and good social adjustment in adulthood. These were the families in which there was little anxious or punitive overconcern with the child's obesity.

In contrast, the follow-up on children whose families showed unrelenting preoccupation with the excess weight and were resistant to reassurance revealed an unfavorable outcome in adulthood, with progressive obesity (40%) or artificially maintained thinness (25%) and poor total adjustment including psychotic reactions in those cases where the psychopathological relationships with the parents had been intense.

Bruch[6] concluded that of practical importance for making fairly accurate predictions concerning the outcome of childhood obesity and for purposes of determining when intensive psychiatric intervention is definitely indicated, the diagnostic evaluation should include the following data: a) an evaluation of the emotional status of the child, b) the child's interaction with the family and in particular the parental attitudes toward the child's obesity, c) an evaluation of the weight curve including its stability or fluctuations.

The need to study the family in depth is also reflected in the results of the following study. Disturbances in family relationships were the rule in those obese adolescent girls in Bullen's, et al.[10] study who were having rather total adjustment difficulties of adolescence. The family relationship disturbances were characterized by a low degree of sociability among family members and by much fighting between siblings. The poorly adjusted obese adolescent girl was more dependent on the family, had conflict over separating from the mother, had a great concern with sex on the fantasy level with a concomitant lack of heterosexual interests at the reality level. They typically used passive responses like avoidance or denial, seemingly clinging to the *status quo,* and gave evidence of disturbances in body image. It would seem imperative then that these psychological symptoms be part of our checklist, since their presence indicates the need for psychotherapeutic intervention which must involve the parents whenever unhealthy emotional parental attitudes concerning the child's obesity are present.

We will proceed now to some other factors for our checklist which specifically have to do with treatment of the obese adolescent. It is clear from the literature that the best treatment for obesity and the accompanying emotional disturbance in 65 per cent of the cases is preventive work done early. Mullins reported that one-third of the adult patients in his survey had a history of juvenile obesity. He also reported that juvenile obesity persisting into adult life tended to be more severe and more difficult to treat than adult onset obesity.[20] It is obvious that the "he'll grow out of his fatness" attitude is false and that much of our previous treatment for the obesities of childhood and adolescence has been less than adequate.

Stunkard and Mendelson[9] attempt to explain why treatment has been inadequate when neurosis and obesity become intertwined. They propose that obesity is the only condition which involves at the same time a disturbance in body image and a disturbance in impulse control. The simultaneous occurrence of both these problems makes each more malignant. In view of this, if we consider the naturally occurring body image changes and impulse control disturbance of the average adolescent state, it is no wonder that the treatment of obesity in adolescents is difficult and that preventive intervention is imperative.

The presence of deviant eating patterns seem to affect prognosis and treatment methods. Stunkard reports that binge eaters are usually able to carry out a weight reduction program successfully. However, obese patients with the night eating syndrome (morning anorexia, evening hyperphagia, and insomnia) are poor therapeutic candidates and frequently become highly emotionally disturbed when they try to diet. Although the obese person with the night-eating syndrome seems fairly resistive to psychotherapy, recent evidence shows that they do respond to antidepressants. Further experimental studies of the "night-eater" may eventually elucidate more clearly the relationship and mechanisms between depression and eating behavior. This night-eating syndrome has not been reported in adolescents, but since its presence has prognostic significance, it should be included in the checklist.

In summary, it seems evident that the use of this proposed checklist with obese adolescents would provide the kinds of data essential for the clinical child psychiatrist's important role as researcher-fact finder in his attempt to differentially diagnose the obesities in adolescence. In addition, such a checklist does appear to provide the clinician also with information useful in determining the indications for psychotherapy.

For the child psychiatrist evaluating obese teen-agers the presence of the following factors obtained from the patient interview and from history-taking would seem, from the literature review, to constitute indications for psychotherapy: evidence of a pathological child-parent relationship; hypercritical family attitudes regarding the patient's obesity; seemingly "compulsive" eating in response to a variety of moods and affects; eating seems to be the only comfort in an otherwise sterile existence; the withdrawal—"hate my body"—increased sensitivity triad is present and seems to represent a way of life; eating patterns include the night-eating syndrome at which time psychotherapy plus antidepressant drug therapy would be indicated; evidence that the teen-ager is not attuned to his own feelings including his own bodily sensations of hunger and satiety; a lack of closeness among family members with coexistent difficulties for the obese teen-ager in separating from the family; an attitude of preference for the *status quo* reflected in delayed involvement with the tasks of adolescence: developing a sense of individual identity, a growing independence and self reliance, involvement in heterosexual orientation, and participation and involvement in the peer culture.

In conclusion, the data reviewed would tend to suggest that there are multiple etiological factors involved in adolescent obesity and that they may be different for obese persons with early age of onset than for those with late onset. In other words, obesity is a symptom which is the end-product of many syndromes:

1. The environment plays a permissive role in that food has to be available in sufficient quantity for a constitutional predisposition to manifest itself.

2. Inactivity seems to be an important factor in the development and maintenance of adolescent obesity.

3. Overeating may be a primary mechanism and may be due to psychological or physiological factors.

4. Inactivity may be the primary mechanism involved and it, too, may be due primarily to physiological and/or psychological factors.

5. It would appear that abnormalities in satiety might be more prevalent in adolescent obesity than difference in hunger.

6. It appears dangerous to underestimate the psychological effects of the pressures of society on the obese child and on the obese female adolescent in particular.

7. It would appear that a psychotherapeutic orientation aimed at proving the psychogenicity of obesity in a teen-ager is contraindicated, ineffective, and out-dated.

It is obvious that in order to understand obesity in adolescence and to understand the obese teen-ager himself the child psychiatrist must approach him in the highly individualized fashion that has traditionally characterized the child psychiatrist's view of the child and his family. But in addition to this helping approach, it is obvious because of the confusion and lack of information in the literature that one of the primary roles of the clinical child psychiatrist with the obese teen-ager is that of fact finder and researcher.

REFERENCES

1. Bruch, H. and Touraine, G.: Obesity in childhood: V. The family frame of obese children. *Psychom Med*, II, No. 2:141, Apr. 1940.
2. Juel-Nielson, N.: On psychogenic obesity in children. II. *Acta Paediat*, 42:133, Mar. 1953.

3. Quaade, F.: On psychogenic obesity in children. III. *Acta Paediat,* 42:191, May 1953.

4. Tolstrup, K.: On psychogenic obesity in children. IV. *Acta Paediat,* 42:289, July 1953.

5. Ostergaard, L.: On psychogenic obesity in childhood. V. *Acta Paediat,* 43:507, Nov. 1954.

6. Bruch, H.: Obesity. *Pediat Clin N. Am,* 613, Aug. 1958.

7. Apley, J. and MacKeith, R.: *The Child and His Symptoms: A Psychomatic Approach.* Blackwell, Oxford, 1961.

8. Stunkard, A.: *Research on a Disease: Strategies in the Study of Obesity.* Roseler, R. and Greenfield, N. S. (Eds.): Physiological Correlates of Psychological Disorder, Chap. 11, Univ. of Wis. Press, 1961.

9. Stunkard, A. and Mendelson, M.: Body image of obese persons. *J Am Dietet Assoc,* 38:328, 1961.

10. Bullen, B. A., Monello, L. F., Cohen, H. and Mayer, J.: Attitudes towards physical activity, food and family in obese and non-obese adolescent girls. *Am J Clin Nutr,* 12, No. 1:1, Jan. 1964.

11. Masterson, J. F., Jr., Tucker, K. and Berk, G.: Psychopathology of adolescence IV: Clinical and dynamic characteristics. *Am J Psychiat,* 120, No. 4:357, Oct. 1963.

12. Shirley, Hale F.: *Pediatric Psychiatry.* Harvard Univ. Press, 1963.

13. Coddington, R. D., Sours, J. A. and Bruck, H.: Electrogastrographic findings associated with affective changes. *Am J Psychiat,* 121, No. 1:41, July 1964.

14. Offer, D., Sabshin, M. and Marcus, D.: Clinical evaluation of normal adolescents. *Am J Psychiat,* 121, No. 9:864, Mar. 1965.

15. Garell, D. C.: Adolescent medicine. *Am J Dis Child,* 109:314, April 1965.

16. Silverstone, J. T. and Solomon, T.: Psychiatric and somatic factors in the treatment of obesity. *J Psychosom Res,* 9:249, 1965.

17. Mayer, J.: Inactivity as a major factor in adolescent obesity. *Ann N Y Acad Sci,* 131, Art., 1:502, Oct. 1965.

18. Monello, L. F., Seltzer, C. C. and Mayer, J.: Hunger and satiety sensations in men, women, boys and girls: A preliminary report. *Ann N Y Acad Sci,* 131, Art., 1: 593, Oct. 1965.

19. Christakis, G., Sajecki, S., Hillman, R. W., Miller, E., Blumenthal, S. and Archer, M.: Effects of a combined nutrition education and physical fitness program on the weight status of obese high school boys. *Fed Proc,* 25, No. 1:15, Jan.-Feb. 1966.

20. Heald, F. P.: Natural history and physiological basis of adolescent obesity. *Fed Proc,* 25, No. 1:1, Jan.-Feb. 1966.

21. Huenemann, R. L., Hampton, M. C., Shapiro, L. R. and Behnke, A. R.: Adolescent food practices associated with obesity. *Fed Proc,* 25, No. 1:4, Jan.-Feb. 1966.

22. Mayer, J.: Physical activity and anthropometric measurements of obese adolescents. *Fed Proc,* 25, No. 1:11, Jan.-Feb. 1966.

23. Seltzer, C. C. and Mayer, J.: A review of genetic and constitutional factors in human obesity. *Ann N Y Acad Sci,* 131, Art. 2:688, Feb. 1966.

24. Masterson, J. F., Jr. and Washburne, A.: The symptomatic adolescent: Psychiatric illness or adolescent turmoil? *Am J Psychiat,* 122, No. 11:1240, May 1966.

25. Lorber, J.: Obesity in childhood: A controlled trial of anorectic drugs. *Arch Dis Child,* 41, No. 217:309, June, 1966.

26. London, A. M. and Schreiber, E. D.: A controlled study of the effect of group discussions and an anorexiant in outpatient treatment of obesity. *Ann Int Med,* 65:81, July 1966.
27. Kessler, J.: *Psychopathology of Childhood.* Englewood Cliffs, N. J., Prentice-Hall, 1966.
28. A. P. A. Committee on psychiatry of childhood and adolescence: Position statement on psychiatry of adolescence. *Am J Psychiat,* 123, No. 8:1031, Feb. 1967.
29. Forbes, G. B.: Weight loss during fasting: Implications for the obese. *Amer J Clin Nutr,* 23:1212-1219, 1970.
30. Wolff, O. H.: Obesity in childhood and its effects. *Postgrad Med J,* 38:629-632, 1962.
31. Lloyd, J. K. and Wolff, O. H.: Childhood obesity. *Brit Med J,* 5245:145-148, 1961.
32. Johnson, M. L., Burke, B. S., and Mayer, J.: Relative importance of inactivity and overeating in energy balance of obese high school girls. *Amer J Clin Nutr,* 4:37-44, 1956.
33. Stefanik, P. A., Heald, F. P., and Mayer, J.: Caloric intake in relation to energy output of obese and non-obese adolescent boys. *Amer J Clin Nutr,* 7:55-62, 1959.
34. Brobeck, J. R.: Neural regulation of food intake. *Ann NY Acad Sci,* 63:6, 1955.
35. Stunkard, A. J.: Physical activity, emotions and human obesity. *Psychosom Med,* 20:366-372, 1958.
36. Bruch, H.: Transformation of oral impulses in eating disorders: A conceptual approach. *Psychiat Q,* 35:458-481, 1961.
37. Bruch, H.: Fat children grown up. *Amer J Dis Child,* 90:201, 1955.
38. Monello, L. F. and Mayer, J.: Obese adolescent girls: Unrecognized "minority" group? *Amer J Clin Nutr,* 13:35-39, 1963.
39. Stunkard, A. J., Grace, W. J., and Wolff, H. G.: The night-eating syndrome: A pattern of food intake among certain obese patients. *Amer J Med,* 19:78-86, 1955.

12

Psychological Observations of Obese Adolescents During Starvation Treatment

Susan Nathan

and

Dorothy Pisula

AN increasingly popular method of dealing with the chronic national health problem of obesity has been total starvation under controlled conditions. Reports of this method have been virtually limited to adults. The only studies of children we have been able to find deal exclusively with *metabolic* aspects of starvation.[8, 15] The availability of a group of young adolescents who undertook two weeks of starvation for control of obesity prompted us to make some observations and examinations with respect to the *psychological* aspects of this experience. Data collected at the time of the fast, and eight to twenty-four months post-fast are presented here with the intention of sharing our experience in this relatively little-tried treatment of adolescents with others who might be considering a similar approach.

In the summer of 1967 a research project was initiated at the Endocrine Clinic of Children's Hospital of Pittsburgh for the study of the treatment of obesity through total starvation. The plan was to admit a child to the hospital for four weeks for a fast which consisted of 1000 calories daily, the first and fourth weeks, and total starvation, the second and third weeks. A principal rationale underlying this treatment was that these chronically obese boys and girls, whose weight was thus reduced, would have direct evidence that weight reduction was possible and that this evidence would motivate them for subsequent control of food intake. Extensive metabolic studies were scheduled during the fast. Because of the immense psychological importance of food deprivation, we requested approval from the project director to make some psychological observations of these children. We wanted to learn what the overall effects of the starvation would be, and more particularly, how a child copes with the stress of total starvation, what motivates a young adolescent to starve in the first place, and whether there are any indications here that further delineate the developmental characteristics of the child for whom obesity is a major symptom. We were, of course, interested in whether starvation would be an effective means of weight control.

Before admission to the hospital, each child and his parents talked with the director of the study. Each child was informed of the procedures involved, what he could expect in terms of weight loss, and what would be expected of him in terms of cooperation in the metabolic studies. Each child was informed that the fast was intended to be voluntary and could be terminated whenever desired. Since most of the children were conspicuously passive, a question arises of whether they agreed to undertake the fasting treatment out of passivity, rather than informed consent. Inquiry around this point indicated that parental attitude was a primary factor determining whether or not the child entered the program. One case is known in which the child wanted to undergo the fast, but could not convince her parents to let her take part. It appears, however, that the majority of the patients agreed to participate because their parents were in favor of it. One boy verbalized this succinctly. Asked what he thought about the program he replied, with a broad smile and without a moment's hesitation. "My mother thinks it's the best thing I ever did." "And you?" "Oh, I agree with her." The program, as perceived by the children, offered them an opportunity to lose weight and hence to be successful in an area in which they had repeatedly experienced nothing but frustration and failure.

As the children were all under eighteen years of age, parental consent constituted legal authorization for the treatment.[6] The psychological tests were offered to the children and their parents as a means of providing a more comprehensive study. All families had the opportunity for discussion of results.

Children were admitted as space became available and families applied. In the summer of 1968, four children participated in the starvation study together. Other than that, the children in this particular study were hospitalized individually. The group consisted of fifteen children, eight girls and seven boys, ranging in age from twelve to sixteen years. Weight range was 164 to 306 pounds. Without exception, the boys and girls came from families where one parent was or had been obese. With few exceptions, siblings were not obese. In a few cases where a sibling was considerably overweight, his obesity did not constitute a distressing symptom to either himself or to his family.

RESULTS

Our data consist of family histories, psychological tests on the day preceding and the day following the fast, post-fast follow-up interviews, informal observations of behavior while the children were in the hospital, and records of weight losses and gains.

Family Histories

The most general characteristic revealed by the family histories is that every one of the children admitted to the total starvation program had been a source of special concern to his family, particularly to the mother. In most cases this stressful relationship had prevailed since early infancy. The mothers described feelings of intense anxiety, frustration, and helplessness in their relations with these particular children. Expressions such as, "He baffles me," "I never know how to deal with her," "She has always been different," "He's not like any of the other children," are but weak verbal intimations of the feelings expressed.

Also common to all of the families was the use of food, feeding, and eating as a major mode of relating. With the four children in whom the onset of obesity had occurred in infancy, there had been periods of forced feeding. It some cases this was reported to be so extreme that the child had been forced to eat until vomiting occurred. The mothers, now twelve to fifteen years after the fact, spoke with feeling about how they *had* to force food into the child. The reason most often given for the forced feeding was effort to maintain life. Death of the baby seemed to be a major anxiety in these families. Their guiding principle seems to have been that the only way they could keep the child alive was by feeding.

These mothers also spoke of the tremendous pleasure they experienced when the child ate lustily. In the nine children whose obesity began in early elementary-school years, gifts of food (from members of the extended family or from parents who had previously been absent) were conspicuous. The underlying premise in these families seemed to be something of the order of to-get-sweet-things-is-to-get-the-attention-of-people. In one of the two boys whose obesity began at eleven to twelve, heaviness, if not actual obesity, seemed to be a general family pattern and value. These were families who ate well, who took pride in "setting a good table."

A rather surprising bit of information revealed by the family histories was the high incidence of life-threatening situations which had occurred shortly before the admission of the child to the starvation program. In two instances, there was a very direct connection between the child's coming to the fast and a sudden death in the family. In another case, a boy came to the hospital on the first anniversary of his mother's sudden mysterious death. One girl came to the hospital during her mother's terminal illness and transacted her final contact with the hospital on the day her mother died.

Five other children had agreed to the fast within a few weeks after the sudden death or, in two cases, threatened death of a person with whom they were strongly identified.

Denial and distortion were prominent in both the parents and the children. This was particularly evident with respect to the subjects of food and body size. One woman said that she had gained only three pounds during her entire pregnancy with the patient. The patient was described as a premature baby with a birth weight of eight pounds. Another woman, talking of preparing her daughter for the hospital, repeatedly referred to getting the girl's *little pajamas* ready. She repeatedly described her daughter as a *little* on the heavy side. This fifteen-year-old-girl weighed 280 pounds. The patients spoke with the same irrationality when discussing their attempts to diet. One girl, weighing 179 pounds when discharged after the fast, said "I thought I was slim now so that I could afford to go off the diet." Another girl, who seemed particularly passive and sedentary even among the obese group, said, in describing her physical activity, "No one is as active as me." This girl thought that no matter how hard she tried, she couldn't get her weight lower than 140 pounds, and she had the peculiar notion that she could lose weight only in the summer.

Psychological Tests

Tests used were the Rorschach and Figure Drawings (administered pre-fast and post-fast), the WISC, and the Embedded Figures Test. The most striking characteristic of test performance was a vague, global, unarticulated approach. While this developmentally primitive style showed up specifically in a striking inability to differentiate and integrate perceptual stimuli, it cut across different areas of functioning.

The outstanding feature of the Rorschach test was a high proportion of amorphous, syncretic responses and inaccurately perceived or poorly structured forms of the type scored F−. The high percentage of whole responses tended to be global and diffuse. There were few well-integrated whole responses, and few attempts to pull together details into accurate forms. The form accuracy of our fifteen patients was below adolescent norms. The mean F+% for our patients was 75 compared with a mean F+% of 92.2 for the adolescent norms provided by Ames *et al.*[1] Specific food responses were present in seven cases. These were direct unequivocal associations of food without any modifying additions or preliminary associations. At the time of the fast this was puzzling, because the food associations seemed to appear capriciously with certain boys and girls independent of socioeconomic status, intelligence, degree of overweight, or mood.

In the follow-up, a relation is suggested between the presence of food imagery in the Rorschach and the pattern of weight gain following the fast. All the direct food responses are concentrated in six patients who gained the most weight between admission and follow-up.

With few exceptions, human figure drawings were primitive and lacking in detail. The figures all contained many erasures and were drawn in a slow, laborious manner, accompanied by many comments by the subjects about the poorness and ugliness of the drawings and their own incompetence. It was not unusual for a subject to require ten to fifteen minutes to complete a drawing. Size varied from tiny stick figures to drawings which filled an entire page. There was no particular emphasis on any particular body organ or area.

All drawings were scored according to the Goodenough-Harris method and norms. Fifty per cent fell below the tenth percentile. This 50 per cent were so primitive and lacking sophistication that in most instances they did not fulfill average expectancy for a five-year-old child.

On the Wechsler Intelligence Scale for Children, mean full scale IQ was 103. Eleven of the subjects (73%) scored an average of 15 points higher on the verbal than on the performance scale.

In the Embedded Figures Test, the subject's task is to locate a simple geometric figure which has been hidden or camouflaged within a larger, more complex figure. Many of our obese subjects found this task extremely difficult, if not impossible. Seven of the children gave incorrect responses to half or more of the figures. The remaining other six subjects seen performed more competently, although not one subject was able to locate all twelve stimuli figures correctly, a task which is not beyond the capacity of adolescents of average intelligence.[20, 21]

Behavioral Observations

During their month in the hospital these patients led a very inactive existence. The daily routine of metabolic tests, school work, and a half hour of physical therapy left the patients with large amounts of free time, most of which was spent watching television or lying in bed, alternately dozing and gazing at activities on the ward. The patients did not come to the hospital prepared to occupy themselves with age-appropriate activities such as reading, knitting, sewing, model building, or recreational games. The few arts and crafts projects they did complete were more suitable for eight to ten-year-old children. Other patients on the research ward were younger, usually infants or preschool children, whom the obese patients occasionally held and amused. Some of the fasting obese patients of both sexes were very effective in assisting ward personnel in feeding babies who otherwise refused to eat. On one occasion, when four obese patients were in the hospital together, daily short batteries of tests (analogies, arithmetic, spatial relations) were administered in order to determine whether continued food deprivation affected performance on tasks requiring intellectual energy and concentration. The patients greeted these tasks unenthusiastically with comments of "Not again!" or "Do we have to?" at the same time making slow motions toward compliance. Although these tests were designed to be completed in twenty minutes, the patients sloughed through them in five to ten minutes. They appeared to check the answers (all multiple choice) randomly and rarely bothered to read, much less think about, the questions. An attempt to organize group therapy sessions with these four patients was met with apathy and indifference and was discontinued.

All fifteen patients were characteristically listless, withdrawn, apathetic, and querulous. They seldom became aroused enough to display joy or direct anger, and approached most persons and situations with an air of passive indifference.

Other indices of pathology, extreme alterations of mood and activity level, hallucinations and delusions, were not observed in any patient during the month of hospitalization. Information on dreams is not available. Children were free to leave the hospital with parents for outings whenever this could be worked into their schedules. Only one boy availed himself of this opportunity. One other boy left the hospital to attend memorial services for his mother on the anniversary of her death. "Bootlegging" food to the children was suspected of two mothers. On discharge from the hospital, most of the children were given completely new outfits of clothing to fit their new sizes. They were all still overweight, even after the fast, and did not show especially noticeable changes in appearance. All children kept daily weight charts, and, during hospitalization, all showed decelerating weight curves, with most rapid deceleration during the middle two weeks.

Follow-up Interviews

By the summer of 1969 (an interval of 8 to 24 months post-fast) all but two of the fifteen boys and girls showed a reversal of the decelerating weight curves which had been established in the hospital. All but four of the children had regained or exceeded their admission weight. One boy, after regaining his admission weight, then proceeded systematically to reduce. The boy's mother had had a coronary attack while the boy was in the hospital. After his mother's discharge, the boy and his mother together reduced their weight. This is also the one child of the group was was in psychotherapy. One girl is reported by her mother to have continued gradually to lose weight after discharge. We were most interested in following this girl's progress, but the family resisted our efforts to arrange more than minimal follow-up.

Denial and illogical thinking were particularly conspicuous in the follow-up evaluation of the fast. Both the children and their parents spoke of the fast in overwhelmingly favorable terms. Most said if the opportunity arose they would be willing to repeat the fast. A few suggested that the fast be lengthened until all of the weight was lost. These positive verbalizations were surprising, considering the amount of deprivation and discomfort involved in the total fast and in light of the fact that the weight so painstakingly lost was so quickly regained. When specifically asked to criticize the program, not one child, and only one parent focused on a point of major importance, namely, that the fast was ineffective for sustained weight loss.

Table 12-I shows the height and weight changes from the time of admission to the post-fast follow-up.

TABLE 12-I

HEIGHT AND WEIGHT CHANGES

Patient	(a) Admission				(b) Discharge		(c) Follow-up				Differences	
	Weight lb	Height in	Overweight %	Overweight lb	Weight	Loss	Weight	Height	Overweight %	Overweight lb	b-c	a-c
AA	227	64	75	47	204	23	197	66	45	61	- 7	-30
AK	221	64	70	91	198	23	250	65	87	116	+52	+29
MK	183	62	76	79	160	23	182	64	52	62	+22	- 1
JL	237	68	48	77	214	23	237	74	26	49	+23	0
OP	306	68	87	142	279	27	291	69	75	125	+12	-15
GS	203	69	23	39	181	27	247	76	25	49	+66	+39
JV	164	62	36	43	146	18	195	68	22	35	+49	+31
GB	243	65	77	106	218	25	246	65	80	109	+28	+ 3
BB	208	66	49	68	194	14	241	67	69	99	+47	+33
JP	231	65	70	95	206	25	235	66	68	95	+29	+ 4
AQ	234	63	86	108	218	16	260	64	100	130	+42	+26
RR	222	65	63	86	198	24	282	66	101	140	+84	+60
LS	192	66	37	52	179	13	198	66	41	58	+19	+ 6
KS	190	67	32	46	172	18	157	67	9	13	-15	-33
BW	189	61	85	87	164	25	175	61	72	73	+11	-14

Percentage overweight was computed by determining the child's ideal weight according to his height and age. Ideal weight was then subtracted from the child's actual weight. A ratio of pounds overweight to ideal weight yields percentage overweight.[11] Both amount of weight change and percentage of overweight are indicated in order to take into consideration the fact that some of the children experienced a height spurt between admission and follow-up. None of the girls grew more than one inch, but some of the boys grew as much as six or seven inches. All children continued overweight at the time of the follow-up, even those who had sustained the weight loss established in the hospital. With the exception of one girl who had reduced her weight to 9 per cent overweight, all of the boys and girls were overweight by 20 per cent or more; two girls were 100 per cent overweight.

We found it of interest that the *amount* of weight, not the per cent overweight, seemed to be important to the family in their evaluation of the child's weight-control problems and appearance. Taking height into consideration, the highest weight-gainers in terms of amount of weight gained between admission and follow-up are not necessarily those who most increased percentage of overweight. GS gained thirty-nine pounds, but the percentage increase in overweight was only 2 per cent. JV, who gained thirty-one pounds, actually decreased percentage overweight because he grew six inches in height. JL, who at the time of follow-up was exactly at his admission weight, actually had a 22 per cent decrease in percentage overweight because he grew six inches. The parents of all three of these boys, however, continued to focus on the child's weight-gain and increased size, with virtually no consideration of the fact that with the increase in height there was a more balanced distribution of weight. Actual weight and clothing sizes seemed to be the major criteria in evaluating the child's success or failure. If he continued to require special-order clothing he was perceived as gaining, regardless of the percentage of overweight. These children were, of course, all except one, 20 per cent or more overweight. Perhaps, in obesity of this proportion, weight redistribution is not readily perceptible.

The difference in scores between weight at the time of admission and follow-up show the children divided into roughly two categories: those who gained twenty-six or more pounds and those who gained six pounds or less or who maintained weight lost in the hospital. The bipolarity of this distribution is striking. We hesitate to speculate about what it might mean, since it may be merely a reflection of our small number of cases and the complex interrelations of the height/weight variables. The categorization is so noticeable, however, that it immediately raises the question of whether related variables might be present in the data which would further differentiate types of obesity and differential responsiveness to weight control through starvation.

DISCUSSION

The pervasive inability of these obese subjects to structure and organize their environment can be conceptualized from a developmental point of view in terms of Werner's[19] orthogenetic principle that development proceeds from a global undifferentiated state, to increasing differentiation, to a final stage of organization and hierarchic integration. The preliminary data suggest that our obese adolescent subjects, although of average overall intelligence, are functioning at an immature developmental level in terms of their ability to differentiate and integrate reality. This tendency toward a vague global perceptual style applies, not only to their perception of test tasks, but also to their perception of their own emotional and physiological states. Typically, our patients could describe the physical, concrete details on TAT cards, but they could not project what the characters might be feeling or thinking. They had great difficulty identifying their own feelings and, if asked to state an opinion, typically gave the opinion of some other person. Pressure on the child to state his own feelings produced signs of discomfort and withdrawal.

The differentiation and interpretation of physiological signals also apparently poses a problem for obese persons. Stunkard and Koch[18] found little correlation for obese persons between subjective reports of hunger and the presence of gastric contractions. For control subjects, however, there was a positive relationship between these two variables. Convinced that obese persons no not eat in response to physiological signals, Schachter *et al.*[12] explored the possibility that eating in obese persons is triggered by such external, nonvisceral cues as smell and taste of food, and knowledge of the time of day. By the use of tampered clocks, Schachter and Gross[13] found that obese subjects ate more when they thought they were eating after their regular dinner time than they did when they thought they were eating before their dinner hour. There was no such effect for normal subjects, whose eating behavior was apparently determined by internal, visceral cues, and who were not dependent on external, body-unrelated stimuli to tell them when they were hungry. The tendency of obese subjects to eat in response to external signals rather than internal physiological cues seems to be one aspect of the passive orientation.

In our efforts to trace out the origins of the amorphous life style of these patients, we find the interpersonal constellation, described by Bruch,[4] of markedly ambivalent attitudes and fluctuating feelings of love and rejection from infancy, compensated by excessive feeding and overprotection. The life histories of our patients were characterized by strong ambivalent parental feelings about the child's survival, and by the use of food as a vehicle of relationship so that feeding and eating became equated with doing. This equation of doing-eating was verbalized graphically by one of our patients who could think of only one complaint about the total fast: that there was nothing to do. The fact of the matter was that it was extremely difficult to get this group of patients to *do* anything. When our patient elaborated on his meaning of "to do," he explained that he meant something "like a thousand calorie picnic."

Reduced motility seems also to be an important aspect of the development of these subjects. The structuring of the body image and of the perceptual environment require motility as an integral determinant. Schilder[14] has emphasized that we do not know very much about our bodies unless we move them, for it is through movement that we gain a kinesthetic awareness of the various limbs and their interrelationships. He stresses that "the body image is not a static phenomenon; it is acquired, built up, and gets its structure by continual contact with the world." As a child moves around in his environment, sensations stemming from multiple perceptions and muscular feedback are integrated into the dynamically developing body image.

Empirical evidence supports the hypothesis of lowered motility in an obese person. Johnson *et al.*,[9] comparing food intake and activity schedules of high-school girls, found that the obese girls spent a strikingly smaller amount of time (two-thirds less) than the controls in physical exercise. Stefanik *et al.*,[17] found the same for obese adolescent boys. Bullen *et al.*,[5] using a photographic technique to estimate caloric expenditure from poses, found unequivocally that obese adolescent girls expended far less energy during scheduled exercise periods than their nonobese counterparts.

Motility plays an essential role, not only in defining the boundaries of the self, but in helping an organism differentiate his total perceptual environment. As an infant explores his environment and contacts and manipulates objects, these objects acquire a functional meaning for him. They become perceptually and functually distinct and discrete and stand out from the unarticulated surrounding. The amorphous, unstructured style of our obese subjects may result largely from their lifelong tendency to observe rather than participate, to passively absorb rather than actively explore. Their passivity interferes with the physical exploration and experimentation necessary for the optimum development of perceptual skills. The global and unarticulated figure drawings of these obese children appear to be at least partially the result of a life style of extreme passivity and lowered motility which deprives them of the kinesthetic sensations necessary for a well-articulated body image.

The pattern of food responses in the Rorschach test suggests that content analysis may be useful in differentiating reasons for obesity and developing indices of ability to fast successfully. All direct food responses were concentrated among the high weight gainers. The other boys and girls gave responses which might be included under the general category of oral content, but they were not responses of the primitive impulsive quality ("watermelon," "egg," "crabmeat," "chicken neck"), where food constituted the primary response, unmodified by any additional or preliminary elaboration such as a person using or preparing the food.

Efforts to relate food imagery and intensity of need or duration of deprivation have not shown a direct correlation.[3] Content of dreams, Rorschach responses, and word associations have not shown significantly increased food imagery with increase in length of deprivation. A clear relation has been shown, however, between length of deprivation and alertness to certain food-associated stimuli. Epstein and Levitt[7] found that hungry subjects learned paired words more rapidly, when the stimulus member of the pair was a food word, than their nonhungry controls. Spence and Ehrenberg,[16] using the word *cheese* as a subliminal stimulus, found that subjects who had not eaten for several hours were more responsive to the stimulus word *cheese* in the recall of words. These findings have been interpreted to support the hypothesis that drives arouse the organism, but do not of themselves provide direction, that for a given direction of influence, the drive must coincide with a relevant stimulus.

With the boys and girls in this study, there was no significant difference in the amount of food imagery pre-fast and post-fast, a not unexpected finding in view of the evidence in the literature, and if, indeed, obese individuals respond primarily to external rather than internal hunger cues. What is more difficult to explain is why some of the subjects gave repeated, direct unadulterated food associations and others did not. McCully *et al.*,[10] in a study of nutrition imagery on the Rorschach in food-deprived patients, found something similar when the most food responses and the least negatively toned food responses came from the patient who least maintained her reduced weight.

Examination of the data of family histories suggests that food, its preparation, acquisition, and use, might have a special meaning in the families of the high gainers that is subtly different from the other families. GS belonged to a family where food and food production was valued highly. The family invested much energy in farming, though farming was not actually the main occupation. His mother related in tones of noticeable satisfaction and pride, that both her husband's and her families had always been close to the land, had always worked at producing food, and that on both sides of the family they had always eaten well. She herself was a large woman, not particularly obese. In JV's family, the integral role of food as a manner of relating was dramatically indicated when on our arrival at the home for the follow-up interview, the mother's first words after the initial greeting were to ask whether we would like, and to urge on us, coffee and pie. This was nine o'clock in the morning. RR and AQ belonged to low socioeconomic families who outspokenly related obesity to poverty. In one of these families there was great surprise at learning that not all the children in the starvation group were from poor families. "I thought only poor people were fat," this mother said. Reminded that any unselected population offered evidence to the contrary, she agreed, then added, "But I thought that when you were poor, there's nothing else you can afford to do like bowling or things, so you eat."

Perhaps in the families of the high gainers the meaning of food, for whatever reasons of deprivation or satisfaction, occupies a position in the value system which makes it in effect a constantly present relevant stimulus. If this is true, then we might expect individuals in this situation to be in a state of hyperalertness to food, and to expect that they would require extraordinary control to inhibit responsiveness in this direction. The success of fasting in these cases might be contingent on the presence or absence of control factors to a greater degree than in other equally obese individuals. In our subjects, at least one index of control, the Rorschach F+%, was lowered for the group comprised of high weight gainers. Among this group, the decrease in F+% was directly proportional to percentage overweight post-fast. AQ and RR, who showed the greatest percentage gain in overweight post-fast, had the lowest F+%; and JV and GS, who showed the least percentage overweight despite actual increase in amount overweight, showed the highest F+%. These data suggest that an individual who shows the combination of reduced capacity for control, as indicated in a low F+% on the Rorschach test, together with the presence of direct food responses on this test and a familial value system in which the meaning of food is paramount, especially if this stems from socioeconomic deprivation, has a poor prognosis for control of obesity through starvation. RR and AQ might perhaps more successfully get their weight under control if the focus of attention were on opportunities for recreation and extended peer-group interaction.

A persisting question is why these particular fifteen boys and girls out of a population of a much larger group who were informed about the fast agreed to the total fast. The first few children who were admitted to the hospital were so exceedingly passive, we were inclined to believe initially that the ones who elected the total fast represent the end point in the passivity-activity continuum. Children admitted to the total fast later, however, did not support this hypothesis. We were impressed by the incidence of deaths of significant people shortly before a child agreed to the total fast, and wonder how this might be related to the child's acceptance of the fast. Bloch,[2] in an extensive treatment of the death wish in psychogenic eating disorders, describes the death wish (in contrast to the death instinct of Freud) as a longing for a reduction of stimuli and tension, an extreme example of which would be a deep sleep. The children who came into the hospital for the total fast certainly exemplify a state of reduced stimuli and tension. They came to the hospital, for the most part, at a time when death was a sudden reality for them. We wonder what ideas of death are stirred up in these boys and girls by the deaths of significant people in their lives. Was there an exaggeration of death wishes? Was there a reaction-formation against fears of death? In many ways, the total fast seems to have been envisioned by the boys and girls and their parents as some sort of magical act.

REFERENCES

1. Ames, L. B., Metraux, R. W. and Walker, R. N.: *Adolescent Rorschach Responses.* New York, Hoeber, 1959.
2. Bloch, R.: Uber die Bedeutung der Todessehnsucht für psychogene Störungen des Ernährungstriebes. *Z Psychosom Med,* 13:63-69, 1967
3. Brozek, J., Gultzkow, H. and Baldwin, M. V.: A quantitative study of perception and association in experimental semi-starvation. *J Personal,* 19:245-264, 1951.
4. Bruch, H.: *The Importance of Overweight.* New York, Norton, 1957.
5. Bullen, B. A., Reed, R. B. and Mayer, J.: Physical activity of obese and nonobese adolescent girls appraised by motion picture sampling. *Am J Clin Nutr,* 14: 211-223, 1964.
6. Curran, W. J. and Beecher, H. K.: Experimentation and children. *J Am Med Assoc,* 10:77-83, 1969.
7. Epstein, S. and Levitt, H.: The influence of hunger on learning and recall of food related words. *J Abnorm Soc Psychol,* 64:130-135, 1962.
8. Garces, L., Kenny, F., Drash, A. and Taylor, F.: Cortisol secretion rate during fasting of obese adolescent subjects. *J Clin Endocrinol Metabol,* 28:1843-1847, 1968.
9. Johnson, M. L., Burke, B. S. and Mayer, J.: The relative importance of inactivity and overeating in the energy balance of obese high school girls. *Am J Clin Nutr,* 4:37-44, 1956.
10. McCully, R., Glucksman, M. L. and Hirsch, J.: Nutrition imagery in the Rorschach materials of food-deprived, obese patients. *J Proj Tech,* 32:375-382, 1968.
11. Nelson, W. E. (Ed.): *Textbook of Pediatrics* (9th ed.). Philadelphia, Saunders, 1969.
12. Schachter, S., Goldman, R. and Gordon, A.: Effects of fear, food deprivation and obesity on eating. *J Pers Soc Psychol,* 10:91-97, 1968.
13. Schachter, A. and Gross, L.: Manipulated time and eating behavior. *J Pers Soc Psychol,* 10:98-106.
14. Schilder, P.: *The Image and Appearance of the Human Body.* New York, International Universities Press, 1935.
15. Spahn, U., Plennert, M. and Pathenheimer, F.: Untersuchungen zur Fastenbehandlung der Adipositas im Kindesalter. I. Das Verhalten des Körpergewichts bei reduzierter Calorienzufuhr und absolutem Fasten. *Z Kinderheil,* 100:160-172, 1967.
16. Spence, D. B. and Ehrenberg, B.: Effects of oral deprivation on the response to subliminal and supraliminal verbal food stimuli. *J Abnorm Soc Psychol,* 69: 10-18, 1964.
17. Stefanik, P., Heald, F. and Mayer, J.: Caloric intake in relation to energy output of obese and non-obese adolescent boys. *Am J Clin Nutr,* 7:55-62, 1959.

18. Stunkard, A. and Koch, C.: The interpretation of gastric motility. *Arch Gen Psychiat,* 11:74-82, 1964.
19. Werner, H.: *Comparative Psychology of Mental Development.* New York, International Universities Press, 1948.
20. Witkin, H. A., Dyk, R. B., Faterson, H. F., Goodenough, D. R. and Karp, S. A.: *Psychological Differentiation.* New York, Wiley, 1962.
21. Witkin, H. A., Goodenough, D. R. and Karp, S. A.: Stability of cognitive style from childhood to young adulthood. *J Pers Soc Psychol,* 7:291-300, 1967.

13

Overcoming Obesity in Adolescents

E. James Stanley
Helen H. Glaser
Dorothy G. Levin
Pauline Austin Adams
AND
Ida Lou Coley

DESPITE the great body of clinical attention that obesity has received,[3, 4, 8, 11, 13–15, 17, 18] long-term treatment as a rule has been relatively unsuccessful.[6, 19]

Seeking guides for formulation of a consistent treatment regimen for adolescents with obesity, we explored the pertinent medical literature. Nowhere did we find any reports of studies in which a group of adolescents, of both sexes, had been admitted to an in-patient setting to be studied systematically and treated intensively, then followed over a long period and restudied. We decided to carry out such a rational treatment plan for these patients.

Obese adolescents tend to grow into obese adults.[1, 10] Adults who have been obese since early life have more distorted body-images[20, 21] and are more refractory to treatment[2] than are those whose obesity is of shorter duration. Thus, correction of obesity in adolescents should reduce its prevalence in adults.

In one recent study, an experimental group of obese high school boys gained an average of 7.7 lb less than did a control group of obese boys after going through a twenty-seven-month program which emphasized nutrition education and physical fitness.[5] Another encouraging report is that of a group of girls from eight to eighteen years old whose weight loss averaged 22 lb during an eight-week summer camp program which stressed recreational activity and dietary education.[16]

GOALS OF OUR STUDY

We proposed to develop a program that would help uncover which characteristics of obese adolescents tend to favor and which tend to hinder success in a treatment program. We desired also to determine those aspects of a complete treatment regimen which would be the most important for those individuals who are successful. Such information might bring everyone closer to a more economical treatment plan for this distressing disorder.

DESIGN OF THE PROGRAM
Preliminary Evaluations

The plans for the program were circulated to local pediatricians. From fifteen referrals, eleven obese white adolescents (five boys and six girls) from middle-income families were selected. We rejected four applicants: one boy because of previous treatment failure at our hospital and three girls who applied late. Although a separate control group would have been of interest we deemed that not essential, inasmuch as each child in the program had a long history of progressive weight gain. In addition, the history of untreated adolescent obesity (beginning in childhood) is almost uniformly discouraging.[9, 20] Each patient, therefore, served as his own control.

Prior to admission, we gave these eleven youngsters psychologic, social work, and physical examinations. The psychologic studies included a complete battery of tests as well as a structured interview. The patients and their families were evaluated extensively by the social service staff. Parents were seen conjointly with their children; in the two-parent families, the parents were interviewed together and separately, and each adolescent separately.

Routine complete blood counts and urinalyses were within normal limits in all instances. Extensive medical endocrine studies were not indicated either for the individual patients or for the purposes of this program. All subjects were over the 97th percentile in weight for their age group (combined Harvard and Iowa Scale). The mean percentage overweight for age was 79 per cent with a range from 49 per cent to 138 per cent.

In-patient Treatment

Following evaluation, the eleven patients were taken into the Stanford Children's Convalescent Hospital. At the time of the study, the hospital had forty beds in two single-story structures on several acres of land near the Stanford University Medical Center in Palo Alto, California. In the hospital the patients underwent a six-week intensive treatment regimen, which included a daily diet of 1,200 calories, dietary education, exercise and activity programs, recreation, and individual and group counseling for children and parents.

Two psychiatric social workers were each assigned four patients and their families, and the remaining three patients and their families were assigned to the staff pediatrician. The individual meetings with patients ranged from one-half hour weekly to one-half hour daily, depending on the degree of difficulty the individual patients experienced in their adjustment to the program. Occasional conjoint sessions were held with some parents and patients, especially as the six-week in-patient period progressed and the strains of separation and divided authority were felt.

The boys met twice weekly in a group conducted by a male Fellow in child psychiatry, while the girls were meeting at the same times with a female psychiatric social worker and a female pediatrician. The parents were seen as couples weekly by either the pediatrician or the psychiatric social worker assigned to them. In addition, two parent groups, in which couples were separated but the sexes were mixed, met weekly. One group session was conducted by the same pediatrician who saw three of the couples individually, while the other group was led by a psychiatric social worker who saw four of the families individually. Attendance approached 100 per cent at all the meetings during the in-patient phase.

Out-patient Treatment

The patients were sent home after six weeks of in-patient care, and separate meetings of the parents' and patients' groups took place at approximately monthly intervals over the next thirteen months. Attendance at these meetings dwindled rapidly toward the end of the program. Seven meetings were held at monthly intervals, but there were only two additional meetings in the last five months. During the last six months the average family attendance at the meetings was four out of eleven. Weight measurements and psychosocial adjustment data were collected during and at the end of the follow-up period.

OBSERVATIONS MADE
Preadmission Evaluations

All families exhibited a high degree of psychologic dysfunction. Divorce had disrupted four of the eleven families, and six of the other seven families had experienced marital problems of a severe degree. Eight of the mothers and five of the fathers were obese at the time of the study or had been obese earlier. Alcoholism was a problem for four fathers and one mother. Four of the fathers had been physically violent with other family members.

All six girls had average to excellent academic records. Two girls had fair to poor social adjustments, whereas the other four girls got along well socially. Of the five boys, one had average grades and a good social adjustment, whereas the rest had done poorly both academically and socially. Among the girls, those with the better academic and social records prior to the study tended to do better with their weight than did the other girls during the fifteen months of our contact with them. No such association

The Psychology of Obesity

TABLE 13-I

WEIGHT CHANGES

Sex	Age (yr.-mo.)	Ht. (Inches) at Beginning of Program	Wt. (lb)	Wt. (lb) after Hospitalization	Change with Hospitalization (lb)	Ht. (Inches) End of Program	Wt. (lb)	Change After 15 Mo. From Start of Program (lb)	Rating: Success, Fail, or Hold *
M	14-11	67	257	237	−20	67	191	−66	S
M	15-11	66¾	237	213	−24	67	179	−58	S
F	13-5	64	157	143	−14	64	153	− 4	H
F	13-2	64	149	138	−11	64	154	+ 5	H
F	13-5	64	153	142	−11	64½	160	+ 7	H
F	14-6	66¾	232	213	−19	67½	241	+ 9	H
M	12-5	60¾	170	147	−23	63	184	+14	F
F	13-4	62½	154	146	− 8	62½	169	+15	F
F	13-11	62¾	185	165	−20	65½	203	+18	F
M	14-5	66¾	264	241	−23	Not obtained	289	+25	F
M	11-9	61¼	147	135	−12	64½	196	+49	F

* The patients are listed in the order of decreasing success at the end of 15 months, with the weight losers at the top and the weight gainers at the bottom. The two boys who lost 66 and 58 pounds each were obviously *successful* (S) in terms of weight loss. We applied the term *hold* (H) to those 4 patients whose weight remained between 4 pounds less and 9 pounds more than the preadmission weights. This group of four patients who held their weight relatively steady during this 15-month period of their adolescence were deemed to have accomplished a moderate success because of the tendency of adolescents to gain weight as they grow older during this age. The five remaining children were rated as *failures* (F) as far as their weight changes were concerned.

was evident for the boys between academic and social record and weight loss. The average WISC* Full Scale IQ of the patient group was 121.

Of the eleven patients, one boy and one girl had obesity of the "reactive type," described by Bruch.[2] Five other patients manifested "developmental" obesity.† Four others could not be classified clearly. The boy with reactive obesity, associated with onset of asthma in the third grade, turned out to be one of the successful weight losers in the program; there was otherwise no relationship between weight loss and obesity type.

* The WISC (Wechsler Intelligence Scale for Children) is an individually administered standardized intelligence test. The sub-tests are: Information Comprehension, Arithmetic, Similarities, Vocabulary (Verbal Scale); Picture Completion, Picture Arrangement, Block Design, Object Assembly Coding (Performance Scale). The Full Scale IQ score is based on the scores from the Verbal and Performance Scales. The mean IQ score of 121 obtained by the patient group is in the Superior range. Bruch also described a high mean intelligence level in her group of obese children.[2]

† "Developmental obesity" is defined as obesity originating at a very early age without any clear, acute precipitant. "Reactive obesity" is obesity starting at a later age, often secondary to some observable stress. Reactive obesity is generally more susceptible to treatment.

Weight Changes During the Program

Table 13-I shows the admission weights, the changes following the in-patient phase, and the changes at the end of fifteen months.

As can be seen from the sixth column, all the children lost weight during the hospitalization. There was no correlation between weight lost during the in-patient phase and the weight change at the end of the program. The subsequent weight changes in either direction were all gradual over the time of follow-up.

To summarize the weight changes, six of the eleven adolescents either lost weight or held their weight relatively steady during a fifteen-month period.

Findings in Adolescent Group Meetings

Both the boys' group and the girls' group used the discussion periods to talk about their feelings about being overweight. The boys reacted to the subject of obesity with solemnity and decreased conversation which indicated feelings of depression about being overweight. They tended to blame their own inactivity for being overweight. They expressed feelings of being victims of "unfairness," in that other people could eat as much or more than they did but did not gain as much. They felt also that their families' emphasis on abnormal eating patterns contributed to their weight problem. Much of the content of the meetings revolved around superficial contacts with girls.

Among the girls, discussions in group therapy often focused on their feelings of worthlessness and lack of importance in the family constellation. The girls expressed many typical adolescent feelings of conflicts, desiring independence from the family while at the same time craving closeness. In respect to their feelings about being overweight, the girls saw their obesity as preventing them from achieving success among the peer group, especially with boys. They thought that society viewed their obesity as evidence of significant emotional problems, and they too expressed feelings of unfairness in this respect, assuring each other that they had good, healthy personalities.

In later sessions, the girls expressed apprehension that excessive eating might actually be a manifestation of loss of self-control similar to alcoholism and excessive sexual activity. It was apparent that they feared that they could succumb to these other excesses as they had to overeating. The girls also expressed strong feelings of resentment toward their mothers, who were slimmer and more attractive than they but who "turned the knife" by claiming to need to lose weight themselves.

The issues discussed both in the boys' and girls' groups were usually brought out after considerable resistance and superficial pleasantries. It was our impression that the presence of others who were fellow-sufferers facilitated these expressions of feeling.

Those who were doing better with weight reduction tended to attend more of the follow-up meetings, though there were several exceptions. It was unclear whether the better attendance was more a cause or an effect of the weight loss.

Findings in Parent Group Meetings

Initially the discussion content of the two parent groups varied in accordance with the orientation of the group leader.[7, 12] The group led by the pediatrician at first focused more on organic aspects such as food and exercise, whereas the group led by one of the social workers (D. L.) tended to talk more of emotions, their connection with obesity, and problems in relationships with people. Soon, however, partly because of consultation between the pediatrician and the social worker (D. L.) the two groups began to deal primarily with the inability of the parents to cope with their children's dependency on them. This difficulty of the parents related clearly to the unsuccessful resolution of their own problems in this area. Thus, instead of being concerned primarily with parent-child conflict over adolescent issues, such as emancipation, peer relations and sexual concerns, the parents seemed preoccupied with the kinds of problems related to earlier childhood. For example, they were deeply involved in issues such as control over food intake, clothes, homework and haircuts of their children. In addition, obvious handicaps in their own functioning, such as alcoholism, physical violence and divorce limited their capacities for dealing with adolescents. These observations were confirmed during individual meetings with the parents. Toward the end of the program, a few of the parents had begun to discuss appropriate adolescent-parent issues.

Changes in Psychosocial Adjustment

At the end of the follow-up period we asked the parents individually by telephone or personal interviews whether or not they had observed any changes in their children's adjustments to the family and to peers.

The parents of six children reported improvement, and five of these were for children who had either lost a significant amount of weight or held their weight steady. This kind of reporting is clearly open to bias. However, we are certain that the weight reduction did not precipitate any significant worsening in familial or social relationships.

To obtain more specific information with respect to the adolescents' adjustment, we inquired at their schools for assessment of changes in school behavior and academic work. Although the changes are spotty (Table 13-II) all of the improvements in school behavior and work were in children

TABLE 13-II

SCHOOL REPORTS OF CHANGE DURING 15-MONTH TREATMENT PERIOD

Academic Achievement	
Positive changes	Failing to above average in one patient S*
	Below average to average in one patient H*
Negative change	Average to below average in one patient F*
School Behavior	
Positive changes	Very poor to good in one patient S
	Good to very good in one patient H
	Very poor to fair in one patient H
Negative change	Fair to poor in one patient F

* As in Table 13-I S = success in weight reduction, H = held weight steadily and F = failure in weight control. Judgments on the teen-agers' school behavior were based on information obtained in interviews with school counsellors. Transcripts were examined to obtain data on school achievement.

who either lost weight or held it steady. The one teen-ager whose academic work declined and the one whose school behavior worsened gained weight.

Three of the patients have become involved in long-term psychotherapy which had been recommended prior to the program but rejected at that time.

Other changes in the families appeared to relate to therapeutic contact with the program. Three families, consisting of girls and their divorced mothers, formed much more appropriate parent-adolescent relationships. Even the least well functioning families showed clear signs of improved relationships recognized by the therapists in group and individual sessions. Without a matched control group one cannot be certain that any of these changes resulted from the program; however, the patients, their families and the staff felt that almost all of the positive changes were related to experiences in the program rather than to growing older or some other factor.

One of the most persistent observations by the therapists was that many of the gains (both in weight loss and adjustment) seemed possible only because of the presence of others with the same problem.[7, 12] The parents as well as the patients derived support in this way. Other studies which have described the highest degree of success have been relatively large group efforts.[5, 16]

Changes in Body-image or Self-image

Stunkard and Mendelson, long-time students of obesity, have stated:[21] "Of the many behavioral disturbances to which obese persons are subject, only two seem specifically related to their obesity. The first is overeating, the second is a disturbance in body-image." The results of two psychologic tests, each given at the beginning and at the end of our program, support the contention that change in the body- (or self-) image is important in regard to weight reduction. The two tests were an adjective check list and the Draw-a-Person test.

ADJECTIVE CHECK-LIST

The test instrument was developed to assess a person's concept of himself. The adolescents were presented a list of sixty adjectives (Table 13-III) and asked to indicate those that are self-descriptive.

The one girl and two boys who at the beginning of the program selected the smallest percentage of positive adjectives to describe themselves were those who later became the only three weight losers in the program. It seemed to us that this choice of fewer positive self-descriptive adjectives represented more of a realistic self-appraisal than an overly harsh self-criticism. However, of equal importance, when the same adjective list was offered at the end of the program, these same three weight losers, plus one other girl who held her weight steady, showed the greatest increases in the percentage of positive adjectives chosen as self-descriptive.

GOODENOUGH-HARRIS DRAWING TEST

In this test[9] the child was asked to draw a picture of a person (the whole person, not just the head), making it as good a drawing as he could. Following the first drawing, a figure of the opposite sex was requested. A maximum score of 73 (71 for drawings of female figures) can be achieved by the complete and accurate representation of body parts, details and proportions. The obtained score is then converted to a standard score for the child's chronological age. A score of 100 would be average at each age.

This test was administered at the beginning and at the end of the program, and was scored on the Harris Point Scale, which yields an index of intellectual maturity. The scores for the same-sex figure were as follows: initial test scores ranged from 81 to 117, and final test scores were from 77 to 121. Four of the patients improved their scores. These were the two boys

TABLE 13-III

ADJECTIVE CHECK-LIST FOR SELF-CONCEPT ASSESSMENT

Accepting, affectionate, aggressive, anxious, artistic, attractive, average, brave, casual, cold, considerate, critical, cruel, dynamic, easy-going, enthusiastic, fearful, feel inferior, feel superior, friendly, generous, gentle, happy, hostile, inconsiderate, intelligent, jolly, kind, mean, nervous, not aggressive, not artistic, pleasant, proud, quiet, rejecting, relaxed, rough, self-centered, self-confident, selfish, socially not well adjusted, socially well adjusted, strong, sympathetic, talented, tense, thoughtful, thoughtless, unattractive, understanding, unfriendly, unhappy, unintelligent, unkind, unpleasant, untalented, warm, weak, worrier.

Note: Prior to the program nine adults rated the sixty adjectives for connotation. On the basis of majority consensus 27 adjectives were considered to be positive, 29 negative, and 4 neutral.

who were successful in their weight program (+32 and +11 points on the test, respectively) and two girls who held their weight steady (+8 points on the test each). In the remainder of the patients the scores at the end of fifteen months had decreased.

We realize that both the small size of the sample and the nature of the tests make any interpretation of the results questionable. Furthermore, we cannot be sure if the changes in the test results represent primarily an effect of the weight reduction or result from a cause or causes similar to the cause of the weight loss. Our guess is, from the literature[20] and from our observations of these adolescents, that the successful weight losers in some way improved their body-image or self-image or both, which in turn helped them to keep their weight down.

Observations by the Occupational Therapist in the Activity Program

All members of the staff had the aim of being able to relate their observations to later success or failure in weight reduction. Thus the occupational therapist had two check-lists on which she rated each patient subjectively during the last week in the in-patient phase of the program. The first list consisted of fourteen "General Behavior Characteristics" shown in Table 13-IV. The second list consisted of six "Work-Behavior Characteristics" which are also shown in Table 13-IV.

The four patients who had the highest general behavior scores included two weight losers and a girl who held her weight steady. Similarly, four of the five highest work-behavior scores were made by two weight-losers and by two patients who held their weight steady.

Even though the small sample size and the subjective nature of the ratings made interpretation of these results open to question, we think that through further refinement and experimentation such a simple evaluation could be developed for use in similar programs to predict the potential for long-term success in weight loss.

TABLE 13-IV

"GENERAL BEHAVIOR" AND "WORK-BEHAVIOR" CHARACTERISTICS USED
BY OCCUPATIONAL THERAPIST TO RATE THE PATIENTS AT
START OF PROGRAM

"General Behavior Characteristics"
Maturity, self-confidence, impulsiveness, unhappy-happy mood, activity level, acceptance of responsibility, reaction to failure and frustration, self-perception, interpersonal relationships with peers, interpersonal relationships with adults, interaction with peers, interaction with adults, dependency, leadership.

"Work-Behavior"
Attention and concentration, perseverance, achievement, work habits in general, motor skill, attitude toward work.

Note: The patients were rated on general behavior and work-behavior characteristics with scales ranging from 1 to 3 on some items to scales of 1 to 7 on others.

COMMENTS AND CONCLUSIONS

These studies have generated some strong clinical impressions even though the data are not fully conclusive. Of considerable importance in our opinion, is the role of the supervised discussion groups held separately with the patients and with the parents. Adolescents rely a great deal on peer support in dealing with many of their difficulties, and obesity seems no exception in this regard. Their parents likewise make use of observations and comments by others with the same problems.[7, 12]

Temporary removal from the home environment, and helping all the patients to lose some weight is very important. Living together for six weeks, our eleven adolescents derived more emotional support from one another than had they simply been attending meetings and living at home. This study was carried out in a chronic disease hospital, but a summer camp or similar temporary communal group-living situation could be as good or perhaps even a better setting for the initial "in-patient" phase. It is difficult to say if six weeks was an optimal time; another successful program keeps the teen-agers eight weeks.[16]

Another important conviction strengthened by our experience is that nonpsychiatrically trained personnel can direct such a program with consultation from an experienced psychiatric social worker, psychiatrist, or psychologist.

More attention should be paid to the issue of body-image and self-image. As shown by two tests (Goodenough Draw-a-Man and adjective check-list) the body-image and self-image improvement was closely related to weight loss. A body-image improvement program would include more sessions on grooming and fashions for the girls, perhaps physical fitness for the boys. A supportive personal relationship with a respected adult could be a step towards improving self-concept.

Regarding the endeavor to predict successful outcome in such a program, we obtained some suggestive data and have developed several convictions. The number of positive adjectives chosen on the self-concept check-list, the "General-Behavior," and "Work-Behavior" characteristics, all turned out to be good predictors of success for this particular group of adolescents. With a slightly larger number of cases and a suitably matched control group, it seems likely that good predictability of outcome is a potential reality. The capacity to select proper candidates in advance would of course be very useful.

A number of changes were noted in the behavior of the adolescents during the program that were related to their weight changes. In each of these aspects (test score improvements, improved school perfomance, group attendance, family and social relationships) the question remains whether these changes result primarily from the weight reduction itself or whether they are affected by some other factor that also helps the weight problem (such as improvement in self-image). The answers to these theoretical questions must await further, more extensive study.

To summarize, eleven obese adolescents and their families were extensively evaluated, treated for fifteen months and then reevaluated. During the first six weeks the adolescents were taken as a group into a chronic disease hospital, where they participated in an intensive treatment regimen including a 1,200 calorie diet, exercise and recreation sessions, and group and individual therapy. Their parents attended group and individual meetings during the in-patient and follow-up phases of the program. At the end of fifteen months, six of the eleven patients had either lost weight or held it steady.

As predictive and treatment methods such as those described here are improved further, a long-term success rate in both weight management and psychosocial adjustment even greater than 50 per cent should be feasible.

REFERENCES

1. Abraham, S. and Nordsieck, M.: Relationship of excess weight in children and adults. *Public Health Rep,* 75:263, 1960.
2. Bruch, H.: *The Importance of Overweight.* New York, Norton, 1957.
3. Bruch, H.: Psychological aspects of overeating and obesity. *Psychosomatics,* 5:269, 1964.
4. Bullen, B. A., Monello, L. F., Cohen, H. and Mayer, J.: Attitudes toward physical activity, food and family in obese and non-obese adolescent girls. *Am J Clin Nutr,* 12:1, 1963.
5. Christakis, G., Sojecki, S., Hillman, R. W., Miller, E., Blumenthal, S. and Archer, M.: Effect of a combined nutrition, education and physical fitness program on the weight status of obese high school boys. *Fed Proc,* 25:15, 1966.
6. Duncan, G. G., Jenson, W. K., Fraser, R. I. and Cristofori, F. C.: Correction and control of intractable obesity. *JAMA,* 181:309, 1962.
7. Glaser, K.: Group discussions with mothers of hospitalized children. *Pediatrics,* 26:132, 1960.
8. Gordon, E. S.: New concepts of the biochemistry and physiology of obesity. *Med Clin N Am,* 48:1285, 1964.
9. Harris, D. B.: *Children's Drawings as Measures of Intellectual Maturity; A Revision and Extension of the Goodenough Draw-a-Man Test.* New York, Harcourt, Brace and World Inc., 1963.
10. Heald, F. P.: Natural history and physiological basis of adolescent obesity. *Fed Proc,* 25:1, 1966.
11. Johnson, M. S., Burke, B. S. and Mayer, J.: Relative importance of inactivity and overeating in the energy balance of obese high school girls. *Am J Clin Nutr,* 4:37, 1956.
12. Luzzatti, L. and Dittmann, B.: Group discussions with parents of ill children. *Pediatrics,* 13:269, 1954.
13. Mayer, J.: Correlation between metabolism and feeding behavior and multiple etiology of obesity. *Bull N Y Acad Med,* 33:744, 1957.

14. Mayer, J.: Physical activity and anthopometric measurements of obese adolescents. *Fed Proc,* 25:11, 1966.
15. Mendelson, M.: Psychological aspects of obesity. *Med Clin N Am,* 48:1373, 1964.
16. Peckos, P., Spargo, J. and Heald, R.: Program and results of a camp for obese adolescent girls. *Post Grad Med,* 27:527, 1960.
17. Reivich, R. S., Ruiz, R. A. and Lapi, R. M.: Extreme obesity psychiatric, psychometric and psychotherapeutic aspects. *J Kansas Med Soc,* 62:134, 1966.
18. Stunkard, A. J., Grace, W. J. and Wolff, H. G.: The night eating syndrome; A pattern of food intake among certain obese patients. *Am J Med,* 19:78, 1955.
19. Stunkard and McLaren-Hume, M.: The results of treatment for obesity; A review of the literature and report of a series. *Arch Int Med,* 103:79, 1959.
20. Stunkard and Burt, V.: Obesity and the body image; II. Age at onset of disturbance in the body image. *Am J Psychiat,* 123:1433, 1967.
21. Stunkard and Mendelson, M.: Obesity and the body image; I. Characteristics of disturbances in the body image of some obese persons. *Am J Psychiat,* 123:1296, 1967.

V
INDIVIDUAL THERAPY

14

New Therapies for the Eating Disorders

ALBERT J. STUNKARD

BEHAVIOR MODIFICATIONS OF OBESITY AND ANOREXIA NERVOSA

IN recent years new and distinctive forms of psychotherapy have commanded increasing attention as evidence mounts that they are more effective than traditional techniques in a variety of disorders. The new treatments, known as behavior modification, behavior therapy, and experimental analysis of behavior, comprise a heterogeneous series of techniques, bound together by the efforts of their proponents to apply the findings and methods of experimental psychology to disorders of human behavior. The most consistent evidence of their effectiveness comes from the treatment of obesity where their superiority over other methods has been demonstrated in nine different studies. This essay reviews these studies, describes the application of behavior modification techniques to obesity and outlines some of the increasingly sophisticated experimental designs which are elucidating the effective elements of psychotherapy. It seems particularly important that psychiatrists know of these developments, for behavior modification has grown up largely outside their purview and, at times, in the face of their opposition. The extent of the leadership exercised by psychologists and social workers is nowhere better illustrated than in the "medical" problem of obesity: physicians participated in only one of nine studies described here.

The distinctive characteristic of the various methods of behavior modification is the belief that behavior disorders of the most divergent types are learned responses and that modern theories of learning have much to teach us regarding both the acquisition and extinction of these responses.[1] Further, proponents of behavior modification have been distinguished by their explicit statements of methods and goals, and their willingness to put their results on the line for comparison with other forms of treatment. Illustrative of these methodological concerns, behavior therapists have been among the first to recognize the power, as a dependent variable in psychotherapy research, of weight change in pounds, and they have turned to the treatment of obesity in order to utilize this measure. It is ironic that psychiatry, so sorely in need of measures to evaluate therapeutic success and

153

failure, has taken so long to recognize the sensitivity, reliability, and validity of weight change as such a measure.

ANOREXIA NERVOSA

The characteristics and potential of behavior modification can perhaps best be introduced by the description of a behavioral approach to anorexia nervosa. Three case reports had suggested that behavioral techniques could modify the undereating of anorexic patients and produce weight gain.[2-4] But not until behavioral analysis had revealed an unexpectedly prominent feature of the disorder was it possible to apply an effective behavioral technology to a series of patients.[5, 6] This feature was hyperactivity, and its use in therapy illustrates the simplicity and power of behavior modification in this chronic, often intractable, disorder.

Pedometer measurements of patients hospitalized for treatment of anorexia nervosa revealed that they walked an average of 6.8 miles per day, as compared with a mean daily value of 4.9 miles for women of normal weight living at home. This observation suggested that opportunity for physical activity might serve as a reinforcement for increased food intake or, as the program came to specify, weight gain. Accordingly, the patient's access to physical activity was made contingent upon weight gain. Specifically, she was permitted a six-hour unrestricted period outside the hospital on any day that her morning weight was at least half a pound above her previous morning's weight. No comment was made concerning the level of activity or food consumption, thus avoiding direct confrontation over eating.

In less than a week after this paradigm was instituted, the first three patients responded with a rapid and consistent increase in body weight. They averaged gains of four pounds per week during six weeks of hospitalization. These results rank with the best reported in the medical literature, including series of patients treated with far more aggressive measures (bed rest, tube feeding, very large doses of chlorpromazine and insulin).[7-14]

The effectiveness of this approach led us to apply it, with modification, in three additional patients, all of whom responded with similarly gratifying weight gains. An instructive example was a seventeen-year-old girl admitted in a state of profound inanition and weighing fifty pounds (height 59 inches). The patient's behavioral repertoire was so limited that a search for a potential reinforcer was at first unsuccessful. Soon after chlorpromazine was started, however, the patient began to complain of its sedative effects. Her complaints suggested a new reinforcement contingency.

We prescribed decreases in chlorpromazine dosage proportional to the amount of weight gained on the previous day: on any day that followed a loss or no change in weight, the patient received 400 mg; a quarter pound gain resulted in a decrease to 300 mg; a half pound gain, a decrease to 200 mg; three-fourths of a pound, to 100 mg; and one pound, to no drug. This patient averaged a gain of six pounds per week, despite the consequent radical decrease in chlorpromazine dosage! Moreover, the results made it clear that the therapeutic efficacy of the behavioral approach did not depend upon hyperactivity or any other specific symptom. Rather, any suitable contingency might serve as the reinforcer in behavioral therapy. This finding was particularly persuasive of the effectiveness of this form of treatment.

OBESITY—FIRST APPLICATIONS

Spurred by the surprising success of a simple behavioral technique in the treatment of a condition as stubborn as anorexia nervosa, and by encouraging case reports of the effectiveness of behavioral modification in obesity,[15-20] I attempted to apply its principles to the treatment of two obese persons. Taking the anorexia nervosa paradigm as my model, I decided to make a small number of reinforcements contingent upon weight changes measured at first once, and later as often as four times a day. In the case of one patient, a cooperative roommate offered to take over such unpleasant chores as doing dishes or taking out the garbage on the day following one during which the patient lost weight. The second patient's wife, herself a psychologist, agreed to make sexual intercourse contingent upon her husband having lost weight that day.

After an initial loss of twenty pounds, the weights of both patients stabilized and they eventually stopped treatment. Paradoxically, it appeared that obesity posed a greater challenge to behavior modification than did the more stubborn anorexia nervosa. Other attempts to apply behavioral therapy to obesity also suggest that the task is more complicated than experience with anorexia nervosa had indicated. Most of these attempts were based on a 1962 paper by Ferster[21] who presented a detailed behavioral analysis of eating, and means of control.

THE BEHAVIORAL PROGRAM

Perhaps it would be well, at this point, to describe a typical behavioral program for the treatment of obesity. Since our program,[22] derived as were most others from Ferster,[21] is similar to them, I will describe it in some detail. Four principles are involved.

Description of the Behavior to Be Controlled

The patients were asked to keep daily records of the amount, time, and circumstances of their eating. The immediate results of this time-consuming and inconvenient procedure were grumbling and complaints. But eventually each patient reluctantly acknowledged that keeping these records had proved very helpful, particularly in increasing his awareness of how much he ate, the speed with which he ate, and the large variety of environmental and psychological situations associated with eating. For example, after two weeks of record-keeping a 30-year-old housewife reported that, for the first time in her life, she recognized that anger stimulated her eating. Accordingly, whenever she began to get angry, she left the kitchen and wrote down how she felt, thereby decreasing her anger and aborting her eating.

Modification and Control of the Discriminatory Stimuli Governing Eating

Most of the patients reported that their eating took place in a wide variety of places and at many different times during the day. It was postulated that these times and places had become so-called discriminatory stimuli signaling eating. The concept of a discriminatory stimulus derives from the animal laboratory, where such stimuli as the flashing of a light or sounding of a tone may signal to an animal that pressing a lever will produce food pellets or other reward. Since the reinforcer never occurs without the discriminatory stimulus, in the language of learning theory, the stimuli come to "control" various forms of behavior. In an effort to decrease the potency of the discriminatory stimuli that controlled their eating, patients were encouraged to confine eating, including snacking, to one place. In order not to disrupt domestic routines, this place was usually the kitchen. Further efforts to control discriminatory stimuli included using distinctive table settings, perhaps an unusually colored placemat and napkin. In addition patients were encouraged to make eating a pure experience, unaccompanied by other activity such as reading, watching television, or arguing with their families.

Development of Techniques to Control the Act of Eating

Specific techniques were utilized to help patients decrease their speed of eating, to become aware of all the components of the eating process, and to gain control over these components. Exercises included counting each mouthful of food eaten during a meal, placing utensils on the plate after every third mouthful until that mouthful was chewed and swallowed, and introducing a two-minute interruption of the meal.

Prompt Reinforcement of Behaviors That Delay or Control Eating

A reinforcement schedule, using a point system, was devised for control of eating behavior. Exercise of the suggested control procedures during a meal earned a certain number of points. These points were converted into money, which was brought to the next meeting and donated to the group. At the beginning of the program, the groups decided how the money should be used and they chose highly altruistic uses. Each week one group donated its savings to the Salvation Army, another to a needy friend of one of the members, a widow with fourteen children.

It has, in the past, been fairly easy to assess any out-patient treatment for obesity because the results have been so uniformly poor and the treatments themselves so obviously inadequate. In-patient treatment, with its potential for greater control of the patient has of course been more successful in weight reduction. Its usefulness has been limited, however, by the almost invariant regaining of weight after discharge.[23, 24] I have summarized my own and my colleagues' results with out-patient treatment quite simply: "Most obese persons will not stay in treatment for obesity. Of those who stay in treatment, most will not lose weight, and of those who do lose weight most will regain it."[25] Attrition rates vary between 20 per cent and 80 per cent. Only 25 per cent of those who enter treatment lose as much as 20 lb; only 5 per cent as much as 40 lb.[26] Against this background, the results obtained by Ferster, whose subjects averaged weight losses of only 10 lb, must be considered poor. Against this same background, moreover, the significance of a report on "Behavioral Control Over Eating"[27] is at once apparent. For in this report, Stuart, using a treatment program based on Ferster's, described the best results yet obtained in the out-patient treatment of obesity.

A LANDMARK IN THE TREATMENT OF OBESITY

Stuart's results depict the weight losses, over a one-year period, of eight patients who remained in treatment (the initial study group had included ten patients). Three, or 30 per cent of the original sample, lost more than 40 lb and six lost more than 30 lb. These results are the best ever reported for out-patient treatment of obesity, and they constitute a landmark in our understanding of this disorder. Even the absence of a control group does not vitiate the significance of the study.

Certain features of the report deserve attention: First, the expenditure of time was not exorbitant. In fact, the study took no longer than a number of others which achieved far poorer results. At the beginning of the treatment program, patients were seen in thirty-minute sessions held three times a week for a total of twelve to fifteen sessions. Thereafter, treatment sessions were scheduled as needed, usually at two-week intervals, for the next three months. Subsequently, there were monthly sessions and finally "maintenance" sessions were provided as needed. The total number of sessions during the year varied from sixteen to forty-one.

The specific behavioral techniques applied by Stuart are similar to those used in the other studies and described previously. One important feature of this study was that the regimen specified a rigid set of "how to do it" instructions for each of the first twelve interviews. Within this framework, however, there was great opportunity for the exercise of creativity by both the therapist and the patient. For example, Stuart noted that for patients suffering from a "behavioral depression," eating may be the only readily available reward or reinforcement. For these individuals, the therapist would have to cultivate a reservoir of positively reinforcing responses. Two patients in the series were helped to develop such responses: an interest in caged birds and in growing African violets respectively. In contrast to the other studies described here, all of which used group therapy, Stuart treated his patients individually.

USE OF NO-TREATMENT CONTROLS

In 1969, Harris reported a well-controlled study which utilized behavioral techniques to control eating in mildly overweight college students.[28] Two treatment groups, of three male and five female students each, were compared with a control group of eight students. In order not to discourage them, and thereby bias the results, the controls were told that they could not enter treatment at once because of a conflict in schedules, but that they would receive treatment later. Treatment sessions were held twice weekly for the first two months and then on a more irregular basis for a second two months.

The mean weight loss for the experimental group was 10.5 lb as compared with a weight gain of 3.6 lb for the control group, a difference that was very highly significant ($p < .001$).

Although the results in the treatment group are clearly far superior to those in the no-treatment control group, they are not as good as others reported in the literature, when judged by the criteria I have mentioned: only 21 per cent of Harris' subjects lost 20 lb and none lost as much as 40 lb. A major reason for these results was that her subjects were less obese than those studied by other investigators.

An interesting and perhaps significant aspect of the study is the note that E (the experimenter) lost 27 lb. As Harris continues, "The modeling effect of E, who went from fat to moderate with the pretest Ss and from moderate to thin with the Ss in the final study, was commented upon by many of the subjects." Harris noted that several variables may have contributed to the outcome besides the planned experimental procedures. She suggests that "a much more controlled study, in which various techniques and combinations of procedures are isolated, would be necessary to discover their differential effects."

Precisely such an investigation was carried out by Wollersheim.[29] Her work is representative of a small but extremely valuable group of studies that are elucidating the effective components of psychotherapy.

THE INTRODUCTION OF ALTERNATE-TREATMENT CONTROLS

Wollersheim's elegant study attempted to disentangle the contributions of various techniques by establishing four experimental conditions:

1. "Focal" (behavioral) treatment.   20 patients
2. Nonspecific therapy.   20 patients
3. Social pressure.   20 patients
4. No-treatment-wait control.   19 patients

The study thus contained three treatment groups (1, 2, and 3) and three control groups (2, 3, and 4) for the behavior modification group. Subjects were, again, mildly (10%) overweight female college students. Four therapists treated groups of five subjects under each of the three treatment conditions. A course of treatment consisted of ten sessions extending over a three-month period.

Wollersheim's findings showed that at the end of treatment and at eight weeks follow-up, the focal group's results were superior not only to the no-treatment control's, but also to those of the other two treatment groups. The "social pressure" group had participated in twenty-minute sessions based upon those of TOPS (Take Off Pounds Sensibly).[30] The sessions included a weigh-in, verbal praise for weight loss and encouragement for failure to lose weight, and the wearing of such TOPS artifacts as a star for weight loss, a sign in the form of a pig for weight gain, and a sign reading "Turtle" for no change in weight. The purpose of this technique is to foster a high positive expectation for losing weight and to develop and use social pressure to help subjects reduce.

The purpose of a "nonspecific therapy" group was to control for the effects of group treatment that resulted from such nonspecific factors as increased attention, "faith," expectation of relief, and presentation of a treatment rationale and meaningful "ritual." The rationale presented to the subjects in this group was that they needed to develop insight into the "real and not readily recognizable underlying reasons" for their behavior and to discover the "unconscious motives" underlying their "personality make-up." Each subject was told that as she obtained insight and better understanding of the "real motives and forces" operating within her personality, she would find it easier to accomplish her goals and lose weight.

In each group, not only weight loss but also responses to an eating-patterns questionnaire were used as dependent variables. Here too, the focal therapy group changed more than the other three, reaching statistically significant results on three of six factors: "emotional and uncontrolled overeating," "eating in isolation," and "between-meal eating."

MORE ALTERNATE TREATMENT CONTROLS:
THERAPY WITHOUT A THERAPIST

Hagen, following up the work of Wollersheim, accepted her finding that behavior modification was the most effective method for the treatment of obesity.[31] He turned his attention to a further refinement—determining whether the results obtained were due only to the specific behavioral techniques used or were dependent also upon the interpersonal influence of the therapist. Hagen constructed an experimental design similar to Wollersheim's. The various treatment groups were compared with each other and with a no-treatment-wait control group:

1. Group (behavioral) therapy.   18 subjects
2. Bibliotherapy (use of a written manual).   18 subjects
3. Group and bibliotherapy combined.   18 subjects
4. No-treatment-wait control.   35 subjects

The ninety subjects in his study were also mildly (10%) overweight female college students. They were randomly assigned to one of four experimental groups in such a way that the groups were comparable in relation to the obesity of their members. Three therapists treated six subjects each in the group therapy and combined therapy conditions. Ten treatment sessions were held over a three-month period.

The greatest weight loss occurred in the group and bibliotherapy combined group, which lost an average of 15 lb during treatment, and regained 2 lb during the four-week follow-up period. However, the difference in weight loss between this group and the other two treatment groups was not statistically significant. There was a significant difference ($p < .01$) between its results and those of the no-treatment group. Wollersheim's eating patterns questionnaire also elicited results from all three treatment groups that were similar to those from her "focal" group, but demonstrated no change in the control group.

Hagen's work showed that it is possible to treat obesity effectively by using a written manual that embodies behavioral therapy principles. Moreover, this treatment is apparently as effective as one that utilizes therapists. These results further confirm the effectiveness of behavioral principles in the treatment of obesity.

A STUDY WITH A CROSS-OVER DESIGN

Stuart has recently completed a study that used the patient as his own control in what is known as a cross-over design.[32] The subjects were divided into two cohorts each containing three moderately obese women. During a preliminary five-week period they kept careful records of their weight and food intake. Group 1 then received twice weekly treatment sessions of about forty minutes, for fifteen weeks. Meanwhile, group 2 was given diet planning materials and an exercise program (both of which were also offered to group 1). Group 1 lost an average of 15 lb while the control group *gained* an average of 4 lb. At the end of the 15 weeks, group 1 continued with the program of its own, while group 2 received fifteen weeks of the same treatment group 1 had received (group therapy plus diet planning and exercise). Under these circumstances, group 1 lost an additional 9 lb, but at a slightly lower rate than when it was under active treatment. Group 2, on the other hand, which had gained weight during the preceding fifteen weeks, lost 15 lb. Both groups continued to lose in the subsequent twelve weeks without further treatment.

TREATMENT OF SEVERE OBESITY

Another dimension of the behavioral approach to obesity was provided by a study of severely obese patients (78% overweight).[22] Two cohorts of eight and seven patients respectively were seen in weekly group therapy sessions lasting about two hours, for three months. The therapists were a male experimental psychologist with a strong background in learning theory but little clinical experience, and a female research technician with no previous experience in therapy. Two control groups received supportive psychotherapy, instruction about dieting and nutrition, and, upon demand, appetite suppressants. Their male and female therapy team consisted of an internist just completing a psychiatric residency, who had had extensive experience in the treatment of obesity, and a research nurse.

The results of treatment of the two cohorts are summarized in Table 14-I. The control group's losses are comparable to those to be found in the medical literature—none lost 40 lb, 24 per cent lost more than 20 lb. By contrast, 13 per cent of the behavior modification group lost more than 40 lb. and 53 per cent lost more than 20 lb. Although the differences between the behavior modification and control groups for weight losses over 20 and 40 lb are not statistically significant, the difference for weight losses over 30 lb is ($p = 0.015$ by Fisher exact probability test). Furthermore, those who

TABLE 14-I

RESULTS OF TREATMENT

| | Per Cent of Groups Losing Specified Amounts of Weight | | | | |
| | *Behavior Modification Groups* *n = 15* | | *Control Therapy Groups* *n = 17* | | *Average Medical Literature* |
	After Treatment	*One Year Follow-up*	*After Treatment*	*One Year Follow-up*	*End of Treatment*
More than 40 lb	13	33	0	12	5
More than 30 lb	33	40	0	29	—
More than 20 lb	53	53	24	47	25

had lost weight during treatment continued to lose weight during the following year.

Two findings should be noted: First, in each cohort the median weight loss for the behavior modification group was greater than that of the control group—24 lb versus 18 lb for the first cohort; 13 versus 11 for the second. Second, there is far greater variability of results in the behavior modification groups ($F = 4.38$, $p < 0.005$). Because of this variability the difference in weight loss between the behavior modification and control groups did not reach statistical significance.

TESTING THE LIMITS OF THE BEHAVIORAL APPROACH

Recently three further studies, on strikingly dissimilar populations, have demonstrated the remarkably wide range of circumstances in which behavior modification may be effective in the treatment of obesity. The first population consisted of chronic schizophrenic patients in a Veterans Administration Hospital,[33] the second of a heterogeneous group of Dutch men and women,[34] and the third, obese women in a general hospital.[35] As in three of the foregoing studies, follow-up data of the first two of these showed significantly greater weight loss among behavior modification subjects than among those who received other forms of treatment.

The first of these studies was carried out to explore the management of the obesity which so frequently develops among schizophrenic patients during prolonged hospitalization.[33] Seven men, matched for degree of overweight, were assigned to each of three groups: behavior modification, group therapy, and diet-only. Treatment was carried out over a six-week period with a four-week follow-up. Behavior modification consisted of a penalty schedule involving forfeiture of part of five dollars weekly allowance for failure to lose weight during the previous week. Weight loss carried no reward other than assuring the patient of his regular allotment. Group therapy sessions were held once a week for an hour, and consisted of weighings with encouraging comments for weight losses and discussion of reasons for gains and losses. Both treatment groups lost significantly more weight than the diet-only group during the six-week treatment period. But the behavior modification subjects lost significantly more weight during the four-week follow-up than did the group therapy subjects.

In the second study the Dutch investigators chose as their subjects university students and others recruited by a variety of means, including advertisements in women's magazines.[34] Two behavior modification groups of fifteen subjects each were compared with fifteen subjects in a traditional diet-therapy group and fifteen no-treatment controls. The program consisted of a four-week treatment period with follow-ups at six weeks and five months. At the end of four weeks, all three treatment groups had lost more weight than those who had received no treatment, and one of the behavior modification groups had lost more than the other two treatment groups. At the five-month follow-up, both behavior modification groups, one of which had continued to lose weight and the other of which had maintained its weight loss, had performed significantly more effectively than the diet therapy group, which had regained most of the weight it had lost.

The results of the third study, reported only briefly, again favored behavior modification.[35] Eleven obese women treated with this modality lost more weight than did nine obese women treated by conventional group psychotherapy (15 versus 6.6 lb). Furthermore, in an interesting parallel to the results reported by Penick *et al.*,[22] this 8.4 lb difference in weight loss was not statistically significant, largely because of the very great variability in the behavior modification group.

CONCLUSION

The studies we have reviewed are an impressive example of the kind of contribution which behavior therapists are making to the scientific study of psychotherapy. These workers have introduced experimental designs of a sophistication and power unprecedented in psychotherapy research: they may well be laying the foundations of a truly cumulative science of psychotherapy.

Two further aspects of behavior modification may be less well appreciated by psychiatrists: the possibility for the exercise of great creativity on the part of both patient and therapist, and the encouragement of patients to assume an unusually high degree of responsibility for their own treatment.

Creativity in Behavior Modification

An unflattering view of behavior modification sees in it mechanistic manipulations to produce trivial changes in overt behavior at the expense of the patient's inner freedom and uniquely human qualities. Such polemics may cite the examples of systematic desensitization of phobias or the conditioned aversion therapy of alcoholism, treatments based upon respondent (Pavlovian) conditioning. Whatever the merit of the criticism of these treatments, it is hardly relevant to behavioral measures such as those reviewed here which utilize primarily operant (Skinnerian) conditioning. A closer look at these measures may help to clarify this point.

A behavioral analysis begins with a careful study of the environmental variables that control the patient's symptomatic behavior. These variables may be divided for convenience into antecedent events, which may precipitate the behavior, and consequent events, which may help to reward and maintain it. For example, understanding a particular episode of binge-eating requires precise information about what was happening to the patient just before the breakdown in eating control occurred. Similarly, it is important to ascertain the immediate effects upon the patient's feelings, on her husband's behavior, and, in fact, upon any significant aspect in her life. Stuart has recently outlined a useful schema for a behavioral analysis,[37] and we have described earlier the kind of therapeutic program which can be constructed out of these analyses of specific behaviors.

I was persuaded of the value of such a method of proceeding as I considered the degree to which it specified techniques for the treatment of obesity which I had evolved empirically over nearly twenty years of treatment of obese persons. It contrasted sharply with the recommendations for treatment derived from psychodynamic theories. Such theories, for example, cautioned against considering with the patient his specific acts of overeating and consequent weight gains. For they saw in these acts merely symptoms of an underlying conflict. Any small benefits which might accrue from concern with these symptoms, it was taught, were likely to be far outweighed by distraction of patient and therapist from their primary task of resolution of the pathogenic conflicts. Such resolution, and only such resolution, could lead to a lasting cure.

Central to a behavioral analysis is the search by patient and therapist for solutions to problems which are at the same time both relatively modest and potentially soluble. By circumscribing therapeutic concern to discrete, clearly specified behaviors, this approach reduces the potentially limitless field of therapeutic encounter and permits patient and therapist to concentrate their efforts on a more limited number of variables than is possible with traditional therapies. By focusing a great deal of attention upon relatively small problems the probability of solving them is greatly increased. The experience of success, even in small matters, encourages the patient to continue the process of defining manageable problems and seeking solutions to them. It is hard to do justice to the remarkable creativity evoked in the course of this endeavor. The few examples described in this review can only suggest the kind of innovative measures which, in remarkable scope and diversity, have been applied to the treatment of obesity.

Responsibility in Behavior Modification

The particular relevance of focusing upon environmental variables in the treatment of obesity is emphasized by Schachter's recent demonstration of the extent to which the eating behavior of many obese persons is under environmental control.[38] He found, for example, that obese persons were far more influenced than nonobese persons by such "external" factors as palatability, time of day, and availability of food, and far less influenced by such "internal" factors as hunger, measured by self report and by length of time after eating.

The high degree of environmental control of the food intake of obese persons may help to explain the failures of both routine medical management and of traditional insight therapy. Obese persons often adapt easily to general medicine's authoritarian-physician-dependent-patient relationship and lose some weight to please the doctor. Failure to deal with the environmental variables which play such an important part in the patient's eating, however, leaves him vulnerable to their influence, and sooner or later he breaks his diet. This transgression strikes at the special qualities of this kind of doctor-patient relationship, which then begins to lose its potency. Overeating recurs and a vicious cycle ensues.

The obese person who enters psychiatric treatment frequently fares little better. Insight therapy, with its focus on inner drives, motives, and conflicts, all-too-often ignores environmental factors in the control of food intake as thoroughly as does general medical treatment. Further, by holding out hope for an eventual solution to obesity through the resolution of conflict, it can foster magical expectations which distract the patient from more mundane concerns of greater therapeutic potential.

In contrast to this neglect by traditional therapies of the environmental influences to which the obese person seems so vulnerable, behavior modification helps him to focus his attention upon them. Not only is he encouraged to observe and make a detailed record of these influences on his eating behavior, but he is also shown how to use this information to plan and carry out tasks to help him gain control over this behavior. The difference between behavior modification and more traditional therapies is particularly notable in the extent of the demands each makes upon the obese patient in the interval between visits to the therapist. In contrast to the limited demands of traditional therapies, behavior modification makes it possible for the patient to invest a great deal of hard work in his treatment. The apparent dependency of successful outcome upon the amount of work invested encourages patients to assume an unusually high degree of responsibility for their own treatment. This increase in the opportunity for the exercise of personal responsibility may prove to be one of behavior modification's major contributions to treatment in psychiatry.

In conclusion, both greater weight loss during treatment and superior maintenance of weight loss after treatment indicate that behavior modification is more effective than previous methods of treatment for obesity. Further, the experimental designs developed to assess these treatments constitute a significant advance in the study of psychotherapy.

REFERENCES

1. Eysenick, H. J.: Editorial. *Behav Res Ther,* 1:1-2, 1963.
2. Bachrach, A. J., Erwin, W. and Mohr, J. P.: The control of eating in an anorexic by operant conditioning techniques. In L. P. Ullmann and L. Krasner (Eds.): *Case Studies in Behavior Modification.* New York, Holt, Rinehart and Winston, 1965, pp. 153-163.

3. Hallsten, E. A., Jr.: Adolescent anorexia nervosa treated by desensitization. *Behav Res Ther*, 3:87-91, 1965.
4. Leitenberg, H., Agras, W. S. and Thomson, L. E.: A sequential analysis of the effect of selective positive reinforcement in modifying anorexia nervosa. *Behav Res Ther*, 6:211-218, 1968.
5. Blinder, B. J., Freeman, D. M. A., Ringold, A. and Stunkard, A. J.: Rapid weight restoration in anorexia nervosa. *Clin Res*, 15:473, 1967.
6. Blinder, B. J., Freeman, D. M. A. and Stunkard, A. J.: Behavior therapy of anorexia nervosa: Effectiveness of activity as a reinforcer of weight gain. *Am J Psychiat*, 126:1093-1098, 1970.
7. Williams, E.: Anorexia nervosa, a somatic disorder. *Br Med J*, 2:190-195, 1958.
8. Dally, P. and Sargent, W.: A new treatment of anorexia. *Br Med J*, 1:1770-1773, 1960.
9. Russell, G. H. and Mezey, A. G.: An analysis of weight gain in patients with anorexia nervosa treated with high calorie diets. *Clin Sci*, 23:449-461, 1962.
10. Crisp, A. H.: Clinical and therapeutic aspects of anorexia. *J Psychosom Res*, 9:67-78, 1965.
11. Crisp, A. H.: A treatment regime for anorexia nervosa. *Br J Psychiat*, 112:505-512, 1966.
12. Dally, P. and Sargent, W.: Treatment and outcome of anorexia. *Br Med*, 2:293-295, 1966.
13. Groes, J. J. and Feldman-Toldedano, Z.: Educative treatment of patients and parents in anorexia nervosa. *Br J Psychiat*, 112:671-678, 1966.
14. Browning, C. H. and Miller, S. I.: Anorexia nervosa: A study in prognosis and management. *Am J Psychiat*, 124:1128-1132, 1968.
15. Erickson, M. A.: The utilization of patient behavior in the hypnotherapy of obesity. *Am J Clin Hypnosis*, 3:112-116, 1960.
16. Thorpe, J. G., Schmidt, E., Brown, P. T. and Castell, D.: Aversion relief therapy: A new method for general application. *Behav Res Ther*, 2:71-82, 1964.
17. Meyer, V. and Crisp, A. H.: Aversion therapy in two cases of obesity. *Behav Res Ther*, 2:143-147, 1964.
18. Cautela, J.: Covert sensitization. *Psychol Rep*, 20:459-468, 1967.
19. Kennedy, W. A. and Foreyt, J.: Control of eating behavior in an obese patient by avoidance conditioning. *Psychol Rep*, 22:571-576, 1968.
20. Wolpe, J.: *The Practise of Behavior Therapy*. New York, Pergamon Press, 204-205, 216-217, 1969.
21. Ferster, C. B., Nurnberger, J. I. and Levitt, E. B.: The control of overeating. *J Math*, 1:87-109, 1962.
22. Penick, S. B., Filion, R., Fox, S. and Stunkard, A. J.: Behavior modification in the treatment of obesity. *Psychosom Med*, in press.
23. Maccuish, A. C., Munro, J. F. and Duncan, L. J. P.: Follow-up study of refractory obesity treated by fasting. *Brit Med J*, 1:91-200, 1968.
24. Swanson, D. W. and Dinello, F. A.: Follow-up of patients starved for obesity. *Psychosom Med*, 32:209-214, 1970.
25. Stunkard, A. J.: The management of obesity. *N Y J Med*, 58:79-87, 1958.
26. Stunkard, A. J. and McLaren-Hume, M.: The results of treatment for obesity. *Arch Intern Med*, 103:79-85, 1959.
27. Stuart, R. B.: Behavioral control of overeating. *Behav Res Ther*, 5:357-365, 1967.
28. Harris, M. B.: Self-directed program for weight control: A pilot study. *J Abnorm Psychol*, 74:263-270, 1969.

29. Wollersheim, J. P.: The effectiveness of group therapy based upon learning principles in the treatment of overweight women. *J Abnorm Psychol*, 76:462-474, 1970.

30. Stunkard, A. J., Fox, S., Levine, H.: The management of obesity: Patient self-help and medical treatment. *Arch Intern Med*, 125:1067-1072, 1970.

31. Hagen, R. L.: *Group Therapy Versus Bibliotherapy in Weight Reduction*. Doctoral dissertation, University of Illinois, 1969.

32. Stuart, R. B.: A three-dimensional program for the treatment of obesity. *Behav Res Ther*, 9:177-186, 1971.

33. Harmatz, M. G. and Lapuc, P.: Behavior modification of overeating in a psychiatric population. *J Consult Clin Psychol*, 32:583-587, 1968.

34. Jongmans, J. G.: *Vermagerings-Therapieen*. Doctoraal Werkstuk Psychologisch Laboratorium van de Universiteit van Amsterdam, 1969.

35. Shipman, W.: Behavior therapy with obese dieters. *1970 Annual Report, Institute for Psychosomatic and Psychiatric Research and Training, Michael Reese Hospital and Medical Center*, Chicago, 1970, pp. 70-71.

36. Shipman, W.: Personal communication.

37. Stuart, R. B.: *Trick or Treatment: How and When Psychotherapy Fails*. Champaign, Ill., Research Press, 1971, pp. 183-194.

38. Schachter, S.: Obesity and eating. *Science*, 161:751-756, 1968.

15

A Three-Dimensional Program
for the Treatment of Obesity

RICHARD B. STUART

WHETHER overweight is determined by gross body weight[40] or skin-fold measurement[52] even when differences in fat as a proportion of body weight are controlled,[19] at least one in five Americans is found to be overweight.[67] The social and economic costs of being overweight are staggering and are complicated by greatly increased vulnerability to a broad range of physical diseases, including cardiovascular and renal diseases, maturity-onset diabetes, cirrhosis of the liver, and gall bladder diseases, among many others.[38] Despite the history of concern with obesity and the magnitude of the problem, little uncontested knowledge has been accumulated with respect to its etiology and treatment. Mayer has suggested that genetic factors may contribute to the onset of a small number of cases, while an additional small number of cases can be explained on the basis of injury to the hypothalamus, hormonal imbalance and other threats to normal metabolism. The exact role of genetic and physiological factors has, however, remained a mystery, and there has been little evidence to countermand an early observation by Newburgh and Johnston[43] that most cases of obesity are as follows:

> . . . never directly caused by abnormal metabolism but (are) always due to food habits not adjusted to the metabolic requirement—either the ingestion of more food than is normally needed or the failure to reduce the intake in response to a lowered requirement (p. 212).

Therefore most obesities can be attributed to an excess of food intake beyond the demands of energy expenditure, and a major objective in treating obesity is a reduction in the amount of excess food consumed.

Just as there is uncertainty concerning the etiology of obesity, there is great confusion over the role of psychological factors in overeating and its management. Some authors have contributed various useful typologies; for example, Stunkard[61] classified eating patterns as night eating, binge eating, and eating without satiation, while Hamburger[24] classified the triggers of excessive eating as either external or intrapsychic. Despite Suczek's[66] observation that "simple psychologic factors may not relate to either degree of obesity or ability to lose weight (p. 201)," other authors have sought to identify specific psychological mechanisms associated with obesity. For example, Conrad[15] postulates that specific intrapsychic factors such as efforts to prevent loss of love and to express hostility or efforts to symbolically undergo pregnancy and to ward off sexual temptations, underlie obesity. In a similar vein, while eating has been seen as a means of warding off anxiety,[32] it has also been seen as a depressive equivalent.[55] Furthermore, while writers have suggested that "depression, psychosis . . . suicide[10] (p. 573)" and other stress reactions have accompanied weight loss[17, 22] other studies have shown that: a) the so-called "depression" associated with weight loss by some people is actually just a function of lowered energy due to reduced food consumption;[8] b) negative psychological reactions are frequently not found;[12, 39] and c) a reduction in anxiety and depression may actually accompany weight loss.[53] Despite this evidence, Bruch's[9] admonition that treatment of overeating which does not give "psychologic factors . . . due consideration (can lead) at best to a temporary weight reduction (while being) considered dangerous from the point of view of mental health (p. 49)" is still influential in dissuading experimenters and therapists from undertaking parsimonious treatment of overeating.

While the research pertaining to physiological and psychological concomitants of obesity has led to some paradoxical conclusions, Stunkard's[63] review of environmental factors related to obesity has demonstrated a clear-cut connection between obesity and socioeconomic status, social mobility and ethnic variables. It is interesting to note, however, that where comparative data are available, the differences ascribed to each of these factors are stronger for women than men. One explanation of this sex difference may be that the physical expenditure of energy in work may reduce the tendency toward adiposity of lower class, socially nonmobile men while the women, faced with relative inactivity, may show a more direct effect of high carbohydrate, low protein diets common at lower socioeconomic strata (Select Committee on Nutrition and Human Needs, 1970).

The literature describing the treatment of obesity is dismal and confusing. One authoritative group noted:

> . . . most obese patients will not remain in treatment. Of those who do remain in treatment, most will not lose significant poundage, and of those who do lose weight, most will regain in promptly. In a careful follow-up study only 8 per cent of obese patients seen in a nutrition clinic actually maintained a satisfactory weight loss.[17]

Failure has been reported following some of the most ambitious and sophisticated treatments (e.g. Mayer;[38] Stunkard and McLaren-Hume[65]), while success has been claimed for some of the more superficial "diet-clinic"-type approaches (e.g. Franklin and Rynearson[21]). The role of drugs has been extolled by many writers, while others have cautioned that their side effects strongly contraindicate their use.[2, 23, 42] Fasting has been shown to have a profound effect upon weight loss (e.g. Bortz;[7] Stokes[57]), but the results have been shown to be short-lived as the patient is likely to quickly regain lost weight when he leaves the hospital setting.[36] Claims of success have also been advanced for individual and group psychotherapy[34, 39, 56, 64, 69] and hypnosis,[25, 35] although these reports are typically not supported by controlled investigation. Finally, positive outcomes have been reported for behavior therapy techniques ranging from token reinforcement,[4] aversion therapy,[41] and covert sensitization[13] through complex contingency management procedures. Illustrative of the latter approaches are the work of Stuart,[58] which has been replicated in controlled studies by Ramsay[48] and Penick and his associates[46] and the work of Harris,[26] which included control-group comparisons in the original research.

It is probably true that behavior therapy has offered greater promise of positive results than any other type of treatment. This paper will present a rationale of and description for the treatment of overeating based upon behavioral principles.

RATIONALE

The treatment of obesity has typically attempted to stress the development of "self-control" by the overeater whose self-control deficit is often regarded as a personal fault. Conceding that behavior modifiers recognize first that self-control is merely the emission of one set of responses designed to alter the probability of occurrence of another set of responses[5, 20, 28, 29] and second, that self-controlling responses are acquired through social learning,[3, 31] most behaviorists still appear to regard self-control as a personal virtue and its absence a personal deficit.[59] For example, Cautela[14] is concerned with the individual's ability to manipulate the contingencies of his own behavior while Kanfer[30] offers among other explanations for the breakdown of self-control "the patient's commitment to change," a presumed index of the patient's degree of motivation, or "the patient's prior skill in use of self-reward or self-punishment responses for changing behavior," a presumed index of the patient's capacity to utilize treatment.

In any event, the relevance of the concept of self-control to the management of overeating may be questioned in the light of many recent studies. The most basic of these is the work of Stunkard[62] who demonstrated that in comparison with nonobese subjects, obese subjects are far less likely to report hunger in association with "gastric motility." Thus the cues for hunger experiences of the obese may be tied to external events. Several ingenious studies have contributed to this possibility. First, Schachter and his associates demonstrated that obese subjects are less influenced than nonobese subjects by manipulated fear and deprivation of food,[49] while they are more influenced by the time they think it is than by the actual time.[51]

In addition it was shown that when the cues of eating are absent, as on religious fast days, obese subjects are more likely to observe dietary restrictions than nonobese subjects.[49] In a similar vein, Nisbett[44] and Hashim and Van Itallie[27] showed that obese subjects are more influenced by the taste of food than are nonobese subjects when the duration of food deprivation is controlled. These varied studies and others suggested that the first of two requirements for the treatment of overeating must stress environmental management rather than self-control because the cues of overeating are environmental rather than intrapersonal.

The second requirement for the management of obesity must be a manipulation of the energy balance—the balance between the consumption of energy as food and the expenditure of energy through exercise. If all of the energy which is derived from the consumed food is expended in exercise, then gross body weight will remain constant. Any excess of food energy consumption over energy expenditure, however, is stored as adiposity at the rate of approximately one pound of body fat for each excessive 3500 kcal.[23, 38] Weight can therefore be lost through: a) an increase in the amount of exercise, holding food intake constant; b) a decrease in the amount of food intake, holding exercise constant; or c) both an increase in exercise and a decrease in food intake.

It has been well-demonstrated that the rising problem of obesity is associated with decreasing demands for exercise. Mayer suggested that "inactivity is the most important factor explaining the frequency of 'creeping' overweight in modern societies," while Durnin and Passmore[19] revealed that food intake is typically not adjusted to reduced exercise. Recent evidence adduced by the Agricultural Research Service[1] demonstrated that the diets of young men in higher-income brackets include 20 per cent more kilocalories than the diets of those with smaller incomes and presumably more physically taxing occupations, and this is most likely to result in some measure of obesity among middle-class males. Increase in the rate of exercise can, however, have a profound effect upon body weight although the amount of exercise necessary is greater than generally expected.* Furthermore, given the fact that an obese person actually expends *less* energy than a nonobese person doing the same amount of work (e.g. a 250 lb man walking 1.5 mph expends 5.34 kcal per min, while a 150 lb man walking at the same rate and carrying a 100-pound load expends 5.75 kcal per min[6]), planned programs for exercise are particularly important. In addition to

---

* Stuart (unpublished data) asked a group of obese women to estimate the amount of exercise required to work off the weight gain attributable to such common foods as donuts, ice cream sodas and potato chips. Comparing their answers with the estimates based upon Konishi's[33] figures for a 150 lb man walking at the rate of 3.5 mph (29, 49 and 21 min respectively), they were found to underestimate the true work required by from 200 to 300 per cent.

aiding in the management of gross body weight, exercise programs for the thin as well as the obese seem definitely to reduce the risk of certain cardiovascular diseases.[37]

Just as it is important systematically to increase the amount of exercise, so too is it important to reduce the amount of food or change the nature of foods eaten. Mayer[38] recommends the following:

> A balanced diet, containing no less than 14 per cent of protein, no more than 30 per cent of fat (with saturated fats cut down), and the rest carbohydrates (with sucrose—ordinary sugar—cut down to a low level) . . . (p. 160).

Apart from its nutritional advantages, it is important to include a substantial amount of protein in the diet because smaller amounts of protein as opposed to carbohydrates produce satiety and because a portion of the caloric content of protein is used in its own metabolism,[23] leaving a smaller proportion as a possible contributor to adiposity. Conversely, it is important to reduce the amount of carbohydrates consumed because a higher proportion of its caloric content is available for adiposity, because at least certain carbohydrates, e.g. sucrose,[71] are associated with increased incidence of certain cardiovascular diseases to which obese persons are vulnerable, and because "carbohydrate food causes the storage of unusually large amounts of water[23]—typically a special problem faced by obese individuals.

The foregoing observations lead to several basic considerations for weight reduction programs. First, it is essential to design an environment in which food-relevant cues are conducive to the maximal practice of prudent eating habits. This is required by the fact that overeating among obese persons appears to be under environmental control. Also, training the patient in the techniques of environmental control will probably reduce the gradual loss of therapeutic effect found in certain[54] but not all other programs.[46] Second, it is essential to plan toward a negative energy balance. In doing this, however, it is essential to avoid exercise or dietary excesses. They are unlikely to be followed, and if they are followed each may result in iatrogenic complications. Excessive exercise might lead to overexertion or serious cardiovascular illness. Unbalanced diets might lead to physiological disease, while insufficient diets might lead to enervation and physiologically produced depression. It is therefore essential to plan gradual weight-loss programs associated with progressive changes in the energy balance, as these are both safer and more likely to meet with success.[70] The exact determination of these levels must be empirically determined for each patient, beginning with tables of recommended dietary allowance,[38] adjusting these for the amount of exercise, carefully monitoring weight and mood changes as time on the program progresses, and being careful to make certain that the degree of weight loss provides sufficient motivation for the patient to continue using the program.

TREATMENT

Translation of the above rationale into a set of specific treatment procedures sometimes requires an arbitrary selection of intervention alternatives derived from contrary or contradictory conclusions in the basic research literature. For example, while Gordon,[23] repudiated his earlier contention that a patient's eating several smaller meals each day would necessarily result in greater weight loss than his eating only the three traditional meals, others[18] have shown that *with caloric intake held constant* patients who eat three meals daily may not only maintain their weight but may actually gain weight, while the same patients dividing their caloric allowance into seven meals lose weight precipitously. As another example, Nisbett and Kanouse[45] demonstrated that obese food shoppers actually buy less the more deprived of food they are while nonobese shoppers increase their food buying as a function of the extent of food deprivation. In contrast, Stuart (unpublished data) demonstrated that when a group of obese women confined their food shopping to the hours of 3:30 to 5:00 pm, they purchased 20 per cent more food than when they postponed their food shopping until 6:30 to 8:00 pm. Thus the therapist reading the Gordon and Nisbett studies would have his patients eat three meals and delay their food shopping until they were at least moderately deprived of food, while the therapist familiar with the work of Debry *et al.* and Stuart would do just the reverse. The therapist familiar with both must decide which recommendations to follow, framing his decision as a reversible hypothesis which can be invalidated in response to patient-produced data.

The treatment procedures which have been used in this investigation fall into three broad categories. First, an effort is made to establish firm control over the eating environment. This requires: a) the elimination or suppression of cues associated with problematic eating while strengthening the cues associated with desirable eating patterns; b) planned manipulation of the actual response of eating to accelerate desirable elements of the response while decelerating undesirable aspects; and c) the manipulation of the contingencies associated with problematic and desirable eating patterns. A sample of the procedures used in the service of each of these objectives is presented in Table 15-I.

Second, an effort is made to establish a dietary program for each patient on an individual basis. The first step in the development of a diet is completion by the patient of a self-monitoring food intake form. Because patients frequently claim to exist on unbelievably small quantities of food, only to lose weight rapidly when their diet is regulated at amounts two or three times greater than originally claimed, it is helpful to provide some social monitoring of the use of the monitoring sheets to ensure accuracy. Procedures such as those employed by Powell and Azrin[47] have proven

TABLE 15-I

SAMPLE PROCEDURES USED TO STRENGTHEN APPROPRIATE EATING
AND TO WEAKEN INAPPROPRIATE EATING

Cue elimination	*Cue suppression*	*Cue strengthening*
1. Eat in one room only 2. Do nothing while eating 3. Make available proper foods only: (a) shop from a list; (b) shop only after full meal 4. Clear dishes directly into garbage 5. Allow children to take own sweets	1. Have company while eating 2. Prepare and serve small quantities only 3. Eat slowly 4. Save one item from meal to eat later 5. If high-calorie foods are eaten, they must require preparation	1. Keep food, weight chart 2. Use food exchange diet 3. Allow extra money for proper foods 4. Experiment with attractive preparation of diet foods 5. Keep available pictures of desired clothes, list of desirable activities
	↓	↓
	Reduced strength of undesirable responses	*Increase strength of desirable responses*
	1. Swallow food already in mouth before adding more 2. Eat with utensils 3. Drink as little as possible during meals	1. Introduce planned delays during meal 2. Chew food slowly, thoroughly 3. Concentrate on what is being eaten
	↓	↓
	Provide decelerating consequences	*Provide accelerating consequences*
	1. Develop means for display of caloric value of food eaten daily, weight changes 2. Arrange to have deviations from program ignored by others except for professionals 3. Arrange to have overeater reread program when items have not been followed and to write techniques which might have succeeded	1. Develop means for display of caloric value of food eaten daily, weight changes 2. Develop means of providing social feedback for all success by: a) family; b) friends; c) co-workers; d) other weight losers; and/or e) professionals 3. Program material and/or social consequences to follow: a) the attainment of weight loss subgoals; b) completion of specific daily behavioral control objectives

helpful. When validated eating records have been obtained for a fourteen-day period, adjustments in food intake can be planned based upon recommended caloric levels, balanced diet planning and adjustments for the level of food intake in light of the patient's exercise. In dietary planning, "food exchange" recommendations are made[60] rather than recommendations for specific food choices. In food exchange dieting, foods in each of six food categories (e.g. milk, fruit, meat, etc.) are grouped according to similar caloric levels (e.g. one egg has approximately the same caloric value as one slice of bread). Selections are made according to food exchanges and this greatly increases the ease and precision of meal planning. Furthermore, when this is done as a means of increasing the probability that the diet will be followed, the unavailability of specific foods frequently leads to a termination of the entire dietary program.

Third, an effort is made to develop an individualized aerobics exercise program based upon walking in most cases.[16] In introducing the need for exercise, the patient is offered a choice between adherence to a punishing diet which may lead to chronic discomfort throughout the day and a more permissive diet coupled with exercise which may lead to discomfort for an hour or less per day. When an exercise program is developed, an effort is made to weave the exercise activity into the normal fabric of the patient's day to increase the likelihood that it will be followed. For example, a patient might be asked to park his car ten blocks from the home of friends he is about to visit, to avoid elevators and walk up to his destinations, and to carry each item upstairs as needed, rather than allowing several items to accumulate, as a means of inceasing the number of steps necessary.

RESULTS

The pilot investigation reported here reflects the treatment of six overweight, married, middle-class women (171 to 212 lb) between the ages of twenty-seven and forty-one. Each woman requested treatment on a self-referred basis. Treatment was offered on an individual basis but women were randomly assigned to one of two cohorts. Both groups of three patients were asked to complete the Sixteen Personality Factor Questionnaire[11] and to keep a five-week baseline of their weight and food intake. The first group was then offered treatment twice weekly (average 40 min per session) for a fifteen-week period, while the second group was asked to practice "self-control" of eating behavior. The self-control subjects were given the same diet planning materials and exercise program that the treatment group was offered. They were not, however, given instruction for the management of food in the environment. At the conclusion of the fifteen-week period, the treated group was asked to continue the treatment program and the second group was offered fifteen weeks of the same treatment. Approximately six months following the termination of treatment of Group 1 and three months following the termination of treatment of Group two, follow-up data were collected including weight, eating patterns and the readministration of the Cattell 16 P.F. Patients in Group 1 lost an average of 35 lb while those in Group 2 lost an average of 21 lb. These results are consistent with the objective set for gradual weight loss approximating 1 lb per week. It will also be seen that the mere collection of baseline self-monitoring data was associated with mild weight loss in both groups, although these gains were dissipated as time progressed for the second group. Finally, comparison of the pre-test and post-test personality test results reveal little change other than small improvement in "ego stability" and tension (Factors C and Q4) of the 16 P.F.

The results provide suggestive evidence for the usefulness of a threefold treatment of obesity stressing environmental control of overeating, nutritional planning, and regulated increase in energy expenditure. The sample size was too small to permit generalization, and the superiority of the initially treated (Group 1) over the initially untreated (Group 2) patients may be due to an inclination among the latter group to be casual about weight reduction. To forestall this possibility, every effort was made to make the treatment appear "official" but no validation of the success of this effort was undertaken. Furthermore, it is perhaps noteworthy that the results were obtained with no evidence of psychological stress in a patient population which was regarded as "well-adjusted" at the start and termination of treatment.

To validate these procedures in any definitive manner, extensive replication is needed using careful experimental control procedures applied to a far more diverse population than was used in this pilot study. Research such as that recently completed by Penick *et al.*[46] has made important strides in this direction. It is only through such experimentation that the vast amount of "faddism and quackery"[23] which characterizes the broad field of obesity control can be replaced by a scientifically validated set of procedures.

REFERENCES

1. Agricultural Research Service, U. S. Department of Agriculture: *Food Intake and Nutritive Value of Diets of Men, Women and Children in the United States, Spring 1965: A Preliminary Report.* (ARS 62-18), Washington, D. C., United States Government Printing Office, 1969.
2. American Academy of Pediatrics, Committee on Nutrition: Obesity in childhood. *Pediatrics,* 40:455-465, 1967.
3. Bandura, A. and Kupers, C. J.: Transmission of patterns of self-reinforcement through modeling. *J Abnorm Soc Psychol,* 69:1-9, 1964.
4. Bernard, J. L.: Rapid treatment of gross obesity by operant techniques. *Psychol Rep,* 23:663-666, 1968.
5. Bijou, S. W. and Baer, D. M.: *Child Development I: A Systematic and Empirical Theory.* New York, Appleton-Century-Crofts, 1961.
6. Bloom, W. L. and Eidex, M. F.: The comparison of energy expenditure in the obese and lean. *Metabolism,* 16:685-692, 1967.
7. Bortz, W.: A 500 pound weight loss. *Am J Med,* 47:325-331, 1969.
8. Bray, G. A.: Effect of caloric restriction on energy expenditure in obese patients. *Lancet* 2:397-398, 1969.
9. Bruch, H.: The psychosomatic aspects of obesity. *Am Pract Dig Treat,* 5:48-49, 1954.
10. Cappon, D.: Obesity. *Canad Med Assoc J,* 79:568-573, 1958.
11. Cattell, R. B. and Eber, H. W.: *Handbook for the Sixteen Personality Factor Questionnaire.* The Institute for Personality and Ability Testing, Champaign, Ill., 1957.
12. Cauffman, W. J. and Pauley, W. G.: Obesity and emotional status. *Penn Med J,* 64:505-507.
13. Cautela, J. R.: Covert sensitization. *Psychol Rep,* 20:459-468, 1967.

14. Cautela, J. R.: Behavior therapy and self-control: Techniques and implications. In *Behavior Therapy: Appraisal and Status* (Ed. C. M. Franks), New York, McGraw-Hill, 1969.
15. Conrad, S. W.: The problem of weight reduction in the obese woman. *Am Pract Dig Treat*, 5:38-47, 1954.
16. Cooper, K. H.: *Aerobics*. New York, Bantam Books, 1968.
17. Cornell Conferences on Therapy: The management of obesity. *N Y S J Med*, 58: 79-87, 1958.
18. Debry, G., Rohr, R., Azouaou, G., Vassilitch, I. and Mottaz, G.: Study of the effect of dividing the daily caloric intake into seven meals on weight loss in obese subjects. *Nutritio Dieta*, 10:288-296, 1968.
19. Durnin, J. V. G. A. and Passmore, R.: The relation between the intake and expenditure of energy and body weight. *Problemes Actuels D'Endocrinologie et de Nutrition* (Serie No. 9), 136-149, undated.
20. Ferster, C. B.: Classification of behavior pathology. In *Research in Behavior Modification* (Eds. L. Krasner and L. P. Ullmann), New York, Holt, Rinehart and Winston, 1965.
21. Franklin, R. E. and Rynearson, E. H.: An evaluation of the effectiveness of diet instruction for the obese. *Staff Meet Mayo Clin*, 35:123-124, 1960.
22. Glucksman, M. L., Hirsch, J., McCully, R. S., Barron, B. A. and Knittle, J. L.: The response of obese patients to weight reduction: A quantitative evaluation of behavior. *Psychosom Med*, 30:359-373, 1968.
23. Gordon, E. S.: The present concept of obesity: Etiological factors and treatment. *Med Times*, 97:142-155, 1969.
24. Hamburger, W. W.: Emotional aspects of obesity. *Med Clin N Am*, 35:483-499, 1951.
25. Hanley, F. W.: The treatment of obesity by individual and group hypnosis. *Canad Psychiat Assoc J*, 12:549-551, 1967.
26. Harris, M. B.: Self-directed program for weight control—A pilot study. *J Abnorm Psychol*, 74:263-270, 1969.
27. Hashim, S. A. and Van Itallie, T. B.: Studies in normal and obese subjects with a monitored food dispensary device. *Ann N Y Acad Sci*, 131:654-661, 1965.
28. Holland, J. G. and Skinner, B. F.: *The Analysis of Behavior*. New York, McGraw-Hill, 1961.
29. Homme, L. E.: Perspectives in psychology: XXIV. Control of coverants, the operants of the mind. *Psychol Rec*, 15:501-511, 1965.
30. Kanfer, F. H.: Self-monitoring: Methodological limitations and clinical applications. *J Consult Clin Psychol*, 35:148-152, 1970.
31. Kanfer, F. H. and Marston, A. R.: Conditioning of self-reinforcement responses: An analogue to self-confidence training. *Psychol Rep*, 13:63-70, 1963.
32. Kaplan, H. I. and Kaplan, H. S.: The psychosomatic concept of obesity. *J Nerv Ment Dis*, 125:181-201, 1957.
33. Konishi, F.: Food energy equivalents of various activities. *J Am Diet Assoc*, 46: 186-188, 1965.
34. Kornhaber, A.: Group treatment of obesity. *Gen Pract*, 5:116-120, 1968.
35. Kroger, W. S.: Comprehensive management of obesity. *Am J Clin Hypnosis*, 12: 165-176, 1970.
36. MacCuish, A. C., Munro, J. F. and Duncan, L. J. P.: Follow-up study of refractory obesity treated by fasting. *Br Med J*, 1:91-92, 1968.
37. Mayer, J.: Inactivity, an etiological factor in obesity and heart disease. In *Sym-*

    posia of the Swedish Nutrition Foundation, V: Symposium on Nutrition and Physical Activity (Ed. G. Blix), Uppsala, Sweden, Almqvist and Wiksells, 1967.
38. Mayer, J.: *Overweight: Causes, Cost and Control.* Englewood Cliffs, N. J., Prentice-Hall, 1968.
39. Mees, H. L. and Keutzer, C. S.: Short term group psychotherapy with obese women. *N W Med,* 66:548-550, 1967.
40. Metropolitan Insurance Company: New weight standards for men and women. *Statistical Bull,* 40:1-8, 1969.
41. Meyer, V. and Crisp, A. H.: Aversion therapy in two cases of obesity. *Behav Res & Therapy,* 2:143-147, 1964.
42. Modell, W.: Status and prospect of drugs for overeating. *JAMA,* 173:1131-1136, 1960.
43. Newburgh, L. H. and Johnston, M. W.: The nature of obesity. *J Clin Invest,* 8: 197-213, 1930.
44. Nisbett, R. E.: Taste, deprivation, and weight determinants of eating behavior. *J Pers Soc Psychol,* 10:107-116, 1968.
45. Nisbett, R. E. and Kanouse, D. E.: Obesity, food deprivation, and supermarket shopping behavior. *J Pers Soc Psychol,* 12:289-294, 1969.
46. Penick, S. B., Filion, R., Fox, S. and Stunkard, A.: Behavior modification in the treatment of obesity. Paper presented at the annual meeting of the Psychosomatic Society, Washington, D. C., 1970.
47. Powell, J. and Azrin, N.: The effects of shock as a punisher for cigarette smoking. *J Appl Behav Anal,* 1:63-71, 1968.
48. Ramsay, R. W.: Vermageringsexperiment, Psychologisch Labratorium van de Universiteit van Amsterdam, *Researchpracticum,* 101:voorjaar, 1968.
49. Schachter, S.: Obesity and eating. *Science,* 161: 751-756, 1968.
50. Schachter, S., Goldman, R. and Gordon, A.: Effects of fear, food deprivation, and obesity on eating. *J Pers Soc Psychol,* 10:91-97, 1968.
51. Schachter, S. and Gross, L. P.: Manipulated time and eating behavior. *J Pers Soc Psychol,* 10:98-106, 1968.
52. Seltzer, C. C. and Mayer, J.: A simple criterion of obesity. *Postgrad Med,* 38: A101-A106, 1965.
53. Shipman, W. G. and Plesset, M. R.: Anxiety and depression in obese dieters. *Arch Gen Psychiat,* 8:26-31, 1963.
54. Silverstone, J. T. and Solomon, T.: The long-term management of obesity in general practice. *Br J Clin Pract,* 19:395-398, 1965.
55. Simon, R. I.: Obesity as a depressive equivalent. *JAMA,* 183:208-210, 1963.
56. Stanley, E. J., Glaser, H. H., Levin, D. G., Adams, P. A. and Cooley, I. C.: Overcoming obesity in adolescents: A description of a promising endeavour to improve management. *Clin Pediat,* 9:29-36, 1970.
57. Stokes, S. A.: Fasting for obesity. *Am J Nurs,* 69:796-799, 1969.
58. Stuart, R. B.: Behavioral control of overeating. *Behav Res Ther,* 5:357-365, 1967.
59. Stuart, R. B.: Situational versus self control. In *Advances in Behavior Therapy* (Ed. R. D. Rubin). New York, Academic Press, in press.
60. Stuart, R. B. and Davis, B.: *Slim Chance in a Fat World. Behavioral Control of Obesity.* Champaign, Ill., Research Press, 1972.
61. Stunkard, A.: Eating patterns and obesity. *Psychiat Quart,* 33:284-295, 1959a.
62. Stunkard, A.: Obesity and the denial of hunger. *Psychosom Med,* 21:281-289, 1959b.

63. Stunkard, A.: Environment and obesity: Recent advances in our understanding of regulation of food intake in man. *Fed Proc,* 6:1367-1373, 1968.
64. Stunkard, A., Levine, H. and Fox, S.: The management of obesity. *Arch Intern Med,* 125:1067-1072, 1970.
65. Stunkard, A. and McLaren-Hume, M.: The results of treatment for obesity. *Arch Intern Med,* 103:79-85, 1959.
66. Suczek, R. F.: The personality of obese women. *Am J Clin Nutr,* 5:197-202, 1957.
67. United States Public Health Service: *Obesity and Health.* (Publication No. 1495), Washington, D. C., United States Department of Health, Education and Welfare, undated.
68. United States Senate, Select Committee on Nutrition and Human Needs: *Nutrition and Human Needs—1970.* Parts I, II and III. Washington, D. C., U. S. Government Printing Office, 1970.
69. Wagonfield, S. and Wolowitz, H. M.: Obesity and self-help group: A look at TOPS. *Am J Psychiat,* 125:253-255, 1968.
70. Wang, R. I. H. and Sandoval, R.: Current status of drug therapy in management of obesity. *Wis Med J,* 68:219-220, 1969.
71. Yudkin, J.: Sucrose and heart disease. *Nutrition Today,* 4:16-20, Spring, 1969.

16

Neurotic Obesity

GUSTAV BYCHOWSKI

CLINICAL observations forming the basis of the present study have been collected in the course of years. While acknowledging the merits of recent publications on the subject, the writer wishes to point out that he arrived at his conclusions independently from other investigators.

As can be easily surmised by any reader familiar with the subject, it is the contention of this study that in a group of cases obesity is a somatic manifestation of a personality disturbance. To be more specific, the writer will attempt to show that in his observation obesity is an expression and a result of autoplastic processes dominated and regulated by unconscious motivations. These processes became possible of materialization, since they succeeded in securing the services of preformed biological and chemico-physical mechanisms.

According to this general thesis the presentation will contain three distinct parts. The first will point out some philosophical premises and implications, the second and main part will present the clinical observations, the third part will indicate some of the underlying biological mechanisms.

As a motto I would like to quote Walt Whitman:

Behold, the body includes and is the meaning, the main concern and includes and is the soul[14]

When we look for philosophical premises for our investigation, we are inevitably attracted by Aristotle. He taught that the soul is the form of the body. The essential feature of the soul, in virtue of which it is the form of the body, is that it makes the body an organic whole, having unity of purpose. In the interpretation of Bertrand Russell whom I follow closely in this brief summary, individuality is connected with the body and the irrational soul, while the rational soul or mind is divine and impersonal.

Entelechy is an essential concept introduced by Aristotle to mean that which realizes or makes actual the otherwise merely potential. In a case of a living organism one may distinguish the mere matter of the organism (as though it were a mere synthesis of inorganic substances), from a certain form or essence or function of inner activity without which it would not really be a living organism at all.[10]

Lamarck in his second law expressed the idea that "the production of a new organ in an animal body results from the supervention of a new want

180

continuing to make itself felt, and a new movement to which this want gives birth to and encourages."[11]

Among modern philosophers Driesch who was originally a biologist taught that the organism is a harmonious equipotential system possessing a vital individualizing entelechy, which works through the matter with a view to the whole.[12]

Psychoanalysis has provided us with a modern version of a theory according to which the body of an individual may be shaped by his instinctual drives. It is in fitting with the essential trend of psychoanalysis that this point of view originated as a bold and profound speculation, based, however, on strictly empirical ground.

The concept of autoplastic materialization was evolved in common by Freud and Ferenczi in their discussions to mean a primitive stage of ego development as opposed to the ulterior stages described as alloplastic. While in the latter the individual attempts to alter reality, in the former own body is used as a medium for expression and alteration. Ferenczi introduces the concept of materialization as characteristic of hysteria: "It might be called a materialization phenomenon, since its essence consists in the realization of a wish, as though by magic, out of the material in the body at its disposal and, even if in primitive fashion, by a plastic representation, just as an artist moulds the material of his conception or as the occultists imagine the 'apport' or the 'materialization' of objects at the mere wish of a medium."[6]

In such pathological manifestations the ego reverts to the old autoplastic stage of development where the protopsyche (Ferenczi) is still extremely close to the soma, that is to the bodily ego.

Under condition of such topic regression charges of libidinal excitation are no longer disposed of in form of mental processes but, by and large, in motoric (hormonal, metabolic) discharges.

In the clinical part I shall present a synthesis of various observations, predominantly of female patients, some of them analyzed thoroughly, others only partially.

Some of the striking characteristics of our patients may serve as an introduction. It is easy to see that their attitude to food and to eating differs from the usual one. There is a definite compulsive feature to their eating; at times they feel that they must eat and overeat even if they know that it is harmful. While being deprived of the possibility to satisfy this compulsive need they may manifest considerable anxiety. In other words they behave like an addict deprived of his drug. This analogy goes even further. Like an addict they react to emotional frustrations with a relapse into or an increase of compulsive eating. Thus in working through transference phenomena we can observe that the patient reacts with depression and overeating to every new difficulty arising between himself and the analyst. He also uses his compulsion as an obvious weapon of resistance and defense against the physician.

Emotional instability, in particular the tendency to reactive depressions, less manifestly to elations, are other important characteristics of our patients.

It is then evident from the very onset that to their subconscious food has a very special meaning. Indeed analysis shows many such implications. Food means strength and serves to strengthen the weak ego. As one of my few belonging to this group of male patients put it: "one has more security when one has the stomach full."

This patient was an active homosexual given especially to oral practices. In his early history severe and constant disappointments in his father made him develop a regressive overfixation and identification with his mother. Homosexuality served as a search for a father substitute and at the same time as a method to replenish his depleted weak ego. With the progress of treatment, with changes in his ego-feeling, his physical ego feeling changed as well. He stopped his overeating and, while working more, he felt less tired and sleepy. Eventually, with a complete change in his sexual attitude, his compulsive need for food subsided completely.

Furthermore, the soothing effect of food as a powerful remedy for frustration and anxiety reveals that its symbolic implication is that of love, predominantly maternal love and breasts as the first distinct objectives of desire and gratification. Accordingly compulsive eating occurs as a direct result of separation anxiety in its various forms and at various levels. As a rule, whenever in analysis we worked through the paternal fixation and frustration, as expressed in terms of transference, there always emerged the preoedipal attachment to the mother, as an ultimate object of libidinal fixation and source of resistance.

One of my patients, whom we shall call Amelia, tense and full of anxiety during her period of depression, remained completely sleepless. Suddenly she would feel an urge to get up and eat, this despite her decision to reduce to which she stuck in the daytime. In analysis she remembered nocturnal fears of her childhood, her sharp craving for love and her terrible longing not to be alone, while she was jealous of all the other family members (parents and two brothers) being together.

The first unconscious implication of compulsive overeating is the securing of the mother in the most primitive but also the most efficient and complete form—introjection, that is cannibalistic incorporation. This desire is obviously a derivative of oral aggressiveness and brings the patient in situation of rivalry, that is hatred of a brother, a sister, or father. Deep ambivalence is characteristic of the relationship to the mother as well as to other family members.

This explains, in very general terms, to be sure, the feeling of guilt accompanying and following the compulsive overeating: the bliss which it accords the patient is never pure, untroubled. This feeling of guilt becomes then one of the determinants of periodic depressions so frequent in our cases, and leads to actions characteristic of a desire for atonement.

Amelia felt nauseated when she happened to witness an autopsy or was offered a bird or a fish to eat. Another patient, Alicia, incurred constant debts while buying gifts for her parents, in particular for her mother. Both patients arranged situations which forced them to remain tied up with their home despite inevitable frustrations and disappointments. Driven by their feeling of guilt and desire for atonement, they carefully avoided possible gratifications on a more mature level and turned their aggressive hatred toward themselves.

Identification through introjection of maternal breast had led to the retention of food in form of fat deposits. They began to appear at early age —period of infantile sexuality—and received a new push at various critical turning points of life history. Thus feminine features in bodily build would appear prematurely, creating a sort of hasty and incomplete feminine pseudoidentification. There was a pseudoidentification physically, since instead of true feminine features there appeared simulated femininity with accumulation of fat around the thorax, covering up underdevelopment of breasts, and around the stomach and the buttocks. Once this excess of fat is removed, one is more often than not surprised at beholding an undeveloped girlish creature emerging from beneath pillows of fat. Another typical element of maternal identification is a phantasy of pregnancy which manifests itself in accumulation of adipose masses in the abdominal region in fitting with the popular concept of the baby being carried "under the stomach."

There are many symptoms indicative of the forbidden character of this mother identification which results in guilt feeling and accounts for anguish and suffering accompanying materialization of this phantasy.

Phoebe, a patient suffering from a severe agoraphobia, used the phobic mechanisms in denying and masochistically distorting the feminine identification which she was unconsciously enacting. Her menstruation which stopped for years reappeared with the progress of analysis only to vanish when the pregnancy phantasy became the center of our discussions and after she finally began to indulge in some purely masturbatory activities with a young man. A memory from her fourth year showed her mimicking a passing-by woman, heavy with a child. This woman was either her mother or a substitute for her mother who at that time was pregnant with Phoebe's sister. Boys with whom she was playing at that time remarked that she should not make fun of the pregnant woman, since one day she would look exactly the same.

Phoebe's posture with her big protruding stomach used to worry her terribly; she considered it as one of her main handicaps preventing her from being attractive to men.

The birth of this sister proved to be one of the most fateful moments in Phoebe's biography, since it deprived her of her extremely privileged position of an only child, cherished by the mother, and spoiled in a senseless way by a psychopathic father.

Intense guilt feeling caused by the pregnancy phantasy had its main sources in oedipal jealousy and in the aggressive impulses aiming at the destruction of the mother's inside and the removal of the baby. Phoebe enacted autoplastically her phantasy of pregnancy and developed at an early age the disturbing posture. However, due to masochistic distortion, this wish fulfillment became fused with punishment and what remained of the initial phantasy was a cause for suffering and anguish. Phoebe fancied herself pregnant, abandoned by the seducer, alone and disgraced. During analysis this phantasy gained so much momentum that it made her fear pregnancy and speak of possible abortion after she had her first heterosexual contacts, involving not even an attempt at penetration and at a time when her menstruation reappeared after many months of amenorrhoea. (It was only natural then that it stopped again shortly after.) Phoebe disclosed that while she was masturbating her lover and was feeling with her hand the ejaculatory movements of his penis she had a very intense phantasy of feeling them inside her vagina.

Ambivalent attitude toward the mother makes feminine patients fear her revenge since they project their own hostility—both preoedipal and oedipal—onto their mothers. It is by no means surprising that in some cases this projection may have also an objective basis and simply serves to overemphasize real hostility and jealousy of the narcissistic mother. Fear of mother's revenge and punishment leads the patients to attempts to curb or to mask the feminine identification, to deny it in various ways. Naturally such attempts gain momentum in all the biological turning points of feminine development and become reactivated at important moments of possible feminine achievement.

Amelia experienced the most striking wave of overeating and gain in weight when she was sixteen. She tried to counter it by dieting and practicing exaggerated physical exercises. She felt very unhappy and unloved. One day she ate up a very sweet prune preserve prepared by the mother for her younger brother who was an apple of her eye. It stunned her since she was never gluttonous. She noticed that she put on weight which was unusual. She begged her mother not to feed her, she did not want to be "round," to which mother replied that it was foolish since she looked anyway like a boy.

At the same time Amelia suffered from her mother's manifesting a hostile attitude toward her sexual development. Of her growing pubic hair, her mother remarked: "You look like a monkey." She brushed off the girl's questions concerning menstruation with the remark that "this is stupid stuff, much too early for Amelia to know."

Amelia made some exhibitionistic overtures toward boys but rejected in indignation any advances which they attempted.

During analysis the hysteric mother developed some pseudoorganic symptoms and started to run from one doctor to another. Amelia thought that she wanted to draw attention to herself since Amelia who recently had had an appendectomy had been the center of family's attention for some time. Amelia knew all the time that her mother's illness was all fake. Yet she reacted with a depression and gain of weight: in making herself unattractive she was giving up the oedipal rivalry with her mother and was clearing the place for her.

Dreams and phantasies disclosed a severe castration fear centered around the mother who allegedly wanted to mutilate her and to damage her feminity. Amelia felt terribly sorry for castrated pigs; their screaming which she had heard in the country resounded for a long time in her ears. She reflected that these pigs when castrated became fat. Thus fat was to her an indicative of castration; at the same time it became a protection against castration since in pretending that one is already castrated, one may avoid true castration. In surrounding herself with a cushion of fat, she was unconsciously attempting to avoid her mother's wrath, since she was eliminating herself as a rival (Oedipus), and her father's anger at her potential relations with other men.

Denial of femininity was, generally speaking, a prominent feature in our cases. In symptomatology it manifested itself by amenorrhoea, homosexual episodes in which the patient played the aggressive rôle, avoidance of feminine grace and apparel. There was a complete vaginal anaesthesia and it was not until a fairly advanced stage of analysis that they "discovered" their vagina (expression of a patient). In deeper analysis it became clear that the patients had developed a deep masculine identification, constantly interfering with their biologically predetermined feminine rôle. Toward men they displayed typical attitudes characteristic of the feminine castration complex and penis envy. In behavior and mannerisms some of them showed distinct trends of masculinization. As an illustration I should like to mention Alicia who, as the only girl, went to a boy's college. Here she tried to imitate as completely as possible her schoolmates, learned to swear and to drink hard liquor. Later on, all throughout her brilliant professional career she managed to preserve those mannerisms, moving along ungraceful, sharp lines and using a biting language. Huge, sharp, and aggressive, she looked at times as if she were all ready to strike.

In the transference situation patients manifest bitter resentment toward the male analyst whose main objective seems to be to humiliate them, especially after he has succeeded in eliciting from them the admission of their femininity. After some stormy manifestations of their feminine desires in transference, they bitterly resent the inevitable frustration, promising themselves and the analyst that never more would they be fooled by false hopes and illusions; it is just not for them to have any share in a woman's happiness.

Similar reactions are likely to occur after therapeutic improvement resulting in first attempts at playing the feminine rôle in relationship to men. Doomed more often than not to failure, those attempts emphasize the inevitable frustration and seem to give right to the "foresight" of the patient who had always known that "love" was not for her and was, therefore, justified in avoiding it.

It is in fitting with the general picture that all those reactions of frustrated love and femininity result in relapses into oral gratification. What then is left after all to an unhappy and unloved female but sundaes, chocolate bars or a substantial order of spaghetti—all this between meals or even at night.

However, in reverting to food our patients not only seek a vicarious gratification and use mechanisms of feminine introjection and pseudo-identification. As much as their denial of femininity may manifest itself in somatic virilization, so in their psychodynamics they display a clear-cut masculine introjection and identification. In this aspect food functions as a symbolic substitute for the paternal or fraternal phallus: thus absorption of food represents a partial incorporation of one of their early male love objects. By the way of this incorporation there becomes established a primitive identification.

As may be expected, such identification occurs in the consequence of an early rejection by father or brother. Moreover, this mechanism becomes enhanced by frustration originating in maternal fixation and rivalry with the opposite sex for the mother. Invariably then the mother seems to prefer the male members of the family, and the little girl in trying to explain this injustice inevitably falls upon their phallic attribute. Consequently in introjecting and retaining the much envied phallus, she hopes to solve so many of her conflicts. Not only food, but another well-known primitive phallic substitute—faeces—becomes regressively overcathected, another factor contributing to the overwhelming predominance of retentive tendencies.

Amelia had displayed the first wave of overeating during early manifestations of the oedipal conflict. At the same time[4, 5] a traumatic event of serious impact had laid further foundations for the desire for annihilation and direct incorporation of the phallus. In one of her innumerable fights with her mother she became upset and vociferous, so that the mother in order to gain a better control of the situation and to punish her more effectively recurred to the help of the neighbor. This individual took Amelia into a separate room, threw her on the bed, beat her up, and put his penis into her mouth, threatening her that the next time he would strangle her.

When around puberty a new wave of overfeeding began to develop, it was in close connection with an apparently harmless yet quite significant occurrence as already mentioned. When the younger of her two older brothers had to study for his examinations, the mother became even more affectionate and demonstrative toward him than usually. Amelia was experiencing this closer union between the mother and the beloved brother as a double rejection and frustration. Everything would be so different she thought, if she too were a boy. One day the mother prepared for the boy a special very sweet prune preserve. Amelia got hold of it and helped herself to a substantial part of the jar. While absorbing it she had a deep feeling of guilt and anxiety and became nauseated. These manifestations became characteristic of her whole pattern of compulsive overeating, preceded by anxiety and followed by nausea and feeling of guilt.

Thus some of the symptoms and their dynamics are reminiscent of Dora, one of Freud's classic case histories. Phoebe, who as already mentioned, suffered from a serious agoraphobia, reacted with nausea and painful globus hystericus to every outside contact, in particular with men. These symptoms became strongly accentuated as a result of some transference situations. Her improvement began when she could admit her femininity: she even began to menstruate after many years of amenorrhoea. It was then that she presented the analyst (she was coming for treatment from out of town) with an unusual and at that time quite precious gift: a big piece of steak.

Incidentally it is not surprising that meat and particularly steak are to some of our patients of portentous importance, exceeding, so it seems at least to one observer, the usual American overestimation of meat.

Till her fourth-fifth year Phoebe had been treated with adulation by her psychopathic father. Unfortunately this "love-affair" ended in an abrupt rejection following the birth of her little sister. After falling from grace the former princess felt like an ugly Cinderella. Her adoration of her father gave way to unbound hatred and caused her to overemphasize her maternal fixation. She wanted to castrate her father and to retain his penis, so that she might play the masculine rôle in the relationship to both mother and sister. From now on she played only with boys; she even tried to match them in their admirable way of urination. She began to grow big and fat, lacking in feminine grace, trying to act manly and yet secretly yearning for women's happiness. This latter attitude, repressed and ever ready to burst forth, has prevented Phoebe from finding a compensation in a career for which her excellent intellectual endowment would have made her eminently fit. Her masculine identification has made her develop a manifest homosexual attitude. She had a regular affair with another young girl, and her latent neuroses broke out after her lover's marriage. For years to come women were her only companions and it was not until the late part of analysis that she was able to accept at first a social and then sexual contact with males.

Alicia had acted out at an early time the unconscious equation between the four elements of the chain: breast-food-penis-feces. In her libidinal regression she became eager not only to partially absorb her early love objects but to retain them as thoroughly as possible. As a little girl she used to devote much time to a characteristic bathroom phantasy. She would sit on the toilet and press with her foot on the floor, imagining that a phantastic Chinaman would either be kept inside or come out. It was a magic way of making the appearance of feces-penis dependent on her will. This phantasy had also an obvious masochistic implication since the appearance of the Chinaman was accompanied by thrilling fear in anticipation of his vague cruelty. This element was further developed in other phantasies. In one a man was carrying a girl upstairs, against her will, in others an undressed couple was tied up with ropes and thus forced to be together.

Since the introjected penis represented the father, it seemed quite naturally of a big size. Consequently Alicia not only felt that she had to be big herself, a direction in which she actually developed, but also could be interested only in big men. They had to be big at first literally, then in a figurative sense. She looked down on most men since they could never live up to her introjected ideal and inevitably appeared as a poor second-hand substitute for the magnificent father. The working through of this problem, in alimentary terms, was well illustrated by the following dream which occurred toward the end of analysis:

"I see turkeys prepared for myself but they are small like chickens."

In her comments and associations Alicia pointed out the shifting from the big paternal penis to somewhat normally sized objects of desire. Apparently she no longer looked upon herself as excessively big nor did she feel in need of a particularly big (important) male. In reality she lost so much weight that her whole appearance underwent a most striking change in the direction of attractive femininity. At the same time she also lost her vaginal anaesthesia; she "discovered her vagina" and became responsive in a normally feminine way to men.

To illustrate the profound changes brought about by analysis and some important aspects of therapy in this case I quote here the letter which she wrote to me four months after the termination of the treatment:

Until I was analyzed my whole approach to life was darkened and obstructed by my excessive obesity. I weighed 186 pounds at the age of 12; 286 at the age of 24. I was perpetually dieting. Every conceivable fad, fancy, or fact which might result in a loss of weight was tried by me. There was a never-ending cycle of losing and gaining.

If I were asked to characterize in one word my reaction to the psychoanalytic process in relation to the physical changes it has caused in me, I should say simply "miraculous." Although four months have elapsed since my last treatment, I cannot quite recover from the feeling of wonder at the changes in me. I find it hard to believe that I am not dreaming. As a matter of fact, I am still unable entirely to see myself as I really am now. I still have a tendency to think of myself in terms of my old girth. I cannot quite grasp that I am normal in size, inconspicuous, the same as other women. Each day brings its special joy in such small but enormously significant things as having some one comment on my slimness, or my good figure. Each day brings with it the continued wonder of being able to do things that were impossible for me hitherto—buying clothes in the misses' department stores, sliding through narrow spaces in crowded areas, using bright colors, wearing styles that were formerly tabu, evoking admiring glances from passers-by.

I find concrete tangible evidence of the success of my analysis in other physical changes such as menstruation. I was always irregular and my periods were preceded by deep depression. Menstruation has now become so regular that I can almost tell to the day and hour when it will start. While the premenstrual difficulty has not been entirely eliminated yet, it too has changed in character. I still feel a sort of malaise, premenstrually, but I have learned to recognize it for what it is and am able to disregard it.

An interesting reaction occurs in friends who see me now for the first time without knowing that I have undergone treatment. The extreme loss of weight is greeted with cries of delight and commendation. Then there follows a look of puzzlement and a groping after some elusive factor. They recognize other physical changes without being able to name them and solve the problem by indicating that I have grown either pretty or prettier, depending on their early estimates of my appearance. Actually, I don't believe that I have grown pretty as a result of analysis. I have never regarded myself as pretty. Nor do I believe, in spite of my high regard for the technique, that even analysis can make a pair of nylons out of sow's ear. My own explanation is that the process of resolving my inner tensions and conflicts has reflected itself in my face. What others see, apparently, is a serenity which was never there before. Since serene faces are rarities in this troubled world no one knows how to describe the phenomenon properly. Resort to existing nomenclature must be had. And so they say I've become good-looking.

I am still adjusting to my change in size. Where once I suffered agonies of embarrassment which had to be controlled forcibly whenever I had to enter a room full of strange people, I am now getting to the point where I don't even think of my appearance. This freedom from self-consciousness has increased my ability to meet and deal with others without preliminary hostility and the old desire to dominate. I can relax and be myself with the result that others find me more acceptable while I need not strain to make an impression.

One of the most important aspects of analysis in relation to the loss of weight, in my opinion, is the reducing process itself. Prior to analysis, I had changed doctors frequently or had embarked on reducing programs as a result of bribes or pep-talks by friends or my own shame. For a while the new relationship with my physicians or the enthusiasm engendered by my own or my friends' desires would carry me along. At one point or another, usually when I was near success (which at that time was considered a level of about 200 pounds) something would occur to upset my equilibrium and I would retrogress. Usually the cause was a feeling that there was too much effort for too little gain. And always I was disappointed at the results because they never came near what I had expected. In analysis all this was changed. The discussions preceding my initiating the diet awoke in me a feeling of shame at my own childish reaction to food and my lack of control in relation to it. In addition, the desire to stick to the regimen was accompanied by a strong desire to appear worthy in the eyes of my analyst of his good opinion of me. Almost from the beginning by some alchemy inherent in the relationship of patient and analyst, the abnormal craving for food abated. When it did recur, from time to time, the complete discussion and analysis of its causes and elements helped considerably in controlling it. The close relationship to my analyst and the knowledge that his strength and understanding were ever present and available to me to help me over the difficult spots did more than anything to keep me rigidly to the reducing program. For the first time in my life I was able to go for a period of six months without a single deviation from the diet and with no accompanying feeling of denial or martyrdom. I was filled with a sense of mastery, of release from slavery to my appetites. For the first time in my life I began to understand what an adult approach to the business of eating was like. After reaching my level of 160 pounds in six months, I was able to remain on a stabilizing diet with little difficulty. When I did go off on occasional rampages, I was always aware of the fact that it was only a temporary deviation and that in short order I would be back on the old routine.

It should be noted that I used no reducing medication during analysis. Prior to that time I had taken tons of pills and quarts of extracts. Although I took off sixty-five pounds in six months I lost proportionately and without becoming haggard or wrinkled. One of the most important results of my analytical dieting is the fact that no one can tell that I was ever obese. No one who has met me for the first time since my loss of weight has believed that I was ever as heavy as I claim to have been. It seems to me, as I review the process, that it was a stripping off rather than a losing program. It is my firm conviction that through no other process except analytical dieting can one attain and retain the results that I have achieved.

In general, my analysis has left me with a sense of renaissance. I regard my last treatment as the birthday of my life. I feel younger than ever before, I have a keener appreciation of my own possibilities and capabilities. I am able in my professional and business relationships to operate successfully at higher levels than ever before. Nothing seems too difficult. Nothing is impossible. I have a deep and abiding sense of security which expresses itself in the feeling that no ill can come to me because I have been provided with strong armor. In my situation involving others, I feel that I have the advantage because I have been analyzed and most others have not. And above all, for the first time in my life, I am at peace with myself.

The following dream illustrates one aspect of this change. "A young man sits on my lap and I become mildly but definitely aggressive toward him." The young man is a substitute for Alicia's only "lover" to whom she remained attached since her childhood. He was particularly fond of her "softness," as expressed in her obesity and enjoyed sitting on her lap like a baby. She was so big and fat that she could remain unaggressive, passive toward him. Now, she anxiously commented, she is losing this great asset, what will happen? Will she really, like in the dream, become aggressive toward males? We see here the shifting from purely maternal attitude toward men to a truly feminine one. The former was maintained in anxious avoidance of incestuous guilt.

Analysis of this patient offered insight into some of the secondary gains derived from adiposity. We found them to a various degree and in various combinations in other cases.

It appears that the adipose cushion served as a protection against masculine aggression and this in a double meaning of a literary protection and in making the young woman possibly unattractive. On the other hand it also helped to protect the patient from her own exhibitionism. She was so ugly that there was nothing to show up and to be proud of. However, in a truly masochistic distortion, through her adiposity, she achieved what she actually wanted to avoid, that is to defend herself against: her wish to be conspicuous and to draw attention to herself. In other words we may say that obesity served to express the idea that the more fat one would put on, the less temptation there would be for exposing oneself and the less danger for being assaulted. One was just a lump of fat and not a female.

Our observations clearly demonstrate the manifold implications of exaggerated absorption and retention of food. However, both medical and psychoanalytical observations point to another important factor of overweight in our patients, namely retention of fluid. Alicia who was most thoroughly observed by Dr. Julia Lichtenstein presented a definite water retention syndrome of high intensity. This could partly account for her increase in weight of 10 to 12 lb in a few days under conditions of emotional frustration and alimentary overindulgence, for instance, in some serious transference crisis or over the weekend. These medical data were paralleled by the following analytical observations. Alicia would weep with utmost facility at a slight emotional provocation. She was aware of this weakness and mentioned that her mother (who certainly had never read Dr. Greenacre's illuminating paper) used to say that she urinated with her eyes.[7]

Since her teens Alicia was an expert in controlling her bladder, urinating rarely, delaying the procedure to the utmost, at times as long as ten hours. She felt that urination was a "dirty and messy business." Her younger brother used to wet the bed "terribly"; she was proud that it never happened to her. In one and a half years of analysis the patient never visited my bathroom; she felt embarrassed, she explained. Moreover, she perspired very little and was proud of it, being particularly sensitive to bodily odors.

In a dream she became all wet, splashing over a water pool in her rush to keep her analytical appointment. It became clear from the whole material that for her urination was tied up with the castration complex and penis envy. Thus delaying of micturition was a manifestation not only of the wish for retention, but also of repression of castration anxiety and of the whole feminine rôle.

The intimate interplay between water retention and psychodynamic factors involving frustration, be it real, anticipated or imaginary, is certainly a striking phenomenon. It becomes perhaps more clear when compared with experimental data on "water balance in the alarm reaction." Selye, Howlett, and S. S. Browne studied animals exposed to conditions of stress and alarm. They found marked water retention and edema formation under the influence of gastric and intestinal manipulation and of histamine injection. Under conditions of experimental stress and danger the animals showed tendency to retention of intravenously injected saliva solution. They developed edema and transudates in the pleura and in the peritoneum.[8]

Those experimental phenomena are a part of what Selye calls the adaptation syndrome. It is important to note that purely functional nervous commotions such as rage and fear may act as strong alarming stimuli and produce the adaptation syndrome in its various forms. There is also some evidence that many if not all the manifestations of the general adaptation syndrome are due to conditioned reflexes.

The following elements of the general adaptation syndrome are relevant to our study. The adaptation syndrome exerts a very marked effect upon carbohydrate metabolism. Lipid metabolism is also affected since marked lipid deposits may suddenly appear in the liver during the course of the alarm reaction.

"During the general adaptation syndrome certain hormones of the anterior pituitary and adrenal cortex are produced in excessive amount in order to increase resistance; this defensive endocrine response is valuable inasmuch as it facilitates adaptation to stress (e.g. infections, intoxications, nervous commotions, and cold) but the resulting hormone overdosage may become the cause of certain cardiovascular, renal, and joint diseases."[13] During the alarm reaction the need for sugar is increased.

In trying to connect these experimental data with our clinical observations we may assume that the ego of the patient, feeling weak and threatened since early childhood has developed a set of somatic reactions based on old, primitive mechanisms reaching deep into the metabolic processes.

Some of these mechanisms were involved in retention of fluid, others in increased production and retention of hormones and certain metabolites, especially fat.

We are now in the possession of certain clinical and experimental data which permit some, even when dim, understanding of underlying biological mechanisms.

Mobilization of adrenalin secretion under the impact of situations involving emotional stress and danger is a well established fact, since it has been demonstrated by the classic studies of Cannon.[3] Moreover, it has been shown that the adrenalin outpour acts as a stimulant increasing greatly within a short time the fatty acids in the blood plasma (Himwich and collaborators).[4] Jones and Fish observed in man a typical rise in the plasma fatty acids after an intramuscular adrenalin injection.[5] Cannon concludes that the adrenal medulla may play a role in the homeostasis of fats in blood.

"Increased adrenal secretion is a more important factor in liberating sugar from the hepatic stores than in the direct action of nerve impulses" (Cannon). In sham rage there occurs an increase of blood sugar which rises to five times of the normal content. However, when glucose is provided in abundance, it is utilized by the organism in preference to fat, so that the burning of fat is almost completely stopped. Excess of glucose is either promptly utilized or it becomes converted into glycogen and stored in the liver and in the muscular system—or it becomes converted into fat.

To all these data we must add significant observations on "correlation between emotions and carbohydrates metabolism in two cases of diabetes mellitus." The authors came to the conclusion that "these food demanding drives, under the condition that nobody is there to satisfy them externally, may turn to an autoplastic satisfaction in a metabolic process which mobilizes glucose out of the glycogen stores of the body."[9]

If we bear in mind the intricate interplay between emotions and the endocrine system, both directly and through the medium of nervous impulses, then the autoplastic expression of prolonged unconscious and, therefore, almost permanent conflicts, defense and compensation mechanisms comes within our grasp.

At the basis of such a development we may conjecture a system of conditioned biochemical reflexes functioning in a circular way. Frustration and threat to the ego makes it reach into the deep somatic resources and mobilize hormones and metabolic processes. It is not long before every occurrence which may acquire the meaning of a threat to the ego acts as such a stimulus. However, because of an increased mobilization and utilization of sugar and possibly other metabolites, the need for a metabolic gratification becomes greater and greater, so that, similar to an addict, more supply is needed to provide both the psychological and chemical gratification. The storage of fat, and possibly retention of liquid, increases according to biochemical mechanisms which we begin to perceive, and along psychological vectors which we have tried to outline.

Moreover, important mechanical and behavioristic factors are at work to add momentum to the physical distortion of the individual. They have been studied particularly well by Hilde Bruch and we can only confirm her observations and conclusions.

The obese child naturally avoids movement and, in so doing, prevents an important outlet for the utilization of fat deposits. Thus he remains more dependent on his environment, especially on the mother who helps to maintain his infantilism. On the other hand, he tries to compensate in mobilizing his growth hormones and in developing an exaggerated bodily size. This contradictory line of development has been well defined by Hilde Bruch who said that "the inordinate expansion reveals the inmost desire of the child to be big and powerful" and pointed out that "this rapid rate of physical development belies all attempts to keep him small and dependent and contradicts his immature and babyish behavior."[2a]

I would like to say a few more words about some psychoanalytical implications of our study. Dealing with our patients we were led to consider problems of oral incorporation of early love-objects. This incorporation we must call a partial one and in our attempt for some theoretical clarification we turn quite naturally to Abraham.[1] It was he who distinguished partial from total incorporation and saw in the former a progress insofar as the incorporating childish ego no longer wants to destroy the object through complete cannibalism but sufficiently cares for it in order to preserve it in its totality, except for the incorporated part. According to our material we would formulate that our obese patients want to incorporate their love-objects in part in order to retain and to preserve them indefinitely. In so doing they strive at the possession of the love-objects, which otherwise, so they feel, would evade them. On the other hand, their aim is to escape from the conflict of ambivalence which is so characteristic of their early love relationships. Instead of either losing the object completely or else destroying it just as thoroughly in their phantasy, they try to avoid the issue by regressing to what Abraham called the preambivalent stage of orality. He equated this stage with sucking, since this kind of interest in the object is naturally free from any hostile-aggressive drives which emerge later. To regress to such a stage requires obviously a great deal of early oral fixation and narcissistic endowment.

The love object itself, when equated with excrements becomes a much more natural object for retention, for which purpose the anal libido is being vigorously mobilized and reinforced.

Identification with the love object on the one hand and its constantly impending loss originating in insufficiently repressed destructive part of ambivalence are responsible for the definitely depressive touch so characteristic of the clinical picture of our patients.

In their desire for incorporation and retention of the love objects, patients try to achieve the impossible ideal of complete self-sufficiency, that is independence from the frustrating and evasive love objects. Finally we may formulate that the autoplastic distortion is a climax of processes aiming at the eternal retention of the main love objects with whom the infantile ego tries to achieve a permanent identification.

Unfortunately in this identification the ego cannot be selective and must absorb the good and the bad objects alike. Its attempts to achieve the bliss of complete introjection and identification are all in vain. Not only does reality contradict such a happy narcissistic solution; what is more, both contradictory identifications struggle with each other. As a result the patients are neither feminine enough nor can they achieve a successful masculine identification. Caught in the trap of their early ego weakness and primitive defenses and compensations, they are too big to impress the environment as lovable females and too soft to strike it efficiently with their aggression.

While bound on retaining their love objects permanently they try to imprison them within themselves so as not to have to face their loss. However, instead of reducing the liberty of the objects, they themselves become compulsively bound to them and thus put fetters on their own freedom.

Thus the autoplastic distortion of physical personality performed by the incorporated love objects is an adequate expression of the distortion of psychological personality.

In conclusion of our study we may formulate:

Neurotic obesity in women is an autoplastic manifestation of various unconscious impulses and ego-defenses. Among the former we find derivatives of oral drives aiming at partial incorporation and retention of both maternal and paternal love-objects. This incorporation, while expressing early fixations which become regressively increased as a result of early frustrations, is the basis for an attempted identification with both parents (or siblings). This double identification interferes with the development of a normal feminine personality and produces a trend toward masculinization. Thus the wish for bigness and exaggerated growth finds its utmost physical expression.

On the side of the defense mechanisms this autoplastic alteration tries to deny femininity and to prevent exogamous heterosexual love relations. The wall of fat serves as a protection against the wish for exhibitionism and for masculine aggression.

In trying to impersonate both the breast and the phallus patients develop to a sort of monstrosity and forfeit their claims to both love and strength. Thus the punishing superego received at least as much gratification as the id.

Obesity may evolve on the basis of early nutritional or endocrinological abnormalities which are being exploited by the subconscious. Overvaluation of food develops in a way of an addiction taking advantage of early established conditioned reflexes connecting the soothing of anxiety and frustration with food. Metabolism is being shifted accordingly toward retention of both fat and fluid. The former is supplied not only by ingestion from the outside but also it evolves, in a truly autoplastic way, from reserves of glucose which are being mobilized out of the glycogen stores of the body.

REFERENCES

1. Abraham, Karl: A Short Study of the Development of the Libido, Viewed in the Light of Mental Disorders. Selected Papers, London Institute for Psychoanalysis, 1942.
2a. Bruch, Hilde: Obesity in childhood and personality development. J Orthopsychiat, 11:1941.
2b. Bruch, Hilde and Touraine, G.: Obesity in childhood: The family frame of obese children. Psychosom Med, 2:141-206, 1940.
2c. Bruch, Hilde: Obesity in childhood: Physiological and psychological aspects of food intake of obese children. Am J Dis Child, 59:739-781, 1946.
3. Cannon, W. B.: The Wisdom of the Body. New York, Norton, 1939.
4. Ibid.
5. Ibid.
6. Ferenczi, S.: Collective Papers. Compiled by Rickman. London, Hogarth Press and Institute of Psychoanalysis, 1926.
7. Greenacre, Phyllis: Pathological weeping. Psychoanal Quart, 14:62-75, 1945.
8. Howlett and Browne: Studies on water balance in the alarm reaction. Am J Physiol, 128:225-332, 1940.
9. Meyer, Bollmeier and Alexander: Correlation between emotions and carbohydrate metabolism in two cases of diabetes mellitus. Psychosom Med, 7:335-342, 1945.
10. Russell, Bertrand: A History of Western Philosophy. New York, Simon and Schuster, 1945.
11. Ibid. and Encyclopedia Britannica.
12. Ibid.
13. Selye, Hans: The general adaptation syndrome. J Allerg, 17:231-239, 289-319, 358-386, 1946.
14. Whitman, Walt: Starting from Paumanok, Stanza 13.

17

Psychological and Physiological Aspects of Marked Obesity in a Young Adult Female

A. Russell Lee

Dr. A. Russell Lee

The case to be presented focuses upon the problems of obesity, in terms of psychodynamics, physiology and treatment.

PRESENTING PROBLEM

Miss B. B., twenty-three years old, single, white, Jewish, 5 feet tall and weighing 340 lb, was admitted to Hillside Hospital in early August 1956, looking tense, fearful, and self-conscious. Coherently and intelligently, she related that in the past two years she had been having "more and more difficulty functioning." She had become unable to hold a job as secretary, or do her housework. In the past six months she had become too self-conscious to leave her house except for a rare automobile ride. She had been "eating compulsively," especially at night, and spent most of the day sleeping, sometimes as much as seventeen hours per day, awakening only to eat. In two years she had gained over 150 lb. During these two years she had been living with a young man. Their relationship was filled with constant bickering, fighting, insults, jealousy, and mutual torment. They were "completely dependent on each other" and she "hated it."

FAMILY BACKGROUND

The patient was born in 1933 in New York City to a family torn with marital strife. She was the younger of two siblings, having a brother four years older. When the patient was four years old, her father left home after an argument with her mother. When the patient was seven, he died of a heart attack.

Her father had been a cafeteria owner and diabetic. Her mother spoke hatefully of him as a "no-good gambler who ran around with young women and only wanted children in order to hurt her." The patient remembers being asked by her mother to spy on him. In contrast to her mother, she remembers him as a "nice man, who liked me, accepted me, and was proud of me." She blames their difficulties on her mother. It is interesting that Mrs. B. (the patient's mother), in her contacts with our social worker, has only spoken highly of her dead husband.

Mrs. B. is fifty years old, well-groomed, heavy but not obese, and bears

197

a strong physical resemblance to the patient. She has always worked in restaurants and has had weight problems herself. She describes her early childhood as emotionally and financially deprived. As the oldest of five sisters and one brother, she assumed responsibilities at an early age. She remarried a few years ago and it ended rather quickly in divorce. She has been inconsistent with her daughter, ranging from overindulgence to screaming arguments and overt rejections. At the hospital she promised the patient new clothes if she lost weight but brought her candy and cake. She does not see the patient as sick, but blames her problem on her obesity and her boyfriend. She weeps that the patient is in a place like this, but welcomes the hospital taking over her responsibility.

The patient sees her mother as aggressive, dominating, inconsistent, stingy, punitive, lying. She blames her for always having made her feel ugly, and giving her the feeling that she could never do anything right.

The patient's brother and only sibling is twenty-seven years old, and has weighed 250 lb. The patient describes him as a "sharpy type, someone to be scared of," but now pities him. They used to go on food binges together when children, looking for hidden or locked-up food and candy and often eating "candy, box, wrapper, string and all." At 8½ her brother made sexual overtures to her, and she very guiltily recalls that they had relations for which she was often bribed with either money or food, when she was between eleven and thirteen. These stopped after he was sentenced to jail for robbery. In the past eleven years he has been almost constantly in jail or on parole, and is now in jail.

EARLY DEVELOPMENT AND HISTORY

According to the mother, the patient was a wanted child. She wanted a girl to name after her own mother who had just died. Her pregnancy and delivery were normal and fairly easy. The patient weighed five pounds at birth. She was bottle-fed, as was her brother, on the advice of the physician. The mother does not remember if she was demand or clock-fed but says that B. was "normal" and immaculate in her eating habits. She walked and talked by fourteen months. Bowel training was easily accomplished by one year, but B. has remained enuretic up to the present despite many efforts at control by the mother. She has only been enuretic at the hospital once or twice.

After the death of the patient's father, her mother returned to work and has worked continuously since. The children were cared for by nurses or relatives but mostly had to fend for themselves. During this early period, B. developed many somatic complaints. A doctor advised that there was nothing physically wrong but that she was seeking attention. The mother solved this by giving her huge and elaborate bandages. When the patient was eight, the children were sent to the same camp and then to the same boarding school for a year, after which they returned home.

It was about this time that food became an issue in this family. Food closets were now locked. Butter and other foods were measured. The night eating pattern was probably established at this time. When her mother returned from work, the children used to gather around, talk, do home-work, and eat. Often several boxes of cookies and three to four quarts of milk were consumed in one evening.

Between thirteen and fourteen the fights with her mother became ex-treme and there were many temper tantrums on both sides. At fourteen she was locked out of the house by her mother and had to live with a ma-ternal aunt. During their many subsequent arguments, the patient would on occasion retaliate by locking her mother out. This has continued up un-til the present. At one time or other she has lived with each of her four aunts and one uncle. She sees these aunts as aggressive women married to weak men. One has been married seven or eight times, and the uncle is called "Sis." At twenty she entered Bellevue Hospital voluntarily for five days to "show her mother that something was really wrong." She was ad-vised that she needed psychotherapy, but her mother interpreted the hos-pitalization as proving that she was a "spoiled brat." Following this, she saw several psychiatrists sporadically, but these attempts were short-lived and characterized by missed sessions and lateness.

School and work records were erratic. She left high school in her third year. At school she was perfectionistic and felt she was not doing well enough. As a secretary she would redo her letters so often that she could not produce enough and was discharged. She was consistently late for work and wanted special permission to report late.

At twenty-one she went to live with K., a passive dependent boy who had followed her around for many years. He brought her sweets and then be-rated her for eating them, thus reestablishing the earlier sadomasochistic relationship. He wanted to marry her but she says this would have "been suicide" for her. However, she gained much satisfaction from being desired by this "handsome" young man. They leaned heavily on each other and she "hated the dependency of it." Since her hospitalization, he has de-compensated a good deal and has been unable to work.

PSYCHOSEXUAL HISTORY

The patient remembers her brother first "trying to fool around with her" when she was eight. At this time also they began to go on "food binges" together. He is the only one with whom she has gone on such a "binge." Under the brother's guidance, and bribed with food and money, their relationship became overtly incestuous when she was eleven. Her brother and her boyfriend K. are the only two persons with whom she has been sexually intimate. With neither one has the experience been pleasurable, nor has she had vaginal orgasm; with them oral sex is the "lesser of two evils." Following sexual activities she feels "repulsive" and eats in order to relieve this feeling. Following an eating binge, she will also have a feeling of repulsion and often is enuretic. Enuresis and eating are also connected in that she remembers having had to restrict liquids at night; when the enuresis persisted, she was deprived of desserts and other foods. Although she denies any fantasies during or after masturbation, her fantasies while eating are of herself as a beautiful, thin woman who can do anything, who is an accomplished pianist and who is ravishingly attractive to men. When she has been eating heavily, she feels less need to masturbate. It is pertinent that the patient speaks with the same reluctant and guilty affect about her excess eating as she does about her sexuality. When asked about this, she said that it was as difficult for her to describe her eating binges as for other people to describe their sexual activities. On dates she was too uncomfortable and embarrassed to eat at all, and would wait until she came home to gorge herself.

The patient's menses began at twelve and were reacted to with shame and guilt. Her periods had been regular until nine months ago. Since then she has been amenorrheic.

MENTAL STATUS

At her initial interview, the patient, despite her great weight, presented the appearance of an attractive young woman, neatly and plainly dressed. Her weight gave her a pseudo femininity which really disguised an adolescent girl. She was tense, apprehensive, self-conscious, and somewhat overly polite. Although she could respond warmly, laugh, and smile appropriately, on a deeper level, she was depressed. She answered questions intelligently and coherently, denied hallucinations and delusions now or in the past. She also denied current suicidal thoughts, but admitted that about two years ago in a fit of jealousy and rage she had swallowed many Dexedrine tablets in an effort to hurt herself. She was correctly oriented, judgment and insight were fair. For years she had hoped that her obesity was "glandular," but had become convinced that it was due to her emotional problems. She was afraid of blood tests, of being enuretic, of going to meals or of meeting other patients (especially males); she feared we would not be able to help her and would "ship her to Kings County"; and that if she argued with any of the staff, she would be discharged immediately. She was too frightened and embarrassed to allow a gynecologist to examine her despite complaints of a groin abscess.

Our psychiatric diagnosis was psychoneurosis, mixed type, with neurotic character traits.

PHYSIOLOGIC SUMMARY

The patient showed a central type of obesity largely sparing her extremities. She was five feet tall and weighed 340 lb on admission. She had purplish striae on her chest, abdomen, and buttocks. She had been amenorrheic for nine months. She was normotensive (130/80). She had no hirsutism. Laboratory examinations reveal normal CBC and normal urinalysis. The Thorn test showed an eosinophile count of 277 per cubic millimeter which dropped to 55 per cubic millimeter after ACTH. A repeat eosinophile count later was 109 per cubic millimeter. BMR was plus 6 per cent. PBI was 4.7 per cent μmg. X-rays of her chest and skull were normal. X-rays of her long bones could not be read for osteoporosis because of obesity. FBS was 83 per cent mg. Blood, calcium, sodium, and potassium were normal. Oral glucose tolerance test revealed a mild diabetic type curve (FBS—90, 30 minutes—179, one hour—153, two hours—132, three hours —126, four hours—77, five hours—100% milligrams). Urinary steroid levels revealed:

1. 17 Ketosteroids—20 mg/24 hours
2. 17 Hydroxysteroids—10.9 mg/24 hours
3. 11 Oxysteroids—2.8 mg/24 hours

All these fractions are elevated and are at least suggestive of a Cushing Syndrome.

COURSE IN THE HOSPITAL

For the first week or so the patient had to be served her meals on the ward which she never left for any activities. She expressed concern over her aching feet and said they pained her too much to walk. Gradually she became more comfortable. She became a kind of ringleader and clown for many of the younger, less psychotic but more emotionally deprived patients. Her room became a meeting place for food, jokes, and card-playing. She was elected housekeeper and president of the ward, so that "she wouldn't have to do any work herself."

The next stage was her gradual activation out of the ward into hospital activities. This was slow and difficulties still exist. At present she is the editor of the hospital newspaper. Although she is unable to delegate responsibility, she has done a rather good job and has derived much satisfaction from this. With the nursing staff she can be rather trying, especially the night staff, where her attempts at night activity create conflict. When provoked she erupts into abusive tirades. At times she manages to disguise her hostility by sarcastic jokes. At still other times, she can be warm and charming. Her main difficulties in interpersonal relations stem from her low frustration tolerance, her resentment of any authority, and her attempts to manipulate her environment to gain special status and privileges.

She varies from a shy, withdrawn, passive, dependent individual to a highly aggressive, outgoing, independent, often hostile, ringleader.

THERAPY

My goal in psychotherapy with this patient has been to establish a relationship and a program, with consistency as its key theme and with a firm reality base. This approach was considered essential in view of her former object relationships which have been intermittent, inconsistent, and paradoxical. In addition, our aims were to help modify her unrealistic goals and provide means for raising her self-esteem, gathering satisfactions and discharging aggression other than by eating.

Strong support and praise have been given for all the group activities in which she has participated. At the same time, I have insisted, without being rigid, that she conform to all hospital regulations.

Her obesity has been treated as of secondary importance. At her request she was prescribed a reducing diet and given 5 mg of Dexedrene three times a day before meals. Against her wishes, but for the sake of consistency, her relatives have been prohibited from bringing her food. They have been advised to bring her cosmetics, clothes or costume jewelry in order to increase her markedly diminished feminine feeling and strivings. When she lost weight, she was praised for it. Here again it was necessary to curb her grandiose self-demands. A weight loss of 2 or 3 lb per week was set as a reasonable goal instead of the 6 or 7 lb per week that she considered the only proof of doing a good job. She has lost about 55 lb since she has been here.

Her relationship with, and her feelings about her mother, father, brother, her other relatives, and her boyfriend are being explored both directly and as manifested in her transference reactions. It is hoped that very gradually her unrealistic self-demands, her low frustration tolerance, her provocation-rejection cycle, and her sadomasochistic trends can be explored and more realistic sublimations and goals established.

SUMMARY AND DISCUSSION

The patient illustrates the background, psychologic and characterologic problems of the neurotic obese. In addition there is evidence of distinct concomitant physiologic dysfunction. She comes from a family background in which there was much marital strife. Her father died when she was seven. Her relationship with her mother was always severely troubled and unstable. Her mother is seen as dominating, aggressive, inconsistent, punitive, lying. Food was the battlefield for much of their difficulties as well as the tie for their good times. There were many early separations from home which have continued to the present. An actual incestuous relationship with her brother existed through her adolescence. Her brother developed the dual problems of the obese and the psychopath. Finally in the last two years she reestablished another sadomasochistic relationship in the course of which she gained over 150 pounds and became "completely unable to function."

Although food began to be an overt battleground for mother and daughter at least as far back as the child's seventh or eighth year, it wasn't until the patient was about sixteen that she became obese. During the early years, food served to pacify the anxiety of her many separations, and food became a "substitute satisfaction of one instinctual urge—hunger—for the satisfaction for another—love" (Anna Freud). These early years seem to have established the prototype of her night-eating so characteristic later.

With the repeated rejections from her highly ambivalent mother, food began to serve the instinctual aggressive urges. When angry, she would "go on rampages" of eating. Thus was established the patient's first sadomasochistic relationship in which the patient could hurt her mother by hurting herself. Now when she goes on a diet, it must be a starvation diet or real torture—eating anything at all is breaking the diet. With the development of her obesity, this narcissistic, exhibitionistic, contradictory patient confirmed her ugliness and her disgust for her body. She now was forced to hide. At the same time, she had developed a fortress of flesh which could be used offensively and defensively and which protected her against both sexuality and hostility. Her thin, megalomanic, grandiose, perfectionistic, driving person was protected by the fat one from having to compete, thereby both assuaging and exaggerating the low self-esteem, lack of self-confidence and self-reliance, guilt feelings and fear of failure of her thin introject. Thus her obesity presents a jolly façade of independence, importance, and prowess which covers a passive, insecure, dependent, helpless child.

Food for this patient has become a polyfactored symbol which results in immediate relief of tension and which feeds her love needs, her aggressive drives, her low self-esteem and her depression.

PSYCHOLOGICAL EXAMINATION

Mrs. Sylvia Markham

The patient, an unmarried, extremely obese woman of twenty-three years, obtained an IQ of 125 on the short form of the Wechsler-Bellevue Intelligence Scale, indicating intellectual functioning on a superior level. The wide scatter of subtest scores ranging from an IQ of 106 (average) in picture arrangement to an IQ of 147 (very superior) in similarities points to such severe disruption of ego functioning that pathology must be suspected. Impairment in judgment in structured situations is indicated (comprehension IQ 110) and suggests an emotional instability of long standing. She experienced difficulty in responding to the questions that demanded common sense. There appeared to be a lapse in attention as her eyes drooped and took on a faraway expression. Her behavior did not reflect as much a disruption of concentration as a tendency toward withdrawal. Actually, her ability to concentrate is being maintained on a superior level as disclosed in the arithmetic IQ of 121. To the question "Why are laws necessary?" she responded, "That's a very good question (laughs) because the government has to make money (this statement was a repetition of a previous response, suggesting some stickiness of thinking). I'm back to the first one. I'm being facetious. Without laws there would be no organization in our lives at all. (We have laws) in order to live and not eat each other up figuratively." Her perception of people as orally devouring creatures who require outside restraint to inhibit their natural cannibalistic instincts is very significant, in the light of this woman's compulsive eating. It also points to her marked trend to project her own orally incorporating urges onto the environment. Paranoid tendencies are likewise disclosed in the patterning of subtest scores in which her ability to abstract and see relationships is very much higher than her ability to anticipate and interpret correctly social and sexual stimuli. She seems to feel that people are out to trick her, and at one point asked the examiner if there was a catch in one of the tests. There are indications of psychopathic-like and manipulating behavior which she attempts to disguise by a jocular, bantering, and sophisticated manner.

Her reactions to the Rorschach reveal an introversive woman who is living largely in her fantasy, as a way of escaping a harsh reality. Relying heavily on constricting and obsessive-compulsive defenses, she is unable to successfully repress the emergence of some autistic fantasy. On Card 4 (father card) of the Rorschach, she responded with a "knocker" to an area often perceived as a phallic symbol. In the inquiry, in a free-associative manner, she described this as a knocker that was on a door of a school that she attended in Tarrytown when she was seven years old. Her father had just died and her mother sent her away to this institution which she hated. She said that it was her first separation from her mother. She went on later (on Card 8) to describe the school as a castle, surrounded by mountains which, despite its frightening and painful memories, attracted her and to which she often returned on a visit. She dreamed of buying this place. She claimed that her experiences in this school was her earliest clear memory. She seems to have experienced this episode as a rejection and a punishment. The expulsion from her home was probably viewed as a punishment for her libidinal feelings for the father, meted out by a mother whom she perceived as a rival. The compulsive need to revisit the scene of all these painful experiences points to strong masochistic tendencies in the patient. She is a woman who suffers tremendous feelings of guilt which she must expiate by turning her aggression toward herself. Her compulsive eating may be viewed in terms of her need to punish herself.

Her affect is not of an explosive or uncontrolled quality but is often inappropriate. She appears to be depressed but makes strenuous efforts to overcome her dysphoric mood, often using humor to pull her out of her doldrums. She experiences difficulty in expressing her hostility and vacillates constantly in giving vent to her destructive urges. After making a highly critical or hostile statement, she regrets it and tries to undo it. She seems to be extremely frightened by the vast store of hate that she harbors. Because of her infantile attachment to the maternal figure, her hostile feelings are so threatening and shattering to her own survival, that she is not able to maintain these negative feelings, nor to explore the depths of these feelings. On the Sentence Completion test she reacted fearfully when her relationship to her brother was touched upon. It would appear that her aggression had always to be expressed in an oblique manner, such as enuresis in childhood. Despite the tremendous hate for her mother, she is constantly seeking her approval.

Having introjected this castrating, critical, punitive maternal figure, she views herself through the eyes of this image. She possesses very low self-esteem, thinks she is a "slob" and is most annoyed by "fat people." Her response on Card 7 (mother card) of "this could be a piece of fried shrimp with a tail" suggests her oral fixation on the maternal image as well as the perception of this image as endowed with phallic strength. She appears extremely confused sexually as indicated by her response on Card 3 of "men because of their penis . . . but I notice that the men have breasts." This breast-penis equation causes her to seek out men primarily as a means of gratifying her tremendous oral needs. She is sexually frigid, frightened of men but must submit to their advances in order to get the ego-bolstering and the oral gratification she needs. Her flight into a heterosexual affair appears to be a defensive maneuver to avoid a homosexual entanglement, as well as a means of dealing counterphobically with a situation which she perceives as a highly destructive act. On Card 5 of the Rorschach she responded with a "stethoscope or some kind of clamp" to which she added in the inquiry, "did you read the Sheppard Case—that's what he was supposed to have clobbered his wife with—I am trying to be completely honest." This response was followed by "a little girl holding their legs together." She still possesses many pregenital sexual urges, including voyeurism, sucking, and masturbation. There is a strong suggestion that some of her guilt is related to masturbatory activity which she unconsciously feels has deformed her body. She also seems to have witnessed primal scenes which she interpreted as sadistic acts. She would like to be able to gratify her sexual demands narcissistically in autoerotic ways but her need for oral supplies forces her to seek out relationships with others. Feelings of inner emptiness and tension which she probably experiences as a sense of boredom are also likely to force her into compulsive eating.

DIAGNOSTIC IMPRESSION

An underlying depression in an orally fixated, masochistic woman who uses obsessive-compulsive defenses to allay her anxiety and her feelings of inner emptiness. She seems moving at present in the direction of a schizophrenia.

SOCIAL WORKER'S REPORT

Mrs. Marilyn (Reiss) Weiss

Social service contacts have been with the patient and her mother. Mrs. B. was first seen by the intake social worker during the admissions process. At that time, Mrs. B. exhibited strongly mixed feelings and attitudes toward patient. She saw the patient's problem mainly in terms of her obesity and her relationship with the boyfriend. Mrs. B. was eager for the patient to be hospitalized so that she could "improve her appearance" and get away from "that man." She in no way indicated that she saw herself as having contributed to the patient's illness, but expressed the feeling that the patient needed her and that she would like to help her daughter.

For the first three months of the patient's hospitalization, there was a delay in the under-care social worker's follow-up with the mother but Mrs. B. did not try to reach the social worker. After the case was transferred to me, I arranged to see Mrs. B. to obtain additional history needed by the patient's psychiatrist and to see if I could help with the difficulties indicated by the mother during the intake process.

Since my initial interview with Mrs. B. in November, I have seen her six times and have had several telephone conversations with her. She is a well-groomed, rather heavily made-up woman who bears a strong resemblance to the patient. Although rather heavy she is not obese. She states that she has always had to control her own weight by dieting, and that overweight is a problem that runs throughout her family. Mrs. B. herself had a financially and emotionally deprived childhood. As the oldest of five children, she had to assume many responsibilities within the family at an early age. Her marriage to patient's father was torn with strife, particularly with mutual accusations of infidelity. They separated when the patient was about three or four years old. The father died a few years later, at which time Mrs. B. resumed work as a bookkeeper to support herself and her children. Interestingly enough, she has always been employed in restaurants. She apparently remarried a few years ago, but we have no information except that it ended quickly in divorce.

I have the impression that Mrs. B.'s own life was so lacking in affection and satisfaction that she was not ready for motherhood. She never really wanted the patient and her guilt feelings over this rejection, while strongly intensified through the patient's illness, actually date back many years. This has led to a marked inconsistency in her relationship with the patient. She is frequently overprotective and overindulgent. When the demands become excessive and Mrs. B.'s inner conflict too great, she erupts into screaming arguments and outright rejection of the patient. Having had little life of her own and little confidence in herself, Mrs. B. has been living out many of her own feelings and desires through her daughter and frequently competes with her.

While Mrs. B. took no initiative in seeking help for herself, her response to our interviews indicates that she wants help in her relationship with the patient. However, she has difficulty in expressing her own feelings and in telling about herself. At first, most of what she said was centered around critical descriptions of the patient's behavior, largely as a means of defending herself. Her denial of her personal difficulties was also seen in her brief and unrealistically positive reference to her husbands and son.

Mrs. B.'s mixed feelings about getting help, as well as her ambivalence toward the patient and her guilt feelings concerning her own contribution to the patient's illness, was shown in her attitude toward the patient's hospitalization. She easily weeps over the idea that her daughter should be "in a place like this," yet she leans heavily on the hospital and seems to welcome our taking over responsibility for decisions regarding the patient.

My emphasis in trying to help this troubled woman has been upon developing a relationship with her in which she will feel important, accepted and liked, as a means toward helping her build up more of a life of her own and recognize her difficulties with the patient in a constructive rather than defensive manner. I felt that she has some strengths upon which to build, primarily as manifested through her ability to function well at employment and to form good interpersonal relationships outside of the home, albeit on a limited basis.

Mrs. B. has been showing an increasingly positive use of help, although her progress has been slow and limited. While she continues to focus her understanding of the patient's illness mainly in terms of her obesity and her relationship with the boyfriend, Mrs. B. has begun to show some insight into the fact that the patient's obesity has an emotional base. Recently, Mrs. B. told me, with awareness, that after she and the patient had an argument during one visiting session the patient "went on a rampage," eating cake, candy, which she had not done in some time. I am contemplating continued interviews with Mrs. B. on a regular basis.

My interviews with the patient have been centered around her desire to have a satisfying occupation and a place to live apart from her mother and boyfriend following her eventual discharge. In her desire for help with these plans, she has been unrealistic, vague, and grandiose in her demands. When faced with reality limitations, she has tended to be easily frustrated and unwilling to work them through. She has readily interpreted any limitations as a rejection, and seems to do much to provoke rejections. She has controllingly expressed objections to my seeing her mother.

Despite the patient's resistances in relation to discharge plans, some beginning steps have been taken. In addition to arrangements for a prevocational educational program here, I have referred her to the New York State Division of Vocational Rehabilitation for guidance and possible training. Arrangements have also been considered for her to be placed in a private family residence via our special residence program with the Jewish Community Services of Long Island.

DISCUSSANTS

Dr. Epstein

This is an exceedingly rich and complex case. Such a case points up a number of very important and very interesting problems. It is possible to discuss a problem like this from a great variety of viewpoints.

Our first discussant is a person who has been interested in and has worked in this field for more than twenty years and who throughout the years has been very much interested in this problem and has a great contribution to make, Dr. Hilde Bruch.

Dr. Hilde Bruch

In the course of my studies, I have come to the conclusion that it is misleading to talk about "obesity" as if it were a disease entity. It is more correct to speak of different types of obesities. There is need to recognize differences in the physiological make-up and the psychological reaction pattern of different obese patients. It has been extensively demonstrated in animal experiments that a variety of metabolic disturbances underlie the different types of animal obesity. No such clear-cut differentiation is possible, at this time, for human obesity, but clinical evidence suggests that there are distinct differences in the weight development and eating patterns of patients suffering from different forms of obesity.

In a follow-up study at Babies Hospital, on 250 fat children, at least four different patterns of development could be recognized. In many children remarkable losses of weight had been achieved and it was expected they would stay slim and have a normal development. This hope was not fulfilled. By following these children into adulthood, it was found that these early efforts did not favorably influence the later development. Externally enforced reducing may interrupt but does not alter the basic pattern of an individual's weight curve. In many cases preoccupation with weight and dieting had become the focal point of serious emotional conflicts. Even though being fat represented a serious emotional and social handicap, it played a definite positive role in maintaining a precarious adjustment to life. The extent of this protective function was fully appreciated only by observing the development over many years.

Psychiatrically the picture is also far from uniform. There is no common personality structure that would apply to all fat people, nor do their manifold symptoms fit into the standard psychiatric classifications. Those who have been fat children with adjustment difficulties continue to have similar problems. People with this type of obesity, which I have come to call *developmental obesity,* have many features in common with borderline schizophrenics and are in danger of developing frank schizophrenia if confronted with life problems that surpass their adaptive capacities. Another group comprises people with what I have called *reactive obesity,* which develops rather suddenly in response to some definite traumatic event. It is my impression that obesity in such cases is an equivalent for a depressive reaction. These patients, and many other somewhat older people in whom no such distinct onset can be recognized, are apt to develop severe depressions when reducing is enforced. Many other psychiatric symptoms that are observed in fat people can be understood only in terms of individual life histories, and quite often they are not directly associated with the development of the excess weight.

My interest in the psychological aspects of obesity was first aroused by observing that the notoriously poor cooperation of fat children was related to emotional problems within the family. A report, *The Family Frame of Obese Children,* was published in 1941. In spite of many differences in the surface picture, it was recognized that the underlying basic problems were essentially similar, namely one or both parents looked upon the fat child as a personal possession to compensate them for the disappointments and frustrations in their own lives, without true regard for the individual needs of the child. This basic disturbance can be traced to several distinct family constellations; in one, a symbiotic involvement with one parent, usually the mother, stands in the foreground; and in the other, hostile rejection of the fat child is more apparent. Those of you who have followed the studies on the families of schizophrenics will recognize the close parallel, not only of the constellation but of the trend in research, namely to abandon the concept of the *one* constellation that would be characteristic for all cases, and to delineate instead different manifestations of severely disturbed family relationships.

In approaching obese patients physicians are often handicapped by sharing the common cultural attitude of contempt for fat people and the assumption that all their problems would be solved if they lost the excess weight. The patient whom we discuss here today is so grostesquely overweight that she must lose a considerable amount before she can function effectively at all. I doubt, however, that it would be possible or desirable to induce her to reduce to a so-called average weight. Once we recognize that obesity is a symptom with a positive function, that it is the manifestation of a variety of underlying disturbances (some of which are accessible to treatment, some not), we are forced to look upon this weight excess in a different light: as an important defense mechanism that should not be removed until the underlying conflicts are resolved. Usually the life situation is so involved that only some aspects can be handled. If we keep in mind that even a heavy person may lead a satisfactory life, we have a more realistic treatment goal.

The traditional task of the discussant at a psychiatric conference is the elaboration of the psychodynamic picture. I am rather reluctant to do so in this case because it implies the making of generalizations beyond the evidence at hand. To give the customary psychodynamic elaboration, the discussant selects some prominent points from the history and relates them to the outstanding symptoms and then attempts to reconstruct the whole dynamics of the intrapsychic and interpersonal development of the patient. To present such a seemingly coherent picture it is necessary to interpret some prominent facts according to certain theoretical presuppositions and to fill in the gaps with knowledge acquired from the study of similar cases.

I have formed a rather skeptical, if not negative, opinion about such discussion of a case, even though I have great admiration for the elegant reasoning it involves. I have come to think of these very clever psychodynamic speculations as something in the line of an invocation, the recital of certain prayers, or public confession of adherence to the prevailing theories. By giving the impression of complete understanding of a case in the beginning of treatment, we are in danger of glossing over unclear spots, loopholes, and contradictions in the history. I consider this a somewhat misleading procedure—and this I shall do here without the customary invocation.

To give an example of drawing conclusions beyond the facts at hand, I might mention one section in the Rorschach report. The patient had interpreted a certain part as a "knocker," which reminded her of the knocker at a boarding school. This was interpreted as indicating her guilt and need for punishment for libidinal impulses toward her father, etc. etc. This is, in my opinion, free association on the part of the interpreter and does not add to the understanding of a patient's problems. In order to be therapeutically effective, it is necessary to listen attentively to what the patient really has to tell us and to become alerted whenever the many details which he will produce do not click. By focusing on the facts, one can generally clarify contradictions and fill in the missing data, and this fact-finding is an essential part of the treatment process.

Indoctrination with psychodynamic formulations may stand in the way of a patient's progress or recovery. I have seen a great many fat people who had been in psychoanalytic treatment with various well-trained analysts but who had failed to make adequate progress. They were able to recite the psychodynamics of their illness and at times sounded as it they had devoured and literally incorporated every psychoanalytic interpretation that had come their way, but the underlying disturbances had remained as beclouded as before. Many other therapists have commented on the fact that this type of patient is singularly unresponsive to interpretative psychoanalytic therapy.

However, these patients are not inaccessible to psychotherapy. I have been fortunate in being of help to quite a few of such patients, even though they were filled to the brim with useless knowledge of psychodynamics, simply by being alert to the minutest discrepancies and confusions in the history and behavior. This implies a very close collaborative effort between therapist and patient and demands from the therapist a continuous alertness to the patient's tendency to reexpress and reexperience past interpersonal patterns (transference) in this minute collaborative examination of the past. This approach represents to the patient a new type of interpersonal experience that is as important for the recovery process as the clarification of the seemingly disjointed life history. I am inclined to view this treatment approach as a continuous formulation and reformulation of various tentative hypotheses, which are offered for scrutiny, verification or disproof, in every treatment session.

If I were to approach this patient therapeutically, I would be most interested in the contradictory father, whom the mother describes as a no-good run-away, a gambler, not interested in her or his family, but of whom the patient has such fond memories. The same applies to the contradictory picture of the mother. I do not want to doubt either the mother's or daughter's conscious intent to be truthful; it is our job to help the patient bring up all the pertinent details and the circumstances under which the different behavior occurred. The same applies to her relationship with the young man. An extraordinary contradiction is expressed in her saying: "We were completely dependent on each other—but I hated it." To take such a statement at face value and to draw interpretative conclusions from it will not help in recognizing what really was going on.

By alerting a patient to the contradictions in his version of his own development, we not only clarify the history but we help him develop an important new tool, a needed equipment to face life in more realistic terms. This girl has grown up in an environment in which there was, in addition to emotional and physical neglect, no opportunity for formulating clear and logical concepts. Having lived under circumstances in which clear perception and rational interpretation of what was going on was not encouraged or was quite impossible, such patients develop a peculiar unclear way of thinking and speaking, for which I have coined the term "counterfeit" communications. It is not an outright lie nor the paralogical double talk of the overt schizophrenic. It sounds all right, but it means something different from what the words indicate.

This lack of truthfulness, the extent and all persuasiveness of the distortions, is quite marked in obese patients. Physicians, on the whole, feel rather impatient, often contemptuous, of fat people, because they accuse them of not telling the truth. Of course, conscious lying does occur, but usually we are dealing with the problem that the patient has simply not learned the difference between fact and misinterpretation. It is of no help to such patients if we gloss over the conflicting data and explain them according to our own theoretical and logical way of thinking. We must become attuned and help bridge the gap between their disturbed thinking and the ordinary logical adult thinking.

When this girl talks about eating the chocolate candy, wrapper and string, it sounds like a joke, but it indicates also something which she really wants to convey. It would be this type of dramatic, seemingly obvious exaggeration with which I might start before going on to the much more subtle use of counterfeit language and communication.

This patient conveys to us, through the very way she gives her history, a feeling of her own helplessness. There again, we are dealing with some glaring contradictions. If she really were so disgusted with the young man and the situation in which she was living, why did she go on with it? If we go along with her story or try to interpret it to her before having clarified all the underlying contradictions, we connive with her misrepresentation of her life and condone that she perpetuate this pattern.

I, for one, am more impressed by the extent to which this patient was capable of creating helplessness in others. She must have been terribly perplexing to her mother, or in a love relationship. I am quite sure that she is perplexing to the hospital personnel, in spite of her rather arty descriptions of how much understanding and insight she has gained. This is part of her maneuvering; her way of getting people on her side and leaving essential things unchanged.

Dr. Lee had described in great detail the multifaceted significance of this girl's food intake, which serves as a façade for a multitude of underlying problems, which cannot be fitted easily, if at all, into the standard psychiatric classification. There are hysterical features, but just as many obsessive-compulsive traits. Some of her behavior may be labeled as psychopathic, but the total trend of her development is in the direction of a schizophrenic adjustment. Quite often the term "depression" was used in the history, whereby it was not clear whether this depression was part of a neurotic or a psychotic development, of schizophrenic or manic-depressive psychosis. I have encounteed this difficulty of applying a meaningful diagnostic label in many cases of obesity.

Another difficulty in the treatment of obesity is the "acting out" aspect of the whole syndrome, which confronts the psychiatrist with a real dilemma. We do not support "acting out," but we are protective of "defense mechanisms." As therapists we have to find our way between these two different aspects of the overeating syndrome.

I have been favorably impressed by what Dr. Lee had to say about his treatment approach, that he has succeeded in creating a consistent attitude and a consistent environment against which this girl's problems can be recognized and in which she can be helped to evolve a more realistic picture of herself in relation to the world. This was well illustrated in the way the diet and the obesity problem were approached as something she can handle when she is ready for it but which is not of the doctor's immediate concern. But one small item may serve to illustrate how extraordinarily difficult it is for a physician to dissociate himself from the cultural attitude, Dr. Lee's encouraging the family to bring cosmetics to make her more aware of her feminine development, and to enhance her charm and appearance. It seems to me that this approach carries a danger in that the patient will feel that the doctor hammers in the same direction as everybody else, that of wanting to make her pretty as if he considered that the essence of her problem.

I am aware that my discussion may have left the therapist with too much awareness of the formidable task ahead of him, the job of helping a person, who in the course of her total development has not had a chance to form clear concepts about herself and her interpersonal relationships, to examine, step by step, the manifestations of her deviant development. I am aware that this is an unglamorous job with little possibility of displaying brilliant thinking, but through this tedious work we have a chance, and a pretty good one, of helping such seriously disturbed people to emancipate themselves from this unfortunate bondage to the distorting early environment. If we have realistic treatment goals and do not try to make glamour girls out of our fat patients, the prospect for successive constructive treatment is favorable.[*]

Dr. Epstein

Thank you very much, Dr. Bruch; it was very enlightening.

Our next discussant is a man who has been interested in psychosomatic

---

[*] Bruch, H. and Touraine, G.: Obesity in childhood: 5. The family frame of obese children. *Psychosom Med*, 2:141, 1940; Bruch, H.: *The Importance of Overweight*. New York, Norton, 1957.

or neurotic problems for quite some time. He has had a great deal of experience in that field. We look forward at this time to hearing from Dr. Bernard C. Meyer.

Dr. Bernard C. Meyer

Let me begin with the perhaps surprising assertion that in a number of respects the case is strongly reminiscent of that opposite extreme of a disturbed nutrition, anorexia nervosa. The case at hand will recall those states of obesity which typically precede the outbreak of anorexia as well as the bouts of bulimia that may occur in the course of the phase of anorexia. I have in mind a former patient of mine, whose "eating binges" bore the unmistakable stamp of a debauch. She would stuff herself to a sickening degree, only to slink home like a penitent alcoholic where she would induce vomiting by inserting into her throat a coil of vaseline-anointed toilet paper, which procedure was thereupon followed by her lying for many hours in a purifying bath. This was the same young woman who created out of her room in the Mount Sinai Hospital a miniature art salon, where she served Chinese tea to a select few in an atmosphere of precious refinement.

There are, moreover, other similarities between these apparent opposites. In both instances, there is the symptom of amenorrhea. Other important elements in common are the highly disturbed relationship with a disturbed, rejecting, and herself rejected mother, the fact that the advent of the menarche, as well as the development of secondary sexual characteristics is met by strongly repellent attitudes. Adult sexuality is deeply disturbing, tends to be regarded in sadomasochistic terms and contains an excessive oral orientation. In fact, as in the present case, sexuality and the process of eating tend to be strongly interconnected: she declared it was as difficult for her to discuss her eating binges as it is for other people to describe their sexual activities. In both cases, the process of eating serves as a means of discharging impulses of primitive instinctual quality, consisting, one would surmise, in aggressive and sadistic attack upon an object, and subjected therefore to an accompanying disturbance in mood as well as by a variety of defensive measures. Thus, our patient of today found it impossible to eat on dates, postponing her eating until she was home alone. I would suspect, furthermore, that the enuresis which followed some of her eating binges represented, among other things, an attempted undoing, an emptying out of the object ingested during the bulimia. For both classes of patients the advent of sexual maturity imposes a nearly unendurable additional burden to young women already struggling with pregenital conflicts. In our experience with anorexia nervosa, we have been struck by the role of an environmental pregnancy in the genesis of this disorder. I wonder whether such a pregnancy, emotionally significant to the patient, may not have occurred in her early childhood, serving as an object of those orally sadistic and cannibalistic impulses which we believe to be implicit in her symptom. In any event, the early death of the father and the almost simultaneous seduction by her brother must have contributed heavily to an already severe struggle against instinctual urges. Parenthetically, we would suspect that despite the overt difference in manifestation, the criminality of the brother contains very similar genetic sources to those of the patient's obesity. The object of these predatory gestures would appear to be the mother herself and perhaps her breast in particular, a striving which if impeded by her pregnancy or by favored siblings may partake of murderous quality.

Typical too of the patient with anorexia nervosa is the obsessional pattern of the personality structure and a fluctuation in mood, ranging from depression to elation. Both of these elements would appear present in the case at hand: she is described as a perfectionist, and the mood of depression has also been clearly indicated although her more recent behavior as ward leader and clown would suggest a hypomanic trend. Seen in this light, the prevailing symptom, be it anorexia or bulimia, must be regarded as only one particularly striking and dramatic manifestation of an underlying disorder whose total extent and range of intensity may be in large part concealed by the symptom itself. In this connection it is instructive to refer to an extremely obese woman described by Seitz. During sixteen hypnotic sessions, when she was told that during the ensuing week she would not overeat, she developed a host of symptom substitutions in which bulimia was replaced successively by finger biting, depression, vomiting, pruritus and excoriation, varied pareses and pain, urticaria, paranoid fantasies, phobias, disrobing compulsions, "accidental" self-injury, insomnia, headache, and so on. This report emphasizes the multitude of both somatic and psychiatric symptom equivalents which may be associated with the bulimia, the relevance of which in the present instance is the emphasis upon the defensive function of the symptom concerning the emergence of underlying psychopathology. In its simplest form, the bulimia may here be regarded as a defense against depression: she eats to avoid despair. In a broader sense the symptom constitutes an overt expression both of underlying impulses and the defenses against them as well as their accompanying affects. A closer inspection of the clinical data would suggest, however, that a still more vital function of the symptom may be a protection against psychotic disorganization. Students of anorexia nervosa, for example, have had reason to suspect that behind the facade of obsessional thinking and on a more fundamental level than the depressive mood, there

lies a grave ego disturbance which may at times assume the form clinically
of a psychosis, probably schizophrenia. Similar suspicions appear warranted here in the present instance. I have in mind not only the self-directed admission to Bellevue Hospital, itself a bizarre act, regardless of its
stated motivation, but also the description of her behavior during the
months preceding her admission to Hillside Hospital: sleeping at times
seventeen hours a day, seclusive, fearful, unable to function and obviously
depressed. Finally, one might call attention to the ego-alien abuse of the
body, through overeating, a practice which must surely be ranked as
morbid and as pathogenic in its way as is the self-starvation in anorexia
nervosa. I would regard the course of the two years preceding her hospitalization as a phase of increasing decompensation in a hitherto precariously
balanced schizophrenic girl. And whereas her relationship with her boyfriend may have aggravated matters secondarily, I would tend to regard
the very establishment of this relationship as a desperate endeavor upon
her part to maintain human contacts. If this be so, one might anticipate that
hospitalization and the establishment of relationships in this milieu would
be accompanied by a loosening of her tie to a man for whom she now has
little need.

As in the case of anorexia nervosa, there is much here to recall to mind
the "oral triad" of Lewin. The wish to eat is the chief symptom in this patient; reference to the wish to sleep has already been made. The wish to
be eaten consists in a psychic elaboration of "the sensation of being en-
gulfed or surrounded by the mother's breast, or of being supported by the
mother during the relaxation that precedes sleep." The wish to be eaten
is, likewise, determined by shifting identifications wherein the object of active oral incorporative impulses becomes identified with the eater himself.
It is evident that the idea of being eaten contains conspicuous phobic implications, evidence for which I would discern in the clinical history, and
which may provide an additional clue for the meaning of the patient's chief
symptom—namely, that the eating compulsion may constitute a counter-
phobic defense against the wish-fear of being devoured.

In summary, we have enumerated the following possible meanings of the
symptom of overeating:

1. Bulimic oral sadistic attack upon the mother, her breast, her pregnant uterus, and the hypothetical younger sibling.
2. As an identification with the object of her aggression.
3. As a defense against being devoured.
4. A defense against depression.
5. A defense against psychotic disorganization.

The question might well arise, if this condition is so akin to anorexia
nervosa, why does she not weigh 72 lb instead of 340? I would not presume
to answer this question with any pretension of certainty. I do not believe

we are in possession of sufficient early data concerning crucial phases of oral development to explain the choice of any "oral" pathology, be it in terms of anorexia, bulimia, asthma or stuttering. There are relatively normal individuals who in the face of depression lose their appetite just as others eat compulsively.

With regard to treatment, I must confess pessimism. Whereas it may be possible for her to lose substantial amounts of weight, I would question the likelihood that it could ever proceed beyond a certain point, a point which would find her still extremely obese. My reason for this opinion is implicit in the above discussion: stripped of this protective armor of fat, she would be assailed by quantities of both anxiety and depression with which she would be utterly incapable of dealing. For the same reason I would doubt that much can be achieved in terms of interpretative insight psychotherapy. Effective help might be looked for in the establishment of some facsimile of that longed-for relationship with an all-giving mother in whose safe embrace the act of eating may become more properly limited to the function of attaining nourishment.

Dr. Epstein

Dr. Meyer raises some very interesting problems. It suggests one or two things immediately, namely, the two-sided aspect of this problem. It would be very interesting, some time perhaps in the near future, to discuss this two-sided aspect, anorexia nervosa on the one side and bulimia on the other, and the relationship to schizophrenia of some of these disorders. It would be interesting to speculate on the possible connection between the two sides of this coin and the problems relating to bulimia and bisexuality.

There is no doubt that in many of these women to be fat means to be feminine, to be ugly, to be pregnant, to be sexual and this has been repeatedly pointed out; whereas to be thin means to be boyish; to be ascetic means to be pure and nonsexual.

I think I might also mention that in 1932 Wolff described a syndrome in which many of these patients seem to fit, characterized by a lengthy discussion of the symbolical meaning of obesity for some of these women and also the symbolical meaning of thinness, but the outstanding characteristics of this syndrome were hysterical manifestations, cyclothymia and addiction; and the close relationship between these problems and the problem of addiction, of course, must be manifest to all of us.

I now would like to call upon our third discussant, who will help to round out this discussion, adding a little more, perhaps, on the physiological or somatic side, Dr. Albert Stunkard.

Dr. Albert Stunkard

Perhaps the most active investigators in the field of obesity at the present time are the physiologists. In the last fifteen years they have made remarkable progress. They have been able to show, within the hypothalamus, discrete areas which mediate feeding behavior. They have been able to map out with some degree of precision the rather complex interactions of these areas: there are two separate types of areas in the hypothalamus, one mediating hunger and one mediating satiety; and, finally, they have been able to confirm this experimentally by actually producing obesity through destruction of the hypothalamic centers. Further, they have been able to demonstrate that in these animals a form of hyperphagia ensues which is characterized by no increase in hunger drive as measured by the usual indices of drive strength. Instead, they have been able to produce rats with the appropriate damage to the satiety centers who present the paradox of an organism eating itself into obesity on the basis of an actual diminished hunger drive. More recently, it has been possible to breed a type of rat which becomes obese soon after birth and the obesity of this animal is qualitatively different from that produced in the animal with hypothalamic damage.

This finding, that there can be different types of obesity in animals, provides evidence that in animals, at least, obesity is not a unitary phenomenon and is not a single disease. Obesity comes about as a result of a disorder in the maintenance of energy balance and any physiological regulation is apt to be a pretty complex mechanism and must contain a good many parts which could get out of order.

Differentiation in the field of human obesity might similarly lead to further advances. Thus, if it were true that obesity in humans too has different origins, it might cast light on two of the most troublesome problems which we face today in psychosomatic medicine: the problem of the choice of neurosis and that of specificity.

I think there is some possibility that the physiologist may in the relatively near future be able to differentiate in obesity five or six different subgroups. In the meantime, two small unique subgroups of obese people have already been differentiated at a physiological level. One of these is the form of obesity which develops in people following some brain damage. It happens very rarely but it is quite analogous to the type of obesity which is produced by hypothalamic damage, and the second type of subgroup which has been recently distinguished is quite analogous to that of the hereditary obesity syndrome in rats. Such people, probably of a fairly small number, can maintain a caloric balance on a diet of 1000 calories; as soon as they got on a standard reducing diet of 1200 calories they begin to gain weight.

These are surely a very small percentage of the vast number of overweight people in our population, but I think they raise the question of how other different types of obesity may still be distinguished and how we, as clinicians, may be able to take part in that.

Dr. Bruch has already described a couple of ways that are being weighed and one particular possibility that has interested me has been that of studying the eating patterns of obese people. Now, I would like to show a slide which indicates the results which have been obtained by this type of analysis in animal work. We see in this slide the eating patterns of four types of rats; patterns A and B show a much larger amount of food consumed per unit of time than either patterns C or D. Pattern D, which is that of a normal rat, shows the slowest rate of food intake of any of the patterns. Pattern C is that of a hereditary obese rat. Pattern A is that of a rat which has had damage to the hypothalamic center, and Pattern B is of a rat made obese by gold glucose. There is almost no difference between the hypothalamic obese rat and the rat who had been made obese by the injection of gold glucose. At the time this work was done the mechanism by which gold glucose produced obesity was quite obscure. No one had any idea how it came about, but it was inferred by the food patterns that the etiology or the pathogenesis might be very similar to that of the animal who is made obese by hypothalamic damage.

Within the last six months this same group of investigators has been able to show that gold glucose produces its action by a chemical destruction of the satiety centers so that from the behavior of the organism inferences apparently can be made back to the pathogenetic factors.

Now, are similar types of patterns present in obese humans? I think they are, and I think they can be identified with some degree of assurance in a relatively small number of people. I want to emphasize that the patterns which I am about to describe are only probably quite a small percentage of the obese population as a whole. Whether there are other patterns in the large number of obese people that we see is, I think, a matter that we are in a singularly good position to discover.

The first eating pattern is one which was present in a man who showed hypothalamic obesity. This was a twenty-year-old man who, at the age of twelve, had a very severe attack of encephalitis with evidence of damage all through the brain. He made a fairly good recovery with few residuals. On his return home, when he was permitted free access to food, he gained weight at the rate of 10 lb a week until he had gained 80 lb. Then his family began to restrict his food intake. Since then, whenever this man is permitted free access to food, he will gain weight, and when it is restricted he will lose it, without any particular uncomfortable consequences. If he was restricted he didn't seem to mind it too much. This is a fairly unique kind of pattern which I do not think I have seen before. I might say that I do not think it has any relation to life or stress. The only relevant variables are the availability of food, and this pattern does not change whether he is emotionally upset or not.

The second type of pattern that I would like to describe is one which I first had occasion to observe in a woman some years after the development of her obesity. She had been closely attached to her mother in a relationship of completely morbid dependency, the mother having spent the last nine years of her life in bed with presumably a cardiac neurosis and having induced the daughter to give up everything to take care of her. Following the mother's death by other causes, the patient got along fairly well until about a year later when she heard from a doctor, who had been taking care of her mother, that he felt that the mother's illness was a neurosis. Thereupon the patient became quite agitated; apparently it was acceptable to her to sacrifice herself for a really sick mother, but since the mother was not really sick she had been defrauded. She left town and put on 200 lb over a period of two years.

The eating pattern during this time was quite characteristic. It would recur at any time later during her life in periods of stress. At such times, she awoke in the morning with no feeling of hunger or no desire for food and would actually reject food if it was ordered for her. She rarely ate before noon and her food intake at lunch and during the afternoon was quite limited. She began to feel a desire for food in the early evening, usually ate a large supper and then, only temporarily sated, she seemed to turn to the kitchen, consuming larger and larger amounts of food at shorter and shorter intervals, assailed all the time by loneliness and anxiety and to lessen her stress at such times she tried to keep someone with her as much as possible. When she was alone she left the door and windows open, played the radio loudly, kept all the lights on. She rarely fell asleep before midnight and usually awoke within an hour, anxious and hungry. She was aware of being hungry at this time. At such times she would eat a pint of ice cream, drink a bottle of Coca-Cola and then, temporarily sated, fall asleep and often awoke three or four times during the night in this way.

Later in her life I had the opportunity of observing this woman actually for the last four years and I was struck by two features of this eating pattern, which Dr. Harold Wolff and I called the "night-eating syndrome." One is the really complete anorexia that the patient feels during the morning hours, not only not wanting food but actually rejecting it; and the other feature was the extreme degree of distress which she suffered during the night. For hours she would pace the corridors, agitated and fearful, intermittently trying to distract herself by reading and knitting and eating anything that she could get by any means, lawful or otherwise.

Another feature of this pattern is the rather complete absence of any expressions of self-condemnation. This particular woman had developed the art of transferring blame to such a very high degree that she had quite a reputation as being an impossible patient. I do not know that this says much about the possible role of guilt in motivating this pattern, but it is in such striking contrast to the next patient that it is worth bearing in mind.

The third patient I would like to describe was a thirty-four-year-old man who generally ate and drank to mild excess a large part of the time and then went on rigid diets so that he was usually somewhat overweight but never really massively obese. Every now and then, however, he overate in a curious and most characteristic fashion. This occurred most commonly following some rather obscure difference with his wife, the meaning of which we have not yet been able to elucidate, and also when he succeeded in getting his hands on some ready cash, either by cashing a check or borrowing money. Now, at such times he was aware that he was likely to overeat; the pattern was quite clear to him; so he used to steel himself against this possibility by repeating to himself all the good advice that he had gotten from his friends and relatives and which he converted into a kind of formula which sometimes worked. But on such occasions, more likely than not, it would not work. Once he suddenly found himself, after having cashed a check, in a delicatessen, having bought an enormous quantity of food, without having any clear idea of how he had gotten into the store. He remembered having seen the store down the street and then the next thing he knew he was in the store and had bought this food, which gave him a sort of frightful, uncanny kind of feeling; but once he embarked on this eating binge, he was quite powerless to resist.

In his most recent episode he loaded his car with about twenty dollars worth of food, took it home and ate it all; then slipped out when he had done that and went from restaurant to restaurant, eating. He did this in a very furtive fashion. He would eat only a very small amount in any one restaurant and he would keep an eye out to see if there was anyone in that restaurant who had seen him in any of the others. He would work his way down the street in this fashion. In this last eating binge he gained 8 lb in a period of twenty-four hours. When he finished he always experienced the most awesome guilt. These eating binges were often followed by a period of dieting.

He said, "I don't know what happened, all of my good intentions just seemed to fade away; they just didn't seem to mean anything any more. I just said, what the hell, and started eating and what I did then was an absolute sin . . . I don't even enjoy it; it just happens. It's like part of me blacks out, just isn't there; when that happens there is nothing there except the food and me, all alone."

We have here therefore three quite distinct and reproducible eating patterns of obese people; the pattern of satiety failure, the night-eating syndrome, and this pattern of binge eating. How many more exist we have no way of telling, nor do we have any information as to the relative frequency with which these patterns are distributed in the obese population as a whole. But these are already questions which, I think, it should be possible to obtain answers to.

In closing, I would like to say again, that I think we are standing on the threshold of great advances in our understanding of obesity. I think these advances will come if we put the appropriate questions to our material and perhaps the richest available material is intensive observation of human behavior which is permitted to us as psychiatrists.

Dr. Epstein

We all feel grateful to Dr. Stunkard for his extremely enlightening and instructive discussion. This is an area of research that cannot be stressed too much, and we more analytically oriented physicians do not always have access to it.

From what Dr. Stunkard says, we should now start to speak of the obesities rather than obesity. There seem to be a number of different disorders. We realize that not everybody who has certain psychological problems develops obesity and, I think, the converse is also true.

This is something which needs to be stressed further, and it is interesting to hear what kind of work is being done. I think it also would be very helpful if we had some better means of intercommunication. The various disciplines, the various approaches to this problem actually tend to work in different little corners and if there is some way of pooling all these different investigations, especially in language which we can mutually understand, I think this would be of tremendous advantage.

One small point comes up, and that is the question of "eating binges." Binges, it should be pointed out, are characteristic not only of food intake; but we, as psychiatrists, have known of such things as drinking binges and sexual binges; so this is not specifically a problem of obesity.

Dr. J. S. A. Miller

I would like to mention briefly the interesting case of a psychopathic young woman in her mid-twenties who was admitted here several years ago and who weighed between 180 and 200 pounds and was a binge eater. She was the daughter of an attorney and her psychopathic behavior was to forge checks and then spend the money on food and in tricking her close friends. The interesting thing about her was that she made a remarkable adjustment in the hospital and was discharged as one of our "prize" cases. She joined the Hillside League of Ex-Patients and became quite a power in that organization, so much so that she was presented before the Women's Division of the Hospital, which we had at that time, as an example of what can be done with rather severe personality disturbances. From there on she manipulated appearances before several meetings of the Women's Division and before the League to such an extent that she became impossible to work with and was thrown out and then reverted again to check forging.

The remarks of Drs. Bruch and Stunkard, particularly in regard to the diversity of syndromes in which overeating and also Dr. Meyer's remarks in regard to anorexia and the relationship to psychiatric syndromes, in which these form symptoms and substitutes for symptoms, of either a schizophrenic or psychotic nature, are extremely important. I would like to remark that while I heartily agree, there are many obesities and there are many factors involved in questions of overeating; there are psychological and particularly psychoanalytical dynamics which seem to offer, at the present time, at least, most of the information concerning the psychological factors of their personal relationships and offer at the present moment the best approach in therapy.

I, too, hope that some day we will be able to and ought to work toward this direction by exchanging the various biological, physiological, psychological data in these problems. Some steps are already being made in this hospital to do this in regard to the manic-depressive reactions, in regard to shock and physical treatment and artificial brain changes, in the physical therapies, in conjunction and in correct dynamic relationship to psychotherapy.

VI
GROUP THERAPY

18

Group Psychotherapy with Obese Women

Herbert Holt

AND

Charles Winick

THIS is a report on psychoanalytic group psychotherapy with a group of obese women over a limited period of time. Obesity is perhaps the most common way of reacting to difficulties and has been extensively studied by many disciplines. The role of obesity in cardiovascular disease, digestive difficulties, joint pains, and other disorders, has been widely discussed. The relative ineffectiveness of most out-patient nonpsychiatric treatment for obesity has recently been documented.[13] It has been established that different types of obesity seem to be associated with different kinds of psychiatric illnesses.[9] One report of a psychotherapy experience with a thirteen-year-old obese girl concluded that obesity can have its dynamic roots on each level of psychosexual development.[6]

Group psychotherapy has been used to treat obesity in groups which appeared to be psychiatrically normal. One therapy group conducted by a psychologist involved fifteen group sessions with women volunteer patients and partially achieved its goal of modifying the attitudes toward eating of the group members.[7] Almost one-third of the patients maintained some weight loss in a follow-up conducted two years after treatment. In another project, a follow-up of a group of women who had sixteen sessions of group therapy from a nurse or dietician two years after the sessions reported that a majority of the patients did report some weight loss.[11]

The current research was undertaken in order to examine the feasibility of psychoanalytically oriented group psychotherapy in the treatment of obesity. The group analytic approach appeared to offer an opportunity to explore obese patients' defenses and group functioning in a depth not previously possible. The study had four hypotheses: a) Group analytic psychotherapy can improve the general adaptation and emotional well-being of obese persons. b) It is possible to predict the patients' weight shifts by the content of the group therapy sessions. c) Patients will lose weight as a result of group analytic treatment. d) Patients would use available ancillary procedures like diet, massage, and relaxation therapy once they begin to get involved in the group process, and their use of these procedures would be related to the content of the therapy sessions.

The therapist was a male psychiatrist. A clinical psychologist evaluated weight gain or loss in implementation of the second hypothesis and participated in research design. The services of cooperating professionals were available at nominal charge to the patients. These included a physician specializing in diet treatment of obesity and a specialist in massage and relaxation therapy. The auxiliary services were offered at nominal charge because it was felt that to offer them free might diminish their possible importance to the patients and might increase their unconscious dependency needs and their resentment against the substitute father image of the analyst.

The group sessions occurred once a week, with each session lasting two hours. The patients met without the analyst in an alternate session once a week. The group met for twenty-two sessions with the therapist and for twenty-two alternate sessions. The content of all office sessions was stenographically transcribed. All patients weighed themselves on the same office scale just prior to each session, so that there would be consistent records of their weight.

THE PATIENTS

The patients were selected from among eighteen women who were referred from various sources. Token fees were charged. The group finally selected consisted of six women, whose age range was from thirty-eight to fifty-four, with an average of forty-five. All were middle-class in income. Three were married, two divorced, and one was separated. The married women lived in suburbs and the others lived in New York City. They averaged 5 ft 3 in in height and weighed an average of 169 lb, or 33 lb above the 1959 national average of the Society of Actuaries for women of their age and height. Every woman had made at least two previous attempts to reduce, which had failed. Every woman's weight was increasing at the time of beginning of the treatment.

Each patient was of average to superior intelligence. One of the patients had a mother who was obese, but the others reported no parents who were unusually fat. The menarche occurred at an average age of 13.4 years, very slightly ahead of normal for the environment. Two patients were older than their siblings, two were middle children, one was the youngest, and one was an only child, in contrast to studies which have reported 70 per cent of obese children being the youngest or only children.[2] Background genetic factors thus appeared to have little relevance to the patient's obesity.

The patients' relationship with their parents was similar to that found in many drug addicts, whose orality has been extensively documented.[14] *Every one* of these patients came from homes in which the mother was overprotectingly rejecting and the father was relatively ineffectual, weak, and submissive. All five of the surviving mothers were relatively attractive women and all had fairly close ties with their daughters, with whom they maintained the same rejecting but solicitous relationship which they had established many years ago. Three of the five mothers were still fairly slim and used to chivy their daughters about the latters' weight. Like mothers of many drug addicts, they overtly wanted their daughters to lose their symptoms, but covertly wanted them to remain ill.

The women in the group were selected because they appeared to offer a real opportunity to explore the usefulness of psychoanalytic group psychotherapy with obese adults. Each patient, in spite of her orality, had demonstrated ability to function on an adult level and to adapt to new situations. They were not like the cases of obesity developed during childhood (developmental obesity), on psychiatric correlates of which there have been recent reports.[3] They became obese in mature adulthood, so that obesity was a relatively recent problem which they were actively concerned in alleviating. Motivation for treatment was fairly high, since each woman had independently sought to lose weight prior to group therapy and each woman's weight had been steadily increasing up to the commencement of group therapy. Each woman was actively interested in her appearance and gave considerable attention to clothing, cosmetics, hair tinting, and other externals, insofar as this was possible within their incomes. Each woman had what appeared to be a fairly good life situation and relationship with reality in terms of vocational or home adjustment. Each woman appeared to be able to profit from group psychoanalytic treatment.

Muriel was thirty-eight, divorced, with two children. She lived with her parents. She had a severe anxiety neurosis. She had been very beautiful and had married a handsome adventurer who was the opposite of her solid and reliable father. Her husband was a ne'er-do-well who never supported her. She got a divorce when she was thirty-four. Her weight had been normal until she reached thirty-five, when she began to overeat. After her divorce, she went back to school, acquired vocational skills, and earned enough to support herself and her children. Her overeating represented an attempt to destroy her beauty so that she would not remarry and would thus remain a burden to her father. As another device to defend herself against meeting possible husbands, she was beginning to fall in love with her already married employer. She weighed 176 lb.

Nancy was a fifty-five-year-old married woman who had an unmarried son of twenty-six. She had fared very well in a business career. Her husband was somewhat older than she was and had been an invalid for some years because of a chronic illness. Although her weight had been normal, she had gained much weight after menopause and weighed 166 lb at the time the group began. The menopause had also made her question the extent to which she had adequately fulfilled herself in her marriage. She was a pseudoneurotic schizophrenic.

Betty was forty-one, married, and had been married twice previously. Betty had elements of both paranoid and schizoid symptomatology. She had a twelve-year-old daughter and a fifteen-year-old son. Her mother was very slender and posed a constant challenge to Betty. Feelings of worthlessness began to be increasingly important in Betty's fantasies, about a year before treatment began. She had begun to have very unpleasant dreams and tried to avoid them by staying awake at night. She did this by having an extra meal around 11:00 PM and her weight had increase to 152 lb.

Mary was divorced, forty-five, with a nineteen-year-old son. She was an attractive woman who had done well in her job, although an ambulatory schizophrenic. She had maintained her great need for closeness by engaging in compulsive and promiscuous sexual relations. Around the age of forty, she began to be less attractive to men. When she realized this, she became panicky and began to overeat. Compensatory daydreams had begun to take up more and more of her time. She weighed 186 lb.

Helen was a forty-year-old professional woman who was separated from her husband, whom she had married because he appeared to be successful in his career and able to take care of her. He turned out to be feckless and much like her relatively weak father. He had married her for the money which he erroneously believed her to have. Helen's mother was a severe disciplinarian who used to beat her constantly. As one result of these beatings, Helen could be said to be "living scared." She had developed some paranoid symptoms. About two years before commencing treatment, she could no longer escape being aware that the husband on whom she had relied was completely ineffectual. She obtained a separation and began to eat more, and to gain weight. She weighed 157 lb.

Ruth was a fifty-four-year-old married woman who had no children and was successful in business. For many years she had maintained a desexualized and brotherly relationship with her husband. They lived in a kind of communal household with several of her unmarried relatives. Ruth was beginning to be concerned about her steadily increasing weight (168 lb), and had begun to feel that she was eating too much. Her husband was opposed to her entering treatment. Ruth's presenting symptoms were probably milder than those of the other patients.

Although the patients came from a variety of ethnic backgrounds, they had few, if any, food preferences which seemed to be related to their weight in what might be any kind of causal or even contributory way. Perhaps the only food preference which they had in common was a preoccupation with desserts. They had knowledge of and ate relatively recondite desserts like profiteroles and baked Alaska. Such special knowledge of "forbidden" foods is not, of course, uncommon in obese patients, who may also know a great deal about reducing regimens, weight norms, and caloric values.

THE SESSIONS

The sessions were conducted on Friday evenings in order to maximize the patients' ability to relax and speak freely and to minimize logistic problems in getting to and from sessions. The alternate sessions were conducted on Tuesday evenings, at the homes of different patients. The analyst made it clear that the group members could discuss anything they wanted, including dreams, daydreams, body sensations, and fantasies. The methods for establishing contact with the cooperating diet and relaxation and massage specialists were made explicit at the first session, and the specialists themselves were introduced and answered questions. The patients were told that these auxiliary services were available at nominal fees. Each patient was encouraged to contact the specialists on an individual basis. The patients were told that they could, if they wished, use the group sessions to discuss their experiences with the specialists, but that the latter's relationship with the patients was completely confidential and individual. In order to emphasize the role of the cooperating specialists and the extent to which other professional disciplines were involved, the project was identified to the patients and referred to as the "Obesity Clinic." Some patients called it "The Club," half jestingly.

The patients were told that the purpose of the Obesity Clinic was to help them to feel better and to lose weight. They were told that the group would meet for at least a half year and that it would be continued if there appeared to be mutual interest in doing so. There was little difficulty in getting the patients to speak freely or in establishing rapport with each other. They enjoyed the feeling of being members of a select group, and the visible obesity of each patient helped to provide a powerful bond which facilitated communication.

After all the sessions were concluded, a content analysis was made of what had been discussed throughout the period of treatment. Each content element was counted as one subject for purposes of the content analysis each time it was mentioned, regardless of how much time was spent on it. A total of 1,331 subjects was discussed in the twenty-two sessions, an average of 60.5 subjects per session. No record was kept of the content of the alternative sessions, which were conducted without the analyst, although sometimes the content of these sessions or of other communications among patients was discussed in the treatment hours.

Although the one thing which the group members had in common was their overweight and interest in food, relatively little attention was paid to such material, as is shown in the analysis of subjects discussed in the group sessions in Table 18-I.

The group members exhibited relatively little of the "dieting depression" often found in adult obese patients whose obesity is reactive and in whom overeating is a response to some traumatic situation.[12] They also exhibited little of the fatigue, irritability, and increased consumption of tea, coffee, and cigarettes which are traditionally found in persons who are reducing.[15] They often did have difficulties in falling asleep, which is a fairly common characteristic of reducers.

TABLE 18-I

CONTENT OF ALL GROUP SESSIONS

Theme	Incidence of Each Theme as Proportion of Total Themes, %
Dreams and other unconscious material	26
Parents and childhood memories	13
Interpersonal relations, exclusive of husbands and other men	12
Fantasies and daydreams	10
Eating and food	9
Relations with own children	8
Weight and appearance	7
Relations with husbands and other men	6
Health and disease matters other than obesity	5
Work	4
Total	100

A typical session would begin with each patient weighing herself on the office scale which was outside the therapy room. The patients usually discussed their weight and their eating activities and problems during the previous few days in the first few minutes of the session. One member might then tell a dream which she had experienced. The analyst would help in clarifying the dream, and other patients might present dreams. Daydreams and fantasies were often produced after or during a discussion of a dream. Some current interpersonal matter might be discussed, often involving friends. The patients' own children and parents were often discussed in terms of some current reality situation. "Therapeutic friendships" among a number of the patients had been formed, and they spoke quite freely about their relationships with each other outside the group analytic situation. Most of the patients met for a "kaffee-klatsch" at a nearby restaurant after each session, and some ate large and high-calorie meals at these sessions in obvious defiance of the analyst and of their own values and purpose.

No two sessions were completely alike. Every single session, however, had at least one patient who reported a dream. In practically every session there was likely to be little return to the subject of weight gain or loss once it had been mentioned at the beginning of each session. This was an obvious avoidance reaction on the assumption that what was not discussed did not exist. The patients' ability to plunge into discussions of relatively difficult unconscious material was a reflection of several factors, including the severity of their emotional illness, their high motivation, their strong identification with the group, and their transference to the analyst and to each other.

The patients seemed to feel that the specifics of diet and ancillary medical activity were less significant than their larger attitudes toward themselves. One patient helped to objectify and clarify the others' attitudes toward food as reflections of other problems by noting how she always felt hungry when she felt it was time to shift from a day to a night activity. She described how hungry she became around midnight, when she began getting drowsy. This discussion, in the second session, aroused so much anxiety among the other patients that the subject of eating became almost dangerous for the patients to talk about. This was doubtless a factor in the patients' devoting so little time to discussions of their obesity, which was the major reason for the existence of the group. When the analyst noted the degree of emotional fright regarding the subject of eating and food, he did not make special efforts to force a discussion of these subjects, because he wished to keep the group's anxiety at a tolerable level.

Most of the patients entered treatment with a relatively simple point of view about the direct causal relationship between caloric intake and weight. They assumed that if they ate less, their weight would decline relatively promptly. They began to become aware that the relationship of food intake to weight was somewhat more complex than they had thought, because of the extent to which the body was a kind of mediating variable and because of the importance of psychological factors in maintenance and establishment of the body image. This awareness helped motivate their desire to "get tuned in to my middle," as one patient put it, and acted as a spur to their motivation for treatment. Attendance at sessions was practically perfect, which was probably a reflection of their high motivation.

In spite of their visceral response to the treatment, with some patients gaining 5 lb in one day and losing 6 lb the next day, there were few somatic complications. Nausea, stomachaches, and headaches occurred often, were usually resistance phenomena, and were discussed as such. Two patients developed urticaria early in treatment, and their symptoms reappeared intermittently throughout the treatment period. They consulted dermatologists but their symptoms disappeared only after they had worked through feelings of anger and hostility in the group.

One unusual response was that of Ruth, who had had a mild chronic case of high blood pressure and visited the family physician who had referred her to the group, midway through the treatment period. He told her that her blood pressure was normal, for the first time in years. She said, "I'm dead." When he took her pressure a few minutes later, it had shot up again. When she mentioned and explored the incident in the group, it became clear that she had had high blood pressure for so long that for her to have normal pressure meant to feel dead. She thus quickly reverted to the accustomed high blood pressure, with which she felt comfortable, in a reverse of a "flight into health."

Another patient who reacted strongly to the uncovering dimension of treatment was Betty, who had a psychotic episode that lasted for a day, about a month after treatment started. It occurred on a Wednesday, on the day after an alternate session and two days before a group session. She had decided that the analyst loved her and that she loved him. She telephoned him twelve times during the day to talk to him about their love. The analyst was able to see her that evening in an emergency individual session. She recovered and her symptoms did not return. The episode was later discussed fully in the group and in a number of further individual sessions with Betty.

The climate of the group was unusually consistent in that all the patients had remarkable abilities to sense each other's mood, to absorb and respond to it, and all the patients were usually in the same mood. A wide range of moods was present in the sessions. On one occasion, for example, the first few patients who came into the office were anxious and depressed. They ignored the chairs on which they usually sat and which were placed around the walls of the rectangular office. Instead, they picked up folding chairs from a pile of such chairs in a corner, and placed them in a circle. As each of the other patients came in, she also picked up a folding chair and joined the circle, which was one way in which the patients expressed their anxiety and need for closeness. This was done before there was any discussion of why the patients felt depressed, or even that they were depressed. During the session, they voiced their anxiety and were able to verbalize their mood and even to note how their circular sitting position reflected their anxiety.

On another occasion, one patient telephoned the analyst a few minutes after a session had begun to say that she would be arriving late for the session. She volunteered the information that she felt very cheerful and in good spirits. The session had just begun, with the patients spontaneously commenting on their cheerfulness and good spirits. This high degree of mutual empathy doubtless helped to create a climate which facilitated therapeutic movement. It is reminiscent of the story told in a 1954 lecture by Dr. Sidney Rose. He reported on a physician who was very successful in treating obesity, although his methods and prescriptions were the usual ones. He had acquired such a good reputation that his waiting room was always very crowded. The patients chatted together while waiting for the physician and thus shared and helped to create an atmosphere of mutual acceptance, confidence in the physician, and friendly competition among each other in losing weight.

FINDINGS

Two of the hypotheses were confirmed and two were not.

General Adaptation and Emotional Well-Being of Patients

The hypothesis that group analytic psychotherapy would improve the emotional well-being and level of adaptation of the patients was confirmed. The role of fantasy in stabilizing their self-systems began to emerge, and their differential use of fantasy was a dimension which they began to face. The group sessions enabled the patients to see that their anxiety was caused less by external reality or even by their interpersonal relations than by the nature of their self-concept and their internalized norms and images. They began to obtain some clarification of the latter. By and large, they engaged in less projection and acting-out behavior. They began to realize the extent to which they had set up situations in which they were associated significantly with persons who exploited, derided, or rejected them for being fat.

Muriel obtained insight into her ambivalent feelings about her father and her desire both to remain a burden to him and to displace her feelings about him onto her employer. She began to feel more acceptance of her role as a self-supporting person who establishes meaningful relationships on her own. Nancy began to clarify her attitudes toward her husband and how she had ended up as the family's breadwinner. Betty's feelings of worthlessness temporarily became intensified during treatment. The tempo of her constructive response to treatment increased after her brief psychotic episode. Betty's relationship with her rejecting mother and selection of husbands who ultimately rejected her were approached during the period of treatment. She realized that she felt her husband was worthless *because* he had married her.

Mary began to develop a more realistic image of herself and one which was less anchored in daydreams and fantasies. Her need to respond in an overintimate manner to men when there was no need for such intimacy became clearer, as did her projections onto her son. Helen began to understand the nature of the mutual fantasies on which her marriage had been based and the extent of her magical thinking. Ruth was helped to see how her home's being geared toward communal living had helped to reinforce her picture of her husband as a brother, with whom she would be having what she would regard as incestuous relations if she engaged in sexual intercourse.

Several of the patients, Muriel, Mary, and Helen, had demonstrated a serious lack of self-assertiveness in their arrangements for divorce or separation. All three women had managed to make their arrangements in such a way that they received neither child support nor alimony payments. Their lack of self-assertiveness toward men was very much like that reported in the patients with "primary obesity" studied by Rascovsky, in whom the ego became fixed at a preambivalent stage of orality.[10] Like many children, they felt so self-sufficient that they did not need anybody's help. As one result of their treatment, Muriel and Helen commenced new legal actions against their former husbands in order to obtain some minimal payment in terms of what was realistically possible, and not for punitive reasons. Mary's son was almost old enough to support himself, so she decided to take no action, although she was helped to understand the reasons for her previous inertia.

These patients realized that they could not previously express their resentment or hostility toward their husbands because they needed to retain every source of approbation and feared disapproval. When their marriages ended, they had begun to express their hostility by overeating, which probably represented an aggressive masculine introjection mechanism.[4] By symbolically placing themselves in competition with other members of the family for solace from their mothers, they began to experience anxiety, which acted as a further spur to overeating. This suggests that the "special vehicle" for coping with tension, reported in Rorschach studies of obese women, is overeating.[8] Since sexual activity was so important to all but one of these patients, they unconsciously began to realize that obesity was one way in which they could reduce the opportunities for sexual activity and thus frustrate themselves further. The patients to whom sexual intercourse meant the most were Muriel, Mary, and Helen, who had no husbands and were thus largely dependent on their appearance for their ability to find sexual partners. The more obese they became, the more difficult it would be for them to find such partners or new husbands.

Betty and Ruth, each of whom had severe sexual problems, were helped to see how they had substituted eating heavily for sexual activity. These patients had grown up with the belief that it was appropriate for a husband and wife to meet on the level of food, but not on the sexual level. Thus, their evaluation of eating was socially reinforced but their image of sexual activity was clearly one with much conflict and negative valences.

These patients differed from the younger patients seen by Bruch, who in their teens clearly used[3] overeating as a protection against more severe mental illness. None of these patients had been overweight until they were well into adult life, even though their psychiatric diagnosis disclosed very severe pathology. They had evidently channeled their illnesses into work and family activity. The extent to which their unconscious and fantasy material was near the surface, as could be seen by their ability to present such material, suggests that one way in which they had maintained themselves was by the healing effect of the dream work itself. In adult life, as a result of some important crisis or situation, the defenses which they had used to shore themselves up against reality began collapsing. They regressed by overeating, which became a major defense. Their overeating represented their body's adjustment to a new situation.

The patients gradually became aware of the extent to which overeating was their major defense against reality, by the extent to which it returned symbolically over and over again in their dreams and other unconscious material. By the end of the treatment period, seven patients had accepted and made terms with their weight and were concentrating their efforts on maintaining their weight. They had developed fairly realistic perceptions of their body image. The other two patients, Betty and Helen, were referred for extended psychoanalytic treatment. Inasmuch as the sessions terminated in July, there was a spurt of interest in weight and eating during May and June on the part of the patients, since they began to think of how they would look in summer clothes and bathing suits.

Prediction of Weight Shifts

It had been hypothesized that the emotional content and tone of each session and the weight loss and gain of individual patients were correlated positively and significantly. The procedure developed to measure this was analogous to that employed by Benedek and Rubinstein in attempts to predict women patients' place on the menstrual cycle from the content of their individual psychotherapy session.[1] The complete transcript of each of the first five sessions was turned over to the research psychologist, who studied the relationship between the affective content of what each patient said and the amount of weight she had gained or lost, if any, in the preceding week. It was possible to form some clear impressions of each patient's "internal clock," which regulated the manner in which she adapted to her intrapsychic and external reality by gaining and losing weight, or by remaining at a stable weight. The transcripts of the last ten sessions were then edited so that all references to weight or weight increase or decrease were removed. These transcripts were then turned over to the psychologist, who attempted to predict, on the basis of what each patient had said during the session, whether she had lost or gained weight or remained at the same weight during the previous week. The psychologist's estimate was then compared with the women's weight shift or nonshift, as measured by her weighing-in before the treatment session. His prediction was right twenty-nine times out of the sixty occasions (6 women for 10 weeks). Since each woman could have moved in any one of three directions, accuracy of these predictions might be expected through chance, one out of three or, twenty out of the sixty times. The critical ratio (t) between the twenty choices that might have been expected by chance and the twenty-nine actually achieved was 2.58, which is significant at the 1 per cent confidence level. There were, of course, sessions during which some women spoke very little, thus making the estimating more difficult. The actual shifts in weight in the 6 patients are shown in Table 18-II. It will be noticed that the last few weeks showed a sharp tendency for patients to gain weight.

It was assumed that any weight gain or loss of up to 2 lb in either direction was not a significant one. Thus, a gain or loss was only computed as such if it was 2 lb or more. During this ten-week period, 49.4 per cent of the changes were losses, 25.6 per cent were gains, and 25.0 per cent involved no weight change. The difference between the losses and gains is significant at the 1 per cent level, as is the difference between the losses and those who remained the same. The difference between those who gained and remained the same is not significant.

One difference between the increase and decrease of weight of these patients is that the average weight decrease per week was 2.3, whereas the average weight increase was 3.8 lb. Some patients gained as much as 7 or 8 lb a week. The ability to predict weight loss or gain was based almost entirely on the patients' feelings and unconscious communication, which had little relation to how much they ate. Some might eat heavily and lose weight, some might eat relatively little and gain weight. There were complex relationships between the achievement of insights and ego strength and weight gain or loss. Some patients lost weight as they improved in their ability to achieve insight. Other patients gained weight as they improved in their ability to obtain insight. These relationships appeared to be idiosyncratic, unique to the individual, and fairly consistent. Muriel, for ex-

TABLE 18-II

DIRECTION OF WEIGHT LOSS OR GAIN OVER CONSECUTIVE
TEN-WEEK PERIOD

Session	Number of Women Who Gained, Lost, or Remained the Same Weight		
	Lost Weight	Gained Weight	Remained Same
13	3	1	2
14	3	2	1
15	4	1	1
16	3	1	2
17	3	1	2
18	4	1	1
19	3	2	1
20	4	2	—
21	1	3	2
22	1	2	3

ample, responded to every insight which she felt herself achieving by punishing herself, by eating more and gaining weight. Her hair had been tinted red, but she decided to dye it black. During one session she realized that she had dyed it black both in order to recall what she had been like as a young brunette and because her employer liked brunettes. This insight represented a real breakthrough in her treatment, but she responded to it by doubling her caloric intake, thus punishing herself.

Special times of the day appeared to be important to some patients in terms of their diets. These times were usually cathected in some way that emerged during treatment. May used to diet very carefully until about 8:00 PM. Around 8:00 she would feel like doing something "ridiculous," and eat "absurd" foods, even though she realized that this was wrong. In anamnesis at the beginning of treatment, she recalled that her father used to play with her when she was three or four years old, around 8:00 PM, just before her bed time. The implications of this became clear to her only later in treatment. Helen often became ravenously hungry around 11:00 PM, and would leave her midtown apartment to go out and visit stores until she found some delicacy that she wanted. After some months of treatment, she recalled that her last quarrel with her husband before their separation had occurred at 11:00 PM on a New Year's Eve and that this time had special meaning for her.

In some patients the reciprocal relationship between eating and other methods of coping with problems became clearly apparent. Muriel, for example, reported that she felt hungry on two occasions: when she read and when she daydreamed. She had supposed that reading and daydreaming were "escape" mechanisms, but that eating was good because it was a counterbalancing mechanism and a tie to what she called "actuality." She thus encouraged herself to eat more so that she would be in closer touch with "actuality." During treatment, she became aware that the reason for her eating when she read or daydreamed was not because eating was a counterbalancing mechanism but because it served some of the same powerful unconscious needs for her as did reading or daydreaming. Taking naps or going to the movies when she felt like gorging herself were temporary procedures by which Muriel attempted to integrate this insight into her daily life.

On the basis of a study of how each patient responded to the stresses and strains of the week, both internal and external, it was thus possible to establish some schematic response of weight loss and/or gain for each patient. These patients were primarily oral, and their major adaptational mechanism was eating and weight gain or loss. During this period of group psychoanalysis, this adaptational mechanism was in full operation. Practically everything that these women did, felt, and thought while they were in treatment was translated into changes in their weight, which was characterized by remarkable lability. The short-term changes in weight experienced by the patients during the period of treatment was far greater than the same women experienced either before or after this period.

Ruth and Nancy, who had undergone climacteric, were more controlled and exhibited less tension, fantasy, and dream activity, as well as markedly less shifts in weight, than did the four women who were still menstruating. The latter usually gained a few pounds just before menstruating. The existence of menstruation seemed to provide opportunities for relatively abrupt and wide ranging shifts of expression in level of aspiration, relations with other people, attitudes toward sexual activity, and feelings about the patient's parents and children.

Dreams about food, candy, and eating occurred from time to time, in most of which there was little displacement or disguise and which needed a minimum of interpretation. Thus, a dream of getting into a supermarket after it had closed and only being able to find low-calorie reducing bread was reported by two patients. A dream of enjoying a luxurious dinner in a restaurant with the analyst was reported by two other patients. Dreams about children, especially in the women who did not have children, were common.

In spite of the well-established difficulties of generalization, even at a low level of abstraction, on the basis of bodily cycles and rhythms,[5] weight seems to be a relatively idiosyncratic but fairly predictable body function, which can be plotted against the patient's communications in group psychoanalytic treatment. It is much less sensitive an indication that the menstrual cycle, which has been shown by Benedek and Rubinstein to correlate almost exactly with patients' communications in intensive psychoanalytic treatment.[1] It is probably a grosser measure than the relative precision made possible by the very nature of the ovarian function. Body weight adjustment is obviously not as schematic and inevitable as the ovarian cycle. It might be possible to take patients in intensive daily psychoanalytic treatment and predict their daily weight shifts on the basis of the content of their psychoanalytic sessions. This would probably be more difficult than doing so on a weekly basis because of the extent to which weight changes may fluctuate greatly from day to day, but present more of a pattern over a period of a week, in a kind of internal smoothing of the curve of weight change.

Loss of Weight

It had been hypothesized that patients would lose weight significantly as a result of treatment. In Table 18-II, in which the trends in weight gain and loss were presented for each of the last ten sessions, the last few weeks of treatment showed a sharp upsurge of weight increases, after a fairly consistent pattern of weight decrease. This probably represents the patients' resentment and concern over the dissolution of a group which meant so much to them, an unconscious request to the analyst not to abandon them, and an attempt to maintain emotional homeostasis. As a result, the patients gained back so much of the weight they had lost that by the last session their weights were very similar to what they had been at the first session. It was felt that the most realistic measure of the effect of the group experience would be to follow the patients up for at least two years. The patients' weights at commencement of treatment and thirty months later are shown in Table 18-III.

All but one of the patients lost weight, although the average loss of 4.3 lb was small in comparison with the starting average overweight of 33 lb. There appeared to be no correlation between severity of emotional illness and weight gain or loss, although the two patients (Betty and Helen) who have continued in treatment lost slightly more than the average. One patient gained a pound, although such a small change is hardly significant. One of the project's major goals, if not the major goal, could thus not be achieved, for a number of reasons.

One reason had to do with what might be called the unconscious climate of the group. The members established a reinforcing unconscious pattern of not losing weight and derived a kind of masochistic delight in not achieving this major goal. They could enjoy feelings of despair, hopelessness, and self-rejection since they confronted each other as heavy middle-aged matrons, while their costumes and make-up belied their age and size. They both wanted to lose weight and wanted not to do so, as one way of maintaining and reinforcing their membership in the group. Their concentrating on subjects other than food and dieting was both a realistic and wise choice in terms of how they wanted to spend their therapy time and an unconscious selection of the less threatening of several alternatives.

TABLE 18-III

WEIGHT OF PATIENTS AT BEGINNING OF GROUP THERAPY AND
THIRTY MONTHS LATER

Patient	Weight at Beginning	Weight at Follow-Up	Net Change
Muriel	178	176	–2
Nancy	166	161	–5
Betty	152	153	+1
Mary	186	175	–9
Helen	157	150	–7
Ruth	168	164	–4
Average Loss			4.3

It was easier for them to discuss unconscious material than to discuss eating. The unconscious feels timeless, but eating occurs today.

Another reason was the analyst's awareness that most of these patients were severely ill and were able to adapt to their difficulties primarily through the medium of eating and food. They were so hungry for contact that the therapy group provided a ready framework within which they could communicate their fantasies and dreams. The closeness to the surface of their unconscious conflicts could be seen in the relative ease with which they were able to communicate dream and unconscious material. The fantasy hunger for affection of these patients was so great that no reality experience could fulfill it. Eating was the way that was most accessible and fulfilling to the patients. The analyst became aware of the dynamic functions served by the patients' overweight and began to restructure the goal of the group as weight maintenance and acceptance rather than weight loss. Both patients and analyst thus began to accept and work toward the new goal.

In one of her earlier attempts to lose weight, for example, Muriel had been on a diet of 1,000 calories a day for six weeks and lost no weight. Other patients had had similar experiences, so that one of the most important insights achieved by the members of the group was the extent to which weight loss or gain was a function of the individuality of each person's body and emotional predispositions. The implications of "making up" one's mind to lose weight, and how this related to caloric intake, were discussed extensively. Weight loss or gain began to be understood by the patients as a process which occurs from the inside out.

Use of Ancillary Facilities

Special diet, massage, and relaxation facilities were made available to the patients in order to provide data on the interaction between the use of each of these facilities and psychodynamic content of group sessions. However, the hypothesis that the patients would make use of such ancillary therapeutic procedures throughout the period of group treatment, and especially once they adapted to their roles as patients, was not confirmed. Four of the six patients expressed little or no interest in such procedures. One patient took a course at a beauty school on posture and dieting and another enrolled at a municipal diet clinic. Both patients made arrangements for enrolling in the courses on their own and told the group after having done so. Only one patient explored the "official" ancillary services, and she lost interest in them after a while.

The analyst stressed that the employment of whatever procedures might be useful for any patient at a given time was appropriate in the quest for self. If a strict regime seemed to be helpful at a given time, there was no reason why a patient might not follow such a regime. It was, however, emphasized that external pressures are hardly likely to be sustained, and that only a reshaping of underlying attitudes can effect lasting changes. When Mary stopped taking even saccharin in order not to give her taste buds or blood chemistry a chance to experience the sugar taste she craved, the analyst pointed out that this was likely to be only a temporary palliative.

The patients preferred to engage in relatively informal diets, on which the analyst was the major resource person. He had had previous experience working in hospital obesity and nutrition clinics, and was thus able to provide realistic diet data. The patients seemed to want to concentrate their efforts on the psychotherapy situation and to feel that they were being disloyal to it or in some magical way violating the unconscious compact they had made as members of the therapy group by using the auxiliary facilities. The analyst discussed and made explicit the possibility that the group felt the analyst might want to hear about unconscious material rather than reports of diet and massage, so that each patient could make a realistic decision on whether to use the auxiliary activities. Even though the cooperating physicians were part of the therapeutic team and had been introduced to the patients at the first group session, the patients did not wish to consult them.

Another possibility is the patients' fear that these specialists might *really* cause them to lose weight, which they both sought and avoided. The possibility that a form of physical therapy might be effective, whereas group psychotherapy clearly was having only a limited effect on weight loss, may have provided a situation which the patients may not have wished to explore further, for fear of losing their confidence in group psychotherapy. None of the patients made any substantial use of these adjuvant therapies in the thirty months after the treatment period.

SUMMARY

Psychoanalytic group psychotherapy was conducted for six months with six obese middle-aged women. There were twenty-two group sessions and twenty-two alternate sessions. Special facilities for diet, massage, and relaxation therapy were available to the patients. The group treatment significantly improved the adaptation, self-awareness, and skills in living of the patients. It was possible to be accurate to a significant extent in prediction of whether each patient had gained or lost weight or remained at the same weight from week to week, from a blind analysis of the transcript of group sessions which had every statement about eating or weight removed. In a follow-up thirty months after the commencement of treatment, the average patient had lost 4.3 lb, compared with an average overweight of 33 lb. The patients made practically no use of the ancillary procedures available.

As treatment uncovered the extent to which eating and obesity were profoundly embedded in the patients' defense systems, the goals of the group were modified in the direction of weight maintenance rather than weight loss. The analyst decided that further group treatment would be unwise, and the sessions were terminated after six months. The two patients who appeared to be able to benefit from more intensive treatment were referred for psychoanalytic treatment.

REFERENCES

1. Benedek, T. and Rubenstein, B. B.: The sexual cycle in women: The relation between ovarian function and psychodynamic processes. *Psychosom Med,* 3:1, 1942.
2. Bruch, H.: Obesity in childhood and personality development. *Am J Orthopsychiat,* 11:467, 1941.
3. Bruch, H.: Developmental obesity and schizophrenia. *Psychiatry,* 21:65, 1958.
4. Bychowski, G.: On neurotic obesity. *Psychoanal Rev,* 37:301, 1950.
5. DuBois, F.: Rhythms, cycles and periods in health and disease. *Am J Psychiat,* 116:114, 1959.
6. Fromm, E.: Dynamics in a case of obesity. *J Clin Exp Psychopath,* 19:292, 1958.
7. Kotkov, B.: Experiences in group psychotherapy with the obese. *Psychosom Med,* 15:243, 1953.
8. Kotkov, B. and Murawski, B.: A Rorschach study of the personality structure of obese women. *J. Clin Psychol,* 8:391, 1952.
9. Meyer, J.: Genetic, traumatic and environmental factors in the etiology of obesity. *Physiol Rev,* 33:472, 1953.
10. Rascovsky, A., Rascovsky, N. W. and Echlossberg, T.: The basic psychic structure of the obese. *Int J Psychoanal,* 31:144, 1950.
11. Simmons, W. D.: Group approach to weight reduction. *J Am Diet Assoc,* 30:442, 1957.
12. Stunkard, A. J.: The dieting depression. *Am J Med,* 23:77, 1957.
13. Stunkard, A. J. and McLaren-Hume, M.: The results of treatment for obesity. *Arch Int Med,* 103:79, 1959.
14. Winick, C.: Addiction and its treatment. *Law Contemp Prob,* 22:9, 1957.
15. Young, C. M., Berresford, K. and Moore, N. S.: Psychologic factors in weight control. *Am J Clin Nutr,* 5:186, 1957.

19

Effectiveness of Group Therapy

Janet P. Wollersheim

ONE of the major difficulties encountered in conducting psychotherapy outcome research is the selection of a dependent variable which not only can be objectively measured, but which also represents a relevant criterion of change. The treatment of obesity involving designation of actual body weight as the dependent variable represents a measure which is not only completely objective, but which also thoroughly defines the criterion, as reduction in body weight represents the primary and specific goal of treatment. Additionally, since obesity is a condition which affects from 23 per cent to 68 per cent of women in the United States,[29] it constitutes a significant health problem which in its own right should merit serious attention.

While psychology and psychiatry have contributed a plethora of theories concerning the cause of obesity, the majority of these theories[1, 5, 10] view obesity and overeating as a symptom of some underlying "psychic abnormality" and imply or directly contend that treatment must focus upon the underlying cause. Emphasis has been placed upon the presumed deviant personality characteristics which distinguish overweight from normal weight individuals. These deviant personality characteristics together with the symptom of overeating are then construed as a basic syndrome which must be treated by dealing with the presumed underlying causes.

Yet, on the basis of a recent review of the relevant literature, as well as from the evidence of an assessment study which they conducted, Wollersheim, Paul, and Werry[31] concluded that while from a physiological point of view, obesity may result from multiple etiologies, overeating has been the only behavioral or personality characteristic consistently distinguishing the obese from the nonobese. In the great majority of cases, successful weight reduction would depend upon reducing the positive energy balance which results from overweight individuals simply *eating too much* for their activity level.

Of the hundreds of papers published on the treatment of obesity, few give even slight attention to specifically helping the client learn to modify his eating practices, although some professionals have stressed the importance of directly focusing upon a change in eating practices.[11, 12] Even more discouraging is the fact that the overwhelming majority of studies fail to

meet even minimal standards of experimental control and scientific reporting, making it impossible to replicate the study or to make definitive statements concerning treatment. In the most comprehensive review of the
treatment of obesity, covering the medical literature for the previous 30
years, Stunkard and McLaren-Hume[25] found that, in general, only 25 per
cent of patients lost a significant amount of weight. A review of group attempts at weight reduction yielded nearly identical results.[26] More precise
estimates of the results of treatment are precluded because of the unfortunate state of affairs characterizing this literature. Investigators have been
further discouraged by high attrition rates showing that from 20 per cent
to 80 per cent of patients beginning weight reduction programs abandoned them before completion.[27]

The theoretical orientation of this study derives from learning principles and views eating behavior and *overeating* as essentially similar to
any other learned behavior patterns in terms of development, maintenance,
and change.[28] While behavior modification techniques derived from learning principles are becoming more popular among psychologists, even within the learning principles framework, experimental studies designed to
establish cause-effect relationships between treatment procedures and
weight loss have been lacking.

The primary purpose of this investigation was to develop a group therapy program for obesity based upon learning principles and to evaluate
the effectiveness of this program in an experimental design including adequate control groups which would control for the effects of time, season,
and intercurrent life experiences (i.e. no treatment); nonspecific effects
of undergoing treatment, such as attention, "faith," rational conceptualiza-
tions, "ritual," and expectation of relief (i.e. nonspecific treatment); and a
control for positive expectation and social pressure, minimizing other nonspecific effects. This latter type of control group is viewed as desirable in an
obesity study as the elements of positive expectation and social pressure
appear to be the major ingredients in the nationwide Take Off Pounds
Sensibly (TOPS) weight-reducing clubs,[25] which, to the best of the investigator's knowledge, have not been evaluated by controlled investigations.

METHOD

Design and Procedure

Seventy-nine motivated, overweight female Ss completed an assessment
battery, including body weight, at the beginning and end of an eighteen-
week base-line period. Following the second assessment, Ss were randomly
assigned from stratified blocks, on percentage overweight, to one of four experimental conditions: a) positive expectation-social pressure (SP); b)

nonspecific therapy (NS); c) focal therapy (FT); d) no-treatment-wait control (C). Since percentage overweight, rather than actual weight, is indicative of degree of obesity, this procedure insured equating the degree of obesity across experimental conditions. Four therapists (two males and two females) each treated one group of 5 Ss in each of the three treatment conditions for a total of ten sessions spanning a period of twelve weeks (mid-October to mid-January). Treatment sessions within all conditions were designed such that any S could miss one session without missing new material. The relative efficacy of the treatments in producing weight loss and changes in eating patterns was then evaluated on the basis of posttreatment and an eight-week follow-up administration of the assessment battery.

Assessment Instruments

The assessment battery administered at the four assessment periods included: height (to the nearest inch without shoes) and weight (to the nearest pound in indoor clothing without shoes) obtained on standard physician's balance scales; an Eating Patterns Questionnaire (EPQ), providing historical data on obesity and yielding six factor scores concerning specific eating practices (Factor 1, emotional and uncontrolled overeating; Factor 2, eating response to interpersonal situations; Factor 3, eating in isolation; Factor 4, eating as reward; Factor 5, eating response to evaluative situations; Factor 6, between-meal eating);[31] modification of Schifferes'[22] Physical Activity Scale, yielding a five-point classification of activity level (1, sedentary, to 5, exceptionally active) based upon reported frequency of six specific types of activities during a twenty-four-hour period; the Pittsburg Social Extraversion-Introversion Scale;[2] the IPAT Anxiety Scale Questionnaire;[7] and ten situation-specific anxiety scales ("Speech Before a Large Group," "Job Interview," "Final Course Examination," "Night Before Big Dance," "Entering Lecture Hall for Large Class," "Discussing College Experience with Parents," "Talking to Attractive Boy at Party," "Chatting with Girlfriends," "Home Watching TV on Saturday Night," "Doing Homework in Study Area"), following the format of the S-R Inventory of Anxiousness.[9] In addition, at the termination of treatment, Ss rated therapist competence and likability.

Therapists

Four therapists (two males and two females), including the investigator, participated in the study. All were PhD candidates in clinical psychology who had completed all clinical training and preliminary examination requirements at the time of the investigation. Each therapist had at least two years of supervised experience in conducting psychotherapy (both individual and group). Their orientations were cognitive-behavioral, with formulations of psychotherapy based upon learning principles being influential.

Treatments

Each S assigned to positive expectation—social pressure, nonspecific, or focal treatment, was treated in a closed group of five. All therapists understood that the criterion of improvement was to be weight reduction. Each of the four therapists treated one group of five Ss within each treatment, for a total of fifteen Ss each, therefore holding constant potentially important effects of therapist characteristics such as sex, personality, and physical attributes.

Prior to treatment contact, each therapist studied four treatment manuals* written for this project by the investigator and met for a total of seven hours of intensive training in the specific treatment conditions. The "Therapist General Orientation Manual for Weight Reduction Study" described the purpose of the investigation, presented an overview of each treatment condition, and detailed procedures common to all forms of group therapy which were to be used in all three treatments.

Besides the General Orientation Manual, therapists were provided with a manual for each of the three treatment conditions which explicitly delineated all procedures to be followed, including the time to be spent in various activities and the rationale to be given Ss. All therapy sessions within each treatment were recorded and monitored weekly by the investigator to insure consistent and appropriate application of procedures.

The Ss in all treatment conditions were presented the same factual information pertaining to obesity, health, nutrition, and weight reduction, and all were told that successful weight reduction depended upon either increased activity or decreased caloric intake. Additionally, Ss in all three treatment conditions were urged to decrease their caloric intake to between 1,000 and 1,500 calories daily, in a manner appropriate to their general living circumstances. They were encouraged to lose 2 lb a week by reducing their caloric intake and were provided with identical booklets listing the caloric value of over 2,600 foods. Students in each treatment were told that they were assigned to the treatment in which they should be most successful, on the basis of personality characteristics. Sessions for the positive expectation—social pressure treatment were limited to 15 to 20 minutes, while nonspecific and focal sessions were 90 minutes each.

---

* The four treatment manuals have been deposited with the National Auxiliary Publications Service. Order Document No. 01251 from the National Auxiliary Publications Service of the American Society for Information Science, c/o CCM Information Sciences, Inc., 909 3rd Avenue, New York, New York 10022.

Positive Expectation-Social Pressure (Group SP)

The main purpose of SP treatment was to foster in Ss a high positive expectation for losing weight and to *foster* and *use* social pressure in helping each S reduce. The rationale presented to Ss assigned to this treatment was that the outstanding variable to which success could be attributed is the motivational one, that is, the fact that S makes a commitment to lose weight and has a group of fellow students and the therapist checking up on the outcome of this commitment in terms of weekly "weigh-ins" before the group. Each session consisted of weighing each S before the group, announcing her weight, and noting her loss or gain from the previous week. The therapist and group administered mild negative reinforcers (e.g. "What a shame!") and encouragement (e.g. "But you'll show us next week, won't you?") for weight gains and positive reinforcers (e.g. "This gal is really going places!") for weight losses. Those who gained weight from the previous week were required to wear a red tag drawn in the form of a pig throughout the session. Those whose weight remained constant wore a green sign reading "turtle," while yellow stars were worn by those who lost weight. The member who lost the most weight that week wore a star and a crown.

After the "weigh-ins," commendations and "playful ribbing" were continued, or group discussions centered upon factual questions relating to obesity, health, nutrition, or weight loss. If Ss began to inquire about specific ways to decrease overeating, the therapist emphasized that the important thing was to reduce daily caloric intake and that each person should do this in a manner appropriate to her particular living circumstances. In the event the group discussion continued on the topic of specific ways to reduce overeating, the therapist diverted attention away from this topic by posing questions or commenting upon factual information concerning obesity, nutrition, or weight reduction.

Nonspecific Therapy (Group NS)

The main purpose of this treatment was, at the minimum, to control for effects of undergoing group treatment resulting from such nonspecific factors as increased attention, "faith," expectation of relief, and presentation of a treatment rationale and meaningful "ritual." The rationale presented to Ss assigned to this treatment was that it would be important for them to develop insight into the "real and not readily recognizable underlying reasons" for their behavior and to discover the "unconscious motives" underlying their "personality make-up." It was explained that as each individual obtained insight and better understanding of the "real motives and forces" operating within her personality, she would find it easier to accomplish her goals and to lose weight.

The first 15 to 20 minutes of these sessions employed the procedures used in the SP treatment. The next 20 to 30 minutes were devoted to a control use of relaxation training following the training procedures reported by Paul and Shannon,[20] with the rationale being to help Ss feel at ease so they could "better develop insight." The remaining 40 to 55 minutes of NS therapy sessions were devoted to discussion focused upon hypothetical *underlying causes* for their behavior, not only in the area of eating, but broadly extending into other areas as well. Historical elaboration was encouraged rather than emphasizing current events. In order to structure this treatment condition to provide an internally consistent conceptual framework which would be maximally specific and acceptable to Ss, therapy procedures utilized a psychoanalytically oriented game model superficially similar to that of Eric Berne's.[4] "Games" were introduced as a way of more clearly conceptualizing the underlying causes of behavior. In the NS treatment, discussions frequently strayed from a game model, obesity, and any current behavior to such topics as movies seen or an experience one had with a grade school teacher. If group discussion turned to specific ways to modify eating patterns, the therapist used his clinical skill in diverting the group's attention away from overt behavior and to underlying causes and historical material. The treatment manual provided twenty-two suggested games as well as specific interpretive principles to be applied.

Focal Therapy (Group F)

The major purpose of this treatment was to identify and shape current eating behavior by applying techniques derived from learning principles. The Ss receiving this treatment were told that their eating practices were learned patterns of behavior. Just as they had learned inappropriate eating patterns, they could, by application of appropriate principles, learn appropriate eating practices which would promote weight loss and make effective maintenance of the loss possible. Extensive use was made of instrumental learning techniques.

Procedures used in the SP treatment were employed during the first 15 to 20 minutes of each session, followed by a discussion period lasting from 40 to 55 minutes. The remaining 20 to 30 minutes were devoted to training and instruction in the use of deep relaxation after Paul and Shannon.[20] Unlike the control use of relaxation in Group NS, Ss were told that learning to become deeply relaxed was a skill, and that as they learned this skill they would be instructed in how to use relaxation to counter tension in many situations which in the past might have typically resulted in eating behavior.

During the discussion phase of the first session, Ss were instructed in methods of recording their eating behavior in a small notebook provided for this purpose. In the following sessions, references were made to the eating records to provide a basis for individual functional analyses of stimuli controlling eating behavior. The first half of the discussion phase in Sessions 2 through 6 was devoted to a review of techniques already presented and discussed in previous sessions, with the second half used to introduce new techniques. The therapist's most important task was to help each S specifically identify discriminative, reinforcing, and eliciting stimuli related to overeating and to implement self-control techniques in the circumstances arising in her individual mode of living. The following is a synopsis of the techniques introduced in each session: Session 1—building positive associations concerning eating control; Session 2—developing appropriate stimulus control of eating behavior and manipulation of deprivation and satiation by shaping and fading; Session 3—rewarding oneself for developing self-control in eating, and developing and using personally meaningful ultimate aversive consequences of overeating; Session 4—obtaining reinforcers from areas of life other than eating and establishing alternative behaviors incompatible with eating; Session 5—utilization of chaining; Session 6—supplementary techniques involving aversive imagery. All techniques were introduced and discussed by the end of the sixth session, with the remaining four sessions devoted to continued discussion of each S's utilization of the techniques and the correction of misunderstanding and misapplications.

No-Treatment-Wait-Control (Group C)

The major purpose of this condition was to provide control for such factors as intercurrent life experiences, time of year, effects of testing, and other potentially influential variables not related to treatment per se. The Ss in this condition followed the same procedures, under the same conditions, as Ss in the treatment groups, with the exception of treatment itself. A few days before their first scheduled group session, Ss were contacted by telephone and told that because of an unexpected increase in clinical and research responsibilities, the doctor, their therapist, was unable to serve in the program. They were assured, however, that treatment would be definitely provided for them the following semester as soon as therapist time became available. At the time of post-treatment assessment, the investigator contacted these Ss by telephone and told them that treatment would be available, but it would first be necessary to again take the assessment battery. After these post-treatment measures were taken, these Ss were given treatment and hence were not available for the eight-week follow-up assessment.

Subjects

A total of seventy-nine female students at the University of Illinois ranging in age from eighteen to thirty-six years ($Mdn = 19$) participated in the study. These Ss were selected on motivation for treatment and percentage overweight from a population requesting treatment for obesity, following announcement of program availability in the university newspaper and bulletin boards. The weight criteria were based upon the 1959 Metropolitan Life Insurance Company norms for desirable weight for women.[29] Desirable weight was determined by taking the lowest weight given for a person of medium frame and 2 in taller than the S in the Metropolitan norms.* A woman was considered overweight only if her actual weight was *at least* 10 per cent above her desirable weight at the time of initial contact (i.e. pre-base line).

Students were further screened for motivation by attendance at pre-treatment assessment and a consequent brief interview (10 to 15 minutes) with the investigator. The purpose of the interview was to establish common expectations for all Ss and to exclude those who felt they did not over-eat, were not sufficiently concerned to attend weekly sessions, or those who were currently receiving any type of psychotherapy or treatment for weight reduction.

The average percentage overweight of the resulting sample of 79 Ss at pre-base line was 28.63 per cent, ranging from 10 per cent to 70 per cent. These Ss reported continuous obesity for 1 to 24 years ($Mdn = 5$ years). All Ss reported unsuccessful attempts to lose weight, with 76 per cent of the sample reporting nearly continuous attempts at weight reduction which resulted in considerable discouragement. In general, these Ss were characteristic of the "hard core" group of obese persons discussed in the literature[16, 18, 32] in that most had been obese since childhood or adolescence and the degree of obesity was considerable with many previous unsuccessful attempts at weight reduction which resulted in significant discouragement. The fact that Ss were all female was also an unfavorable prognostic indicator.[25]

RESULTS

Attrition

Of the seventy-nine Ss participating in the study at pre-treatment (20 Ss in each of the treatment groups and 19 Ss in the control group), seventy-

---

* The lower end of the weight range was appropriate for determining desirable weight since the Metropolitan norms are for women over age twenty-five who are expected to weigh more than the younger women in the present sample where only three were age 25 or over. Two inches were added to height as the Metropolitan norms are based upon height measurements taken with shoes on and S's height was measured with shoes off in the present study. This procedure tended to make the estimate of the degree of obesity conservative.

six remained at post-treatment (Group F lost 2 and Group C 1). The attrition rate was less than 4 per cent for the total sample. The amount of attrition was not significant, as evaluated by Fisher's test of exact probability for all possible combinations of the four experimental groups (all $ps > .21$). At follow-up, only three treated Ss (2 from Group SP and 1 from Group NS) were lost as they had left school. The Ss not available for post-assessment were dropped from all subsequent analyses, with the consequent N for the total sample being 76. The N for each group was as follows: SP = 20; NS = 20; F = 18; C = 18. Analyses involving follow-up data involved a total N of 55 (SP = 18; NS = 19, F = 18).

Comparative Treatment Effects: Weight

Detailed analyses of actual weight and percentage overweight demonstrated that the four experimental groups were equated on these variables at pre-base line and pre-treatment and that there were no significant changes in these measures over the base-line period.[30]

Major analyses on actual weight and the other assessment measures were performed on the basis of residual change scores for each S, consisting of the difference between the obtained score at post-treatment and that predicted on the basis of multiple linear regression from pre-base line and pre-treatment, thus providing a base-free measure of change.[8] Since the sample of Ss changed from post-treatment to follow-up because of the loss of control Ss and three treated Ss, separate residual change scores were computed for post-treatment and follow-up data, using pre-base line and pre-treatment to predict post-treatment scores with a sample of seventy-six and using pre-base line and pre-treatment to predict follow-up scores with a sample of fifty-five.

The means and standard deviations of the four groups on actual weight at pre-base line, pre-treatment, post-treatment, and follow-up are presented in Table 19-I. Results from the one-way analysis of variance on treatments on postresidual change scores are presented in Table 19-II. The treatment effect for actual weight was highly significant ($p < .001$), indicating differential changes between groups. For the measures of actual weight, ratings involving rate reduction, and the factor scores on eating practices, differences between treatment means were tested with a more refined analysis utilizing Duncan's multiple-range tests, corrected for unequal Ns[15] with $\propto$ equal to .05, using one-tailed comparisons for differences in the hypothesized direction. (The hypothesized order of treatment effects for weight was that most weight reduction would be shown by Group F, then Group NS, then Group SP, and then Group C. For factor scores on eating practices, the hypothesized order of treatment effects was that most reduction in reported frequency of eating behaviors would be shown by Group F, followed by Group NS or SP and then Group C.)

TABLE 19-I
MEANS AND STANDARD DEVIATIONS OF EXPERIMENTAL GROUPS
FOR ACTUAL WEIGHT ACROSS ALL TIME PERIODS

Time	Group											
	Social Pressure			Nonspecific			Focal			Control		
	M	SD	N	M	SD	N	M	SD	N	M	SD	N
Pre-base line	157.80	21.15	20	161.35	25.29	20	154.11	18.70	18	157.72	22.58	18
Pre-treatment	160.15	23.91	20	159.20	25.13	20	153.61	19.06	18	156.39	22.54	18
Post-treatment	154.75$_a$	22.44	20	152.30$_b$	21.03	20	143.28$_{ab}$	16.69	18	158.78$_{ab}$	28.40	18
Follow-up	156.61$_a$	23.24	18	152.68$_b$	18.72	19	145.00$_{ab}$	16.11	18	—		—

Note: Subscript symbols refer to means which differ significantly in residual change score analyses. If any two means within a row share the same symbol, it means that significantly different changes from pre-treatment were revealed ($p < .05$, Duncan's multiple-range test).

Duncan's tests on postresidual change score treatment means showed that all three treatment groups evidenced significant weight reduction in contrast to Group C. Additionally, Group F differed significantly from Group NS and Group SP, while the latter two did not differ significantly from each other.[30] An additional analysis of variance demonstrated that therapist and therapist-by-treatment effects were nonsignificant.[30]

Further analyses showed a slight increase in weight for all groups from post-treatment to follow-up. However, from post-treatment to follow-up, there were no significant differential weight changes by treatments or therapist-treatment groups.

Residual change scores of treated Ss at follow-up were subjected to a two-way analysis of variance, summarized in Table 19-III. With the control group absent, and treatment effects of the SP and NS groups similar to each other, the analyses of variance revealed no significant effects. However, Duncan's multiple-range tests performed on the means of the treatment groups revealed that while Groups NS and SP did not differ significantly, Group F was significantly different from *both* of these treatments, indicating that at the time of the follow-up, Ss in the focal treatment condition still showed a significantly greater weight loss from pre-treatment than either of the other two treatment groups. The results of the Duncan's multiple-range tests for the analyses on residual change scores are indicated in Table 19-I

TABLE 19-II

ONE-WAY ANALYSES OF VARIANCE ON POSTRESIDUAL CHANGE SCORES FOR ACTUAL WEIGHT, EATING PATTERNS QUESTIONNAIRE FACTOR SCORES, AND PHYSICAL ACTIVITY SCALE (PAS)

Measure	Source	Analyses df	MS	F
Weight	Treatment	3	524.64	11.58‡
	error	72	46.49	
Factor 1 (Emotional and uncontrolled overeating)	Treatment	3	527.09	6.01†
	error	72	87.65	
Factor 2 (Eating response to interpersonal situations)	Treatment	3	23.18	1.46
	error	72	15.92	
Factor 3 (Eating in isolation)	Treatment	3	107.99	9.87‡
	error	72	10.95	
Factor 4 (Eating as reward)	Treatment	3	25.10	3.49*
	error	72	7.20	
Factor 5 (Eating response to evaluative situations)	Treatment	3	2.19	.29
	error	72	7.46	
Factor 6 (Eating between meals)	Treatment	3	33.53	4.38†
	error	72	7.65	
PAS	Treatment	3	.89	2.08
	error	72	.43	

Note: N = 76.
* $p < .05$.
† $p < .01$.
‡ $p < .001$.

TABLE 19-III

TWO-WAY ANALYSES OF VARIANCE ON FOLLOW-UP RESIDUAL CHANGE SCORES FOR ACTUAL WEIGHT EATING PATTERNS QUESTIONNAIRE FACTOR SCORES AND PHYSICAL ACTIVITY SCALE (PAS)

Source	df	Actual Weight		Factor 1		Factor 2		Measure Factor 3		Factor 4		Factor 5		Factor 6		PAS	
		MS	F	MS	F	MS	F	MS	F	MS	F	MS	F	MS	F	MS	F
Treatment	2	137.49	2.89	236.94	1.78	8.28	.39	75.41	6.08*	19.22	2.16	.82	.12	15.44	1.73	.53	1.17
Therapist	3	97.08	2.04	208.48	1.57	12.56	.59	18.50	1.49	6.86	.77	4.14	.61	2.43	.27	.93	2.07
Treatment × Therapist	6	27.87	.59	98.96	.74	6.43	.30	8.70	.70	14.11	1.59	7.60	1.12	6.19	.69	.17	.39
Error	43	47.63		133.11		21.22		12.40		8.89		6.77		8.94		.45	

Note: N = 55.
* p < .01.

with reference to raw score means, since raw score means and mean changes in raw scores are more meaningful from an interpretive point of view than residual change scores.

From pre-treatment to post-treatment, Group C gained 2.39 lb, Group SP lost 5.40 lb, Group NS lost 6.90 lb, while Group F showed a 10.33 lb reduction. From pre-treatment to follow-up, weight losses were less than those at post-treatment for all groups, but Group F still maintained a significantly greater weight loss from pre-treatment than the other groups, with weight loss for Group F being 8.61 lb, for Group SP, 3.44 lb, and for Group NS, 6.52 lb.

Individual Subject Improvement

Because clinical workers are frequently more concerned with percentage improvements in individual cases than with mean group differences and because negative treatment effects would be more easily identified from data on individuals, all data concerning weight reduction were further evaluated on the basis of individually significant change scores. In evaluating significant change in weight from pre-treatment to post-treatment, an individual case was classified as showing a "significant loss" if the pre-treatment-post-treatment reduction in weight was 9 lb or more. Likewise, an individual case was classified as showing a "significant gain" if the pre-treatment-post-treatment increase in weight was 9 lb or more. These criteria were derived empirically in the following manner: a cumulative frequency distribution was made of *absolute* change in weight for each S from pre-base line to pre-treatment ($N = 76$); absolute change in weight at the ninety-fifth percentile was 12 lb (absolute change in weight at the fiftieth percentile was 3 lb) over the 18-week base-line period, meaning that the change in weight of 95 per cent of the Ss was less than ⅔ lb/week; treatment (pre-treatment—post-treatment) extended over 12 weeks, so 95 per cent of the Ss could be expected to show less than an 8-lb weight change; hence, 9 lb was used as indicating a significant change in weight.

Improvement rates from pre-treatment to post-treatment are presented in Table 19-IV. Particularly striking is the finding that not a single case in any treatment group evidenced a significant weight gain, while 11 per cent of the control Ss did. Only 6 per cent of the control Ss showed significant weight reduction, while 25 per cent of Ss in Group SP lost a significant amount of weight, contrasted with 40 per cent in Group NS and 61 per cent in Group F. A Kruskal-Wallis one-way analysis of variance by ranks on these data over the four groups revealed that the differences in cases showing a significant gain, loss, or no change were highly significant ($H = 23.71$, $p < .001$).

Table 19-IV also presents the percentage of cases who still met the 9-lb criterion of significant loss or gain in weight from pre-treatment to follow-

TABLE 19-IV

PERCENTAGE OF CASES SHOWING SIGNIFICANT CHANGE IN ACTUAL WEIGHT
FROM PRE-TREATMENT TO POST-TREATMENT AND FROM
PRE-TREATMENT TO FOLLOW-UP

Time		Treatments*		
	SP	NS	F	C
Pre-treatment-Post-treatment				
Significant loss	25	40	61	6
No significant change	75	60	39	83
Significant gain	0	0	0	11
Pre-treatment-Follow-Up				
Significant loss	33	21	50	—
No significant change	61	79	50	—
Significant gain	6	0	0	—

Note: From pre-treatment to post-treatment, Ns = 20, 20, 18, and 18, respectively, for Groups SP, NS, F, and C. From pre-treatment to follow-up, Ns = 18, 19, and 18, respectively, for Groups SP, NS and F. Classifications were empirically derived from base-line data (see text).

* Numbers given are percentages.

up. At follow-up, the highest improvement rate was still obtained by Group F (50%), while only 21 per cent of the Ss in Group NS and 33 per cent in Group SP had lost 9 lb or more from pre-treatment to follow-up. A Kruskal-Wallis one-way analysis of variance by ranks on these data over the three groups showed that the differences in percentages were highly significant ($H = 9.79, p < .01$).

Comparative Treatment Effects: Eating Behavior and Physical Activity

Results from the one-way analyses of variance on treatments on the post-residual change scores for the factor measures and the physical activity scale are presented in Table 19-II. The following four factors showed significant treatment effects: Factor 1, emotional and uncontrolled overeating ($p < .01$); Factor 3, eating in isolation ($p < .001$); Factor 4, eating as reward ($p < .05$); and Factor 6, between-meal eating ($p < .01$). Analyses by means of Duncan's tests revealed that on Factors 1, 3, and 4, Group F showed a significantly greater reduction in the defined eating behaviors than did any of the other three groups whose changes did not differ significantly from each other. On Factor 6, the reduction for Group F was again significantly greater than that of the other three groups and Group SP showed a significantly greater reduction than Group C, although the reductions shown by Group SP and Group NS did not differ significantly from each other. No differential changes occurred in reported level of physical activity. Thus, while all treated groups showed significant pre-treatment-post-treatment weight reduction in contrast to the control group, only Group F showed systematic reduction in the reported frequency of various eating behaviors as defined by the factor scores.

Next, follow-up residual change scores on the factor measures and activity scale were subjected to two-way analysis of variance summarized in Table 19-III. Only the treatment effect on Factor 3, eating in isolation, reached statistical significance ($p < .01$), with Duncan's tests showing that Group F showed significantly greater reduction than the other two groups whose changes did not differ significantly from each other. Duncan's tests were also performed on Factors 1, 4, and 6 since these measures showed significantly different changes among treatment groups at post-treatment. These analyses at follow-up revealed no differential changes on Factors 1 and 6, but on Factor 4, eating as reward, Group F showed a significantly greater reduction than either of the other two groups whose changes did not differ significantly from each other.

Supplementary analyses[30] for therapists and therapist-treatment combinations indicated that the differential changes in reported frequency of eating behaviors which did occur were the results of the different treatments rather than different therapists or therapist-treatment combinations, with focal treatment resulting in significantly greater reductions in the reported frequencies of various eating behaviors than the other groups from both pre-treatment to post-treatment and from pre-treatment to follow-up.

Generalization Effects of Treatment and "Symptom Substitution"

Although none of the other personality or anxiety scales in the assessment battery were concerned with the specific target behaviors of treatment, they were included to aid in identifying the sample and to check on the generalization effects of treatment or, conversely, "symptom substitution." From the learning framework underlying focal treatment, no change or mild positive changes would be expected on the measures of these secondary variables. The *disease-analogy* model, however, would interpret the reduction in weight achieved by Groups F and SP as merely symptomatic and the result of suggestion or positive transference.[19] This model would also expect Groups F and SP to manifest harmful results as a result of "symptomatic weight reduction." In addition, the disease-analogy model might possibly predict "symptom substitution," not only for these two groups but for Group NS as well, since in this project Group NS was not designed to be truly representative of traditional psychodynamic treatment but instead served as a control condition, adding to social pressure elements nonspecific factors such as presentation of a treatment rationale and a "ritual" meaningful for Ss. In this investigation, the measures of extraversion, general anxiety, and situation-specific anxiety (SR scales) served to check on the "symptom substitution" hypothesis.

Analyses of variance of the residual change scores of these secondary measures at post-treatment and follow-up revealed no evidence for "symptom substitution."[30] Additionally, detailed correlational analyses indicated that reduction in weight and in reported frequencies of eating behavior were related to reductions on anxiety measures. Thus, rather than providing evidence for "symptom substitution," the data supported the learning framework model which would expect specificity of treatment effects with perhaps some degree of generalization of positive effects.

Subject Ratings

An analysis of variance (Treatment × Therapists) of Ss' ratings of therapists on the scale of likability (unlikable, likable, or very likable) revealed no significant differential effects. All therapists were rated as "likable" or "very likable" by every one of their clients. Ratings of therapists on the competency scale (incompetent, competent, very competent) revealed a significant treatment effect ($p < .05$), while treatment and Therapists × Treatment effects were nonsignificant. While every S rated her therapist as competent or very competent, Ss in Group SP rated their therapist competent more often than very competent, while Ss in the other two groups rated their therapist as very competent more often than competent.

Prediction of Improvement

The ability to predict which persons respond to treatment was not of major interest in this investigation. However, as such information would be of considerable value in both clinical practice and future research, possible relationships between the pre-treatment assessment measures and weight reduction were investigated. Each pre-treatment measure was correlated with post-treatment and follow-up residual change scores for weight. The results of these correlational analyses were totally nonsignificant. Of the thirty-eight coefficients computed, not even one attained significance at the 5 per cent level. Thus, for the sample included in the present study, measures of extraversion-introversion, general anxiety, situation-specific anxiety, physical activity, and reported frequencies of various eating behaviors were all unable to predict specific responsiveness to treatment.

DISCUSSION

The results of the present study demonstrate the superiority of focal treatment based on learning principles over nonspecific and social pressure treatment. Focal therapy produced greater weight loss and greater reduction in reported frequencies of various eating behaviors, not only at the termination of treatment but at an 8-week follow-up as well. Evidence for symptom substitution was totally lacking. While significant differential, weight reduction occurred for the various treatments, it did not occur for the different therapists or for the various therapist-treatment combinations. It is quite possible that when treatment techniques are explicitly specified and that when skilled therapists are trained in the therapeutic procedures and consistently apply them, treatment outcome becomes more a function of the treatment techniques utilized rather than the therapists using them. In addition to developing a feasible group therapy for obesity and demonstrating its effectiveness, the present study, in contrast to the weight reduction studies reported in the literature, was characterized by an extremely low attrition rate. Making acceptance into treatment contingent upon a firm commitment to attend sessions regularly and emphasis throughout the sessions of the importance of attendance to their own success and the success of their fellow group members were seemingly the factors most responsible for preventing "drop-outs."

The specificity of effects with focal treatment is considerably enhanced by comparison with the effects of nonspecific treatment which contained both social pressure and "placebo" elements. Not only did focal treatment produce significantly greater weight reduction, but it also produced significantly greater reductions in reported frequencies of various eating behaviors over the control group. The findings suggest that while Ss in Group F were systematically reducing the frequencies of their eating behavior, Ss in the NS and SP groups were generally not changing their eating behavior in any systematic way. The weight loss of these latter two groups may well have resulted from erratic, temporary, and fluctuating caloric intake. Yet, the weight losses of both of these groups were as good as and even better than many of the losses reported for therapy groups in the literature. It should be further noted that Group C did not constitute a "pure control" in the sense that a no-treatment, no-contact group would have. Group C received extra attention in the form of four telephone calls, a short interview, and participation in three testing and weighing sessions. If no-treatment control groups are actually therapy groups as stated by some investigators,[3] then the control group in the present study represents a conservative control measure. The finding that all three treatments produced significant weight loss in contrast to the control group is encouraging in an area so characterized by pessimism[25] and in view of the fact that the sample of Ss in the present investigation were characteristic of the "hard core" group of obese persons described in the literature.

To the investigator's knowledge, the present study represents the first group psychotherapy study concerning weight reduction designed with the controls necessary to establish cause-effect relationships between therapeutic techniques and treatment outcome. Two studies published after the completion of the present investigation[13, 14] and a report of eight case studies[23] all strongly point to the potential effectiveness in the utilization of learning principles in the treatment of obesity. These studies together with the present investigation reported rates of weight loss which would be considered highly favorable by members of the health professions.[29] The results for Group F in the present study are among the most carefully validated and successful results reported to date in the psychological treatment of obesity. These results take on even greater significance when it is realized that both psychologists and physicians[17, 21] have pointed out that the psychological treatment of obesity, although discouraging, is impressive when compared to other methods of treatment such as dieting alone or endocrine therapy.

Groups NS and SP deserve further comment. Since Group NS did not lose significantly more weight than Group SP, seemingly it would be of questionable value to treat obesity in relatively lengthy nonspecific therapy sessions when using 15 to 20-minute sessions of positive expectation—social pressure seems to be just as effective. The social pressure treatment of the present study is highly similar to the nationwide TOPS weight reducing groups. Usually, however, TOPS groups employ a more complex reinforcement system for weight loss than does the social pressure group (e.g. monetary fines for weight gain, slogans and songs, local and national conventions). TOPS groups, however, average about 30 persons per group.[27] Although to the investigator's knowledge, the effectiveness of TOPS has not yet been scientifically investigated, it is suspected that it would be about as effective as Group SP in the present study in promoting weight loss of members who do not drop out. At any rate, from a clinician's viewpoint, weight loss may be just as great for a client who is referred to TOPS as for one who is involved in nonspecific forms of psychotherapy.

The most notable limitation of the present investigation is that the treatment period was relatively short in relation to the degree of the Ss' obesity. Weight loss requires time and should be gradual if it is to be sound from the viewpoint of physical health. Since Ss in this study were considerably obese, even the majority of those who lost a significant amount of weight during the treatment period still were considerably overweight. When treatment terminated, group reinforcement for weight loss also terminated, and perhaps most Ss had not lost enough of their excess weight to warrant sufficient reinforcement from their own appearance, family, and friends to motivate them to endure the hardships of continued caloric restriction. It is suspected that all groups would have evidenced better maintenance if they had continued to meet at regular intervals after the tenth session merely for 15 to 20 minutes for use of the positive expectation—social pressure techniques alone. Ten sessions appeared to be adequate in instructing Ss in focal treatment in the implementation of learning principles, but subsequent additional sessions involving only social pressure techniques and social reinforcement would most likely have promoted further weight loss.

Two further limitations of this study deserve comment. The first revolves around the fact that the focal treatment herein developed and evaluated represents a treatment *package* including many techniques derived from learning principles. Only subsequent research can specifically delineate the more potent elements of this package. For example, research is not in progress to test the hypothesis that the use of deep relaxation could be subtracted from the focal treatment package without decreasing its effectiveness. Second, the extrinsic validity[6] of the present investigation would be extended by employing nonlearning theory-oriented therapists in the implementation of the techniques of focal therapy.

In conclusion, in that the present investigation obtained carefully validated and highly positive results in an area so characterized by failure, replication certainly seems warranted. Beyond its specific contribution to the treatment of obesity, this study represents an attempt to contribute to more sophisticated therapy outcome research by focusing upon the establishment of cause-effect relations between therapeutic techniques and treatment outcome.

REFERENCES

1. Alexander, F. and Flagg, G. W.: The psychosomatic approach. In B. J. Wolman (Ed.): *Handbook of Clinical Psychology.* New York, McGraw-Hill, 1965.
2. Bendig, A. W.: Pittsburg scale of social extraversion-introversion and emotionality. *J Psychol,* 53:199-210, 1962.
3. Bergin, A. E.: The effects of psychotherapy: Negative results revisited. *J Counsel Psychol,* 10:244-250, 1963.
4. Berne, E.: *Games People Play: The Psychology of Human Relationships.* New York, Grove Press, 1964.
5. Bruch, H.: Disturbed communication in eating disorders. *Am J Orthopsychiat,* 33:99-104, 1963.
6. Campbell, D. T. and Stanley, J. C.: *Experimental and Quasiexperimental Designs for Research.* Chicago, Rand McNally, 1966.
7. Cattell, R. B.: *The IPAT Anxiety Scale.* Champaign, Ill., Institute for Personality and Ability Testing, 1957.
8. DuBois, P. H.: *Multivariant Correlational Analysis.* New York, Harper, 1957.
9. Endler, N. S., Hunt, J. McV. and Rosenstein, A. J.: An S-R inventory of anxiousness. *Psychol Mono,* 76(17, Whole No. 536), 1962.
10. Fenichel, O.: *The Psychoanalytic Theory of Neuroses.* New York, Norton, 1945.
11. Ferster, C. B., Nurnberger, J. I. and Levitt, E. B.: The control of eating. *J Math,* 1:87-109, 1962.
12. Goldiamond, I.: Self-control procedures in personal behavior problems. *Psychol Rep,* 17:851-868, 1965.
13. Harmatz, M. G. and Lapuc, P.: Behavior modification of overeating in a psychiatric population. *J Consult Clin Psychol,* 32:583-587, 1968.
14. Harris, M. B.: Self-directed program for weight control: A pilot study. *J Abnorm Psychol,* 74:263-270, 1969.
15. Kramer, C. Y.: Extension of multiple range tests to group means with unequal numbers of replications. *Biometrics,* 12:307-310, 1956.

16. Mendelson, M.: Psychological aspects of obesity. *Int J Psychiat*, 2:599-611, 1966.
17. Meyer, V. and Crisp, A. H.: Aversion therapy in two cases of obesity. *Behav Res Ther*, 2:143-147, 1964.
18. National Dairy Council: Obesity and its management. *Dairy Council Digest*, 36: 13-18, 1965.
19. Paul, G. L.: Insight versus desensitization in psychotherapy two years after termination. *J Consult Psychol*, 31:333-348, 1967.
20. Paul, G. L. and Shannon, D. T.: Treatment of anxiety through systematic desensitization in therapy groups. *J Abnorm Psychol*, 71:124-135, 1966.
21. Rynearson, E. H. and Gastineau, C. F.: *Obesity*. Springfield, Ill., Thomas, 1949.
22. Schifferes, J. J.: *What's Your Caloric Number*. New York, Macmillan, 1966.
23. Stuart, R. B.: Behavioral control of overeating. *Behav Res Ther*, 5:357-365, 1967.
24. Stunkard, A. J.: The dieting depression. *Am J Med*, 23:77-86, 1957.
25. Stunkard, A. J. and McLaren-Hume, M.: The results of treatment for obesity: A review of the literature and report of a series. *Arch Intern Med*, 103:79-85, 1959.
26. Suczek, R. F.: Psychological aspects of weight reduction. In E. S. Eppright, P. Swanson and C. A. Iverson (Eds.): *Weight Control: A Collection of Papers Presented at the Weight Control Colloquium*. Ames, Iowa State College Press, 1955.
27. Toch, H.: *The Social Psychology of Social Movements*. New York, Bobbs-Merrill, 1965.
28. Ullmann, L. P. and Krasner, L. (Eds.): *Case Studies in Behavior Modification*. New York, Holt, 1965.
29. United States Department of Health, Education, and Welfare: *Obesity and Health: A Sourcebook of Current Information for Professional Health Personnel*. Arlington, Va., United States Public Health Service, 1967.
30. Wollersheim, J. P.: The effectiveness of learning theory-based group therapy in the treatment of overweight women. Unpublished doctoral dissertation, University of Illinois, 1968.
31. Wollersheim, J. P., Paul, G. L. and Wherry, J. S.: Correlates of Obesity: Clarification and Suggestions for Treatment. Unpublished.
32. Young, C. M., Berresford, K. and Moore, N. S.: Psychologic factors in weight control. *Am J Clin Nutr*, 5:186-191, 1957.

VII
HYPNOTHERAPY

20

Systems Approach for Understanding Obesity

WILLIAM S. KROGER

MANAGEMENT BY BEHAVIORAL MODIFICATION
THROUGH HYPNOSIS

ONCE the methodology for understanding the cause and treatment of "obesity" was to investigate various disparate mechanisms. But such studies indicated that the nosological entity of obesity referred to a descriptive overlapping of many syndromes. Therefore, the multifactoral causation of obesity and its therapy shall be presented from a *systems approach*—a discipline that does not segregate the various responsible factors, but rather studies these holistically to understand the *"gestalt."* I shall explain how behavioral modification through conditioning under hypnosis involves the planning of objectives, coordinating and controlling various psychoneurophysiological mechanisms for production of symptomatic relief, characterological change and relevantly permanent weight loss. With these goals and the space limitations in mind, I have brought together a recent cross-disciplinary exchange of information from the fields of general medicine, psychoneurophysiology, genetics, learning theory and conditioning under hypnosis in an attempt to provide a unified field approach for an understanding of obesity and its management.

It is generally agreed that obesity is a disease of mutually contradictory theories as to its causation, prevention, and effective therapy. A vast literature implicates numerous causes ranging from neural regulation of the feeding and satiety centers, glucostatic mechanisms associated with control of the appetite, and aberration of lipid and adipose metabolism. Also, psychologic factors for obesity have been posited as increased anxiety and depression and denial of hunger for reasons of social approval.[40] More recently it has been considered that overweight is a manifestation of a behavioral deficit.[2] Overeating also has been attributed to specific personality profiles characterized by immaturity, passivity, and strong dependency strivings—the so-called mechanism of orality, a symbolic "return to the breast." However, it has been noted that most of these dynamisms occur in thin persons. Even the dictum that overweight occurs when caloric intake exceeds caloric output, but is corrected when this imbalance is reversed, has been challenged. These reasons will be discussed more fully below.

The high relapse rate with all types of diets and therapeutic regimens indicates that permanent weight loss cannot be maintained without nutritional education, long-term physical fitness training, and removal of maladaptive eating habit patterns. These goals are best achieved by the systematic application of scientifically verified laws of learning. The long-term results have been obtained on an obese population sample composed chiefly of individuals refractory to standard therapy.

The spate of lay articles has apprised everyone that excessive weight gain is a predisposing factor to cardiac disease, hypertension, arthritis, diabetes, and other degenerative diseases. Therefore, such warnings only reinforce their faulty eating habits. Few change their eating behavior; nearly all want a magic formula, thus not having to forego the pleasures of gluttony. The myriad of fads and contraptions used in "treatment" attest to this attitude. Many are peripatetic "medical shoppers"; some are looking for an endocrine "label" which seldom accounts for their obesity.

PREVENTION

Prevention is particularly effective during the early years of life. This is especially important for fat children having a defective capacity for dealing with specific foods. Even though their metabolic rate is not increased, they apparently more readily convert carbohydrates into stored fat. And, too, many of these have more fat storage cells in their tissues proportionate to their body weight than those whose weight remains constant. Both can have a similar caloric intake and energy expenditure, indicating the chronically fat have an excess of storage over use. The *biochemical* reasons will be detailed more fully below.

However, learning to minimize intake of specific foods is important if initiated during the early years of life. This is best accomplished by reeducation of the family, since fat children generally adopt the eating patterns of their parents and/or culture. As adults, they continue eating the wrong foods. With advancing years, the quantity is not decreased even though their work and exercise require less food intake. Females, especially, should be watched carefully at adolescence, during pregnancy, and postmenopausally. In an affluent society, significant changes begin from maturity and increase up to middle age when energy requirements are reduced by 10 per cent and may even reach 30 per cent after age 60. In middle age and thereafter, the ready availability of transportation further cuts down on energy expenditure.

TREATMENT

Before initiating therapy, all organic factors should be ruled out, even though they rarely account for obesity. During the initial visit usually the patient is ill at ease. For better history taking, I sit in front of my desk alongside the patient, using two chairs of similar construction and height. This fosters closer rapport and helps allay anxiety. I take no notes, nor do I interrupt, realizing how difficult it is to talk when one is writing or not focusing his full attention on another person's verbal and nonverbal communications. I follow the old adage that "if one opens his mouth enough times he will put his foot into it." I do not ask routine questions, because routine questions yield only routine answers. Nor, as mentioned, is there any need to pontificate on the harmful sequelae of overeating.

A quiet and understanding attitude elicits more honesty and cooperation, and facilitates more spontaneous elaboration of the patient's emotional conflicts. The few questions I ask consist of the kind of food habits since infancy, the current economic status, vocational and social environment. I note signs of discomfiture as nonverbal behavior often reveals more of the patient's emotional overlay than can be obtained from talking. I listen with the "third ear" for "hot material." Important are the kinds of interpersonal relationships within the family and with friends and members of the opposite sex. Of more importance, the motivation for losing weight should be evaluated. Often I pay more attention to what the patient does *not* say.

The usual rationalizations for overeating are anxiety, boredom, and everyday pressures. Common subterfuges are the following: "It's my glands," "I eat like a bird," "I was born heavy." The majority who ardently protest that they "would give anything to lose weight" as a rule actually want to cling to their hedonism. A facetious, sarcastic, or brusque attitude only alienates and aggravates self-disgust, mobilizes guilt, and increases rejection. Too often, the obese person is driven by ridicule to seek help only to find, to his dismay, a physician with contemptuous attitudes toward his problem.

After completing the history taking, I discuss the diet in detail. I mention that all diets are good, but *they are good only in the way that they are followed*. I emphasize that the word "diet" does not mean restriction of food; rather, the patient can eat gourmet food, even six times daily, but it must be smaller portions and *of the right type*. A well-balanced, high-protein and animal fat, low carbohydrate, high potassium, and low-sodium diet is recommended. With minor adjustments it is ideal for those eating most of their meals in restaurants. It consists of about 2500 calories. I no longer stress the use of safflower, corn, soybean, and cottonseed oil as a substitute for animal fats. But I do emphasize that *what* a fat person eats is more important than *how much*.

Though science was not then aware of faulty genetic factors, the concept that even small amounts of starches and sugars are converted to adipose tissue while proteins and animal fats are not was first postulated in 1862 by

William Banting; he learned it from his physician, William Harvey. The Banting diet allows one to eat to the limit of his appetite. Recently Pennington (1968) has revised the theory that obesity often is caused by an inability to convert carbohydrates into fat. He obtained excellent results on an unrestricted calorie, high-fat, high-protein diet. It is believed that as the result of an inborn error of metabolism and deficiency of specific hormones, large quantities of pyruvic acid are blocked, and therefore, since carbohydrates cannot be used for energy, they are stored as fat. Also, the pyruvic acid block prevents mobilization of fat from fat storage depots by inhibiting oxidation of fatty acids.

MEDICATION

Diuretics are not used, since the causes of fluid retention are often due to excess carbohydrate reserves (sugar holds three times its weight of water and is eliminated when the sugar is burnt up). Electrolyte imbalance is most important. Reduction of sodium and increase of potassium induces diuresis. Enteric KCl, with the edge bitten off to facilitate absorption and lessen gastric irritation, is advised in 0.5 to 1 gm doses after each meal. At least two quarts of water must be drunk daily. This is the best diuretic known to man. The initial weight reduction due to fluid loss acts as a reward stimulus and facilitates keeping the serum potassium level high and sodium intake low. The ready availability of low-sodium dietetic foods makes the regimen less monotonous. I seldom see apathy or depression due to salt restriction *per se*. I never insist on calorie counting as this aggravates the problems that bedevil the obese.

I no longer prescribe amphetamines or other so-called anorexogenic agents. These have no direct action on the feeding and satiety centers, but rather are mood elevators. The rationale for their use has been that less depressed individuals supposedly eat smaller amounts of food. As yet there is no known drug that exerts a selective action on the feeding centers.

I have done random, cross-over, and doubleblind studies on several amphetamines.[23, 24] The placebo reactor rate is exceedingly high when the data are subjected to rigid analysis. I used to prescribe these for their morale-boosting effects but noted that most became "amphetamine veterans" and refractory to the drug. Nor do I use "shots," such as human chorionic gonadotropin (HCG). In a well-controlled series I found a placebo to be as good as the HCG. Others have noted the ineffectiveness of HCG in treatment of obesity.[13] The fact that obese patients were coming to the office, paying a fee, having to be weighed, were on a restrictive diet, and receiving supportive psychotherapy helped produce weight loss.

Thyroid and its derivatives are helpful for some refractory obese, even when euthyroid. If a patient weighs over 200 lb I prescribe 2 or 3 gr of desiccated thyroid U.S.P. Armour's, even if his P.B.I. is within normal limits.

Determination of the free thyroxin, T_3 and T_4 levels are not important except in patients with known coronary disease and hypercholesteremia. The recently completed Framingham heart disease study casts doubt on the widely held belief that the cholesterol level is dependent on the fat in the diet. In apparently healthy fat people the blood cholesterol is not important as by itself it does not account for obesity. Many fat people have low blood-cholesterol levels and many thin persons have a high cholesterol. Carbohydrates, especially refined sugars, can raise it. Emotional tension *per se* can elevate serum cholesterol up to 35 mg in an hour. In the extremely overweight individual the dosage can be raised to 4 gr daily, provided he is seen weekly for physical evaluation. I am aware that the 1966 edition of *New Drugs* discourages the use of desiccated thyroid and points out that it increases appetite. The report states, "The net result is to make the program of weight reduction more unpleasant and perhaps to prevent its success." This, generally, has not been my experience. Nor am I convinced that thyroid administration suppresses endogenous thyroid excretion in all patients. This may be true in animals, but the limbic system and higher levels of neural integration are different in humans than in animals. Furthermore, one should not extrapolate research findings like the "rat psychologists" from animal studies to humans. I am not implying that thyroid administration is the answer to obesity, as I prescribe it for less than 10 per cent of my patients. Empirically, I have noted that a high percentage of this group are able to tolerate thyroid and initially show significant weight loss. Their motivation to continue is thus enhanced. Naturally, those who have an elevated diastolic blood pressure, coronary disease, hyperthyroidism, or nervous tension are not given thyroid.

PSYCHOTHERAPY

Frank[14] states that more than 60 per cent of emotionally ill persons get better irrespective of the therapy utilized. Thus, a large placebo effect obviously is operating in all types of psychotherapy—"suggestion and/or hypnosis in slow motion." The latter is the acme of scientifically applied suggestion. Words, thoughts, and feelings act as conditioned stimuli when specific reactions are elicited even though the original stimulus has been forgotten. We can therefore regard "suggestion" as the simplest form of conditioned reflex.

The experimental basis for conditioned reflex therapy was established by Pavlov and Thorndike at the turn of the century. Watson and Mowrer launched the applied science of behavior modification, and in 1950, Wolpe[41] demonstrated that the counter-conditioning method he called systematic desensitization when utilized during hypnosis was remarkably effective in neurotic disorders. About the same time, Skinner demonstrated he could modify behavior by operant conditioning. Treating obesity and alcoholism with aversive drugs or instrumental conditioning was sporadically attempted but has not caught on in these fields.

Before describing my therapeutic approach in detail, I should like to define the term "hypnosis." However, before I do this, may I state what this age-old art and science is *not*. Hypnosis is not a "trance," "state of unconsciousness," nor is it remotely related to "sleep." Nor can one state that hypnosis is due to suggestibility or that suggestion produces hypnosis. Unfortunately, this type of circular reasoning has been used to explain hypnosis for the past century. Reification of theoretical formulations and continual redefining of hoary shibboleths associated with outmoded concepts about higher nervous system activities has only produced a welter of confusion. The reason is that what we observe is not necessarily the *way things are*.

Operationally, hypnosis is the art of influencing people without their realizing they are being influenced. The techniques are similar to those used by advertising, propaganda, and religious rites. All of these have a misdirection of attention which consists of a ritual or "smoke-screen" producing an appropriate inhibitory mental set. If strong motivation precedes the inhibitory set, the formula for attaining hypnosis is as follows: motivation + the inhibitory mental set + misdirection of attention + increased suggestibility at various levels of awareness = compounding of belief → faith → "programmed" conviction → conditioned internal inhibition (neutralization of harmful conditioned or unconditioned stimuli). Such a linear set of happenings facilitates readier acceptance of suggestions. I have (Kroger, in press) discussed hypnosis from a physical-machine simulation model involving the comparison of sensory processing of information and control in human functioning with that of the activity patterns of servomechanisms (automata)—a brain/computer analog model of neuro-behavioral functioning.

The *raison d'etre* for the adjunctive use of hypnosis in psychotherapy is to enable the patient to transcend his normal volitional capacities and thus more effectively modify maladaptive behavior. Everyone possesses this ability but does not know how to achieve it. The *leit motif* of the above brief discussion is that hypnosis *(internal inhibition)* is a brain mechanism whose function psychiatry must ultimately incorporate if one wishes to potentiate modification of behavior by conditioning techniques.

During the past twenty-five years, I have employed *interoceptive conditioning* under hypnosis for changing eating behavior to produce weight loss. By "inner speech" based on "scene visualization" of past experiences (sensory imagery conditioning), greater mastery of autonomic systems (ANS) functioning can be obtained. This task is more readily accomplished if control of the inborn, nonconditioned reflexes such as thermal sensations is first taught. These ideosensory responses do not have to be learned and are functions of the primary signaling system so well described by Pavlov. They are closely related to other primary signaling system activities such as hunger and appetite.

Patients under autohypnosis are trained to develop "heat" by imagining their foot being placed in a tub of hot water and "cold" by their hand being put in a glass of ice water. After both of these hallucinations or sensory imagery responses are achieved, more complex responses such as satiation or aversion for specific types of food are readily developed by recalling the representations of disgusting thoughts and feelings. Such symbolic activities are part of the secondary signaling system of higher nervous elaboration. This method is not new but differs from the classical-type Pavlovian conditioning initially produced by external stimuli—*exteroceptive conditioning*.

The approach is similar to the extraordinary "mind-body" responses provided by Yoga, Zen, and other Eastern therapies. Such methodologies indicate that the ANS is not as autonomic as believed and that some portions of it can by appropriate training come under volitional control. However, Western scientists are trying to compromise the Christian view (a minority group) with Yoga and Zen training. This is a serious mistake. If Yoga and Zen conditioning could be examined objectively within our own culture and compared with current empirical psychotherapies, their applications could better be understood.

Recent data[36, 37] indicate that conditioned reflexes established under hypnosis are more durable and less likely to go into extinction. I have taken this type of conditioning one step further by employing sophisticated hypnotic techniques with reinforcement to establish corrective behavioral changes. The close interaction between therapist and subject fills "the space between" and more readily taps the "forgotten assets" and hidden potentials for changing such compulsions as ungovernable eating drives. The punishment and reward alternatives implicit in behavioral and operant conditioning can be incorporated when hypnosis is employed, particularly if posthypnotic suggestions (PHS) are oriented around the patients' needs.

Most of these techniques have been described by Erickson.[11] The first is *symptom substitution*. Through PHS, one can "trade down" to other eating behaviors such as chewing gum, or become intensely interested in the taste of organic or dietetic foods. In *symptom transformation*, the overeating can be transferred by appropriate PHS to other behaviors such as physical exercise, shopping, child raising, P.T.A. meetings, and interest in community affairs. Although seemingly similar to symptom substitution, dissolution of excessive eating occurs by transformation of the symptom into a less noxious one without directly attacking the character of the symptom itself. In *symptom amelioration* the overeating is reduced. First, it is deliberately increased by PHS on the supposition that if this is done volitionally it eventually can be decreased. *Symptom utilization* consists of encouraging, accepting and redefining cooperative activity of an aversive nature toward the faulty eating patterns. This differs from symptom removal by direct suggestion. Any one or all can be used in various combinations in conjunction with imposing a "double bind." In a typical double-bind maneuver, a patient's insistence that he cannot help himself to stop overeating is *accepted* rather than opposed. He is directed in such a way that he must stop behaving in the way he does or stop denying that he is behaving in that way.

"Glove anesthesia" is yet another valuable dynamism for appetite control. It is extremely useful for minimizing hunger contractions. The patient places the hand "made numb" over the epigastrium. This technique has been employed in dentistry, for amelioration of pain in cancer, with surgical and obstetrical patients.[20, 21, 22, 25, 26, 32] The technique for glove anesthesia is as follows:

Imagine that your right or left hand is in a pitcher, jug or bowl of ice water. You can practically feel the imaginary ice cubes bumping your hand. At first you will notice a numb, tingling sensation in the fingertips. As you imagine your hand in that cold, chilling ice water, the colder and more numb your fingers will become. So, if you wish to develop this numbness in your hand, just lift it toward the side of your face. If you wish to increase the numbness, suggest to yourself that with each motion of your hand toward your face it will get more numb and more woodenlike. (At this point the hand continues to move upward.) After each movement, pause to give your hand a chance to feel the suggestions of numbness. (The hand continues to move a short distance of an inch or two at a time, and to move steadily toward the side of the face.) If you wish more numbness of the hand, notice that the closer it approaches your cheek the more numb it will get. And when it finally reaches your cheek, just let the palm of your hand rest lightly against your cheek. Then allow the numbness to be transferred from your palm to the side of your cheek. After you are certain that your cheek has become very numb, only then will your hand drop to your side, and it will feel normal. However, the side of your face will feel just as if a dentist had injected novocaine into your gums. Remember how leathery and stiff one side of your face feels following an injection?

Such suggestions make full use of subtle techniques leaving the patient no alternative but to make the side of his face feel completely "anesthetized." After feeling the glove anesthesia he is convinced that the numbness of the cheek is genuine. This suggestion is given as follows:

Whenever you feel the onset of hunger, you can stop it by placing the anesthetized hand over the pit of your stomach to control the hunger pangs.

During subsequent sessions, the patient is informed:

"This is your mind, your body, and your problem. You got yourself this way, and what the mind can do it can undo."

I generally follow this by saying:

"Don't you ever tell anyone that I helped you to stop overeating. That would not be true. I can only show you how you can remove the habit. Furthermore, when I see you in a year or so, and you have changed your eating patterns and lost weight, please do not thank me."

These are extraverbal suggestions concealing the direct suggestion, "you will not be overeating a year from now." Hence, it is not the hypnosis that actually achieves the therapeutic results, but rather how it is used to catalyze behavior dynamics within a psychologic methodology. This is of the utmost importance.

"Age regression" is useful if the patient is a somnambule. If not, "pseudo-revivification" can be used. I suggest that he think of himself in the body image he once possessed. Or hypnotic pseudo-orientation in time (age progression) also can, by fantasy evocation, create the necessary thoughts and feelings associated with the desired body image. I have described the interesting applications of this technique in other fields.[25, 26] Use of "time condensation" or "time expansion" as described by Cooper and Erickson[10] can speed up the effectiveness of the autohypnotic suggestions or slow them down to allow for fuller absorption of their import.

If one wishes to use psychoanalysis under hypnosis (hypnoanalysis), the genesis of the eating behavior can be studied longitudinally by age regression. The hypnoanalyst also can use a vertical exploration of a specific aspect of the symptom by first giving a PHS that associative material germane to the overeating will be revealed in dreams as well as future therapeutic sessions. An amnesia for the PHS is engrafted. The spontaneous verbalizations during the hypnotic sessions can be cross-checked against dream material for validation. I seldom use this technique (the "interim phenomenon") because it is too time consuming and requires training in deep hypnosis.

Since I have a reputation for successful treatment of obesity by hypnosis, patients come in with a favorable mental set. This promptly establishes good rapport. Appropriate explanations inform them that if they wish help they will have to "stick out" a program requiring hard work and practice. Though not difficult, the techniques of autohypnosis and the following of PHS can be mastered by most. Those poorly motivated soon become disillusioned when they realize that changing their eating behavior is *their* responsibility.

Hypnosis is not a doctor-directed tool but rather a patient-centered, autonomic, adaptive response mechanism on the sleep-wakefulness continuum.

The sensory processing, control, storage, and retrieval of information in hypnosis is characterized by hyperacuity—*selective attention* to the signal input environment with *selective inattention* to irrelevant stimuli.[34] From a biomedical frame of reference, whenever a system adjusts its feedback networks to the psychophysiologic parameters so as to increase the signal to noise ratio, it is functioning in homeostasis, in negative feedback, or in dynamic equilibrium—optimally. Improvement in behavior occurs when the system switches from maladaptive (positive feedback) to adaptive performance.

I explain that the organism, like a nonliving system, responds better when associated with hypnosis. The relaxation and increased concentration result in greater receptivity and better response to heterosuggestions or autosuggestions. Looking at the self and meeting one's needs in any kind of therapeutic situation is of the utmost importance and yet often difficult to achieve. Since one of the characteristics of hypnosis is the pinpoint specificity in response, the subsequent evaluation of faulty needs for overeating allows the engrafting of beneficial behavioral patterns. It is stressed that hypnosis *per se* is *not* a therapy and that only suggestions of an acceptable nature will be followed. Thus a patient is treated *in hypnosis, not by hypnosis.*

The average subject usually requires about two sessions to obtain a suitable depth of hypnosis. The next one or two sessions are directed toward deepening the hypnosis. For deepening it, the "elevator" technique is useful. The individual imagines himself descending past one floor after another; and as he looks at the automatic panel, the numbers get smaller and smaller as he passes each floor. By the time he fantasies that the elevator has reached the lobby floor, he usually has achieved moderate relaxation. If he wishes to go deeper, he can "descend" into the basement or sub-basement. At this point, I suggest:

You will have the same suspended feeling as if you have reached the bottom of an elevator shaft.

At this very relaxed level, suggestions are "imprinted" on the neural circuits and are more likely to be acted upon.

Full use of mnemonic material (reviving past experiences that are similar to those he would like to achieve) via the imagination is employed to relax progressively the eyelids, toes, feet, chest, trunk, and head. It is axiomatic that whenever the imagination (the experiential background) and the so-called "will" come into conflict, the imagination always "beats the will to the draw." Therefore, the "battle of the bulge" is going to be won or lost on the field of imagination.[35] If full control of simple feedback sub-systems (the "how am I doing" error correcting information transmission mechanisms) producing relaxation is learned, then more complex and larger systems such as taste, smell, and sight become amenable to at least semi-volitional regulation. Harry Emerson Fosdick once stated, "Hold a picture of yourself long and steadily enough in your mind's eye and you will be drawn toward it. Great living starts with a picture, held in your imagination, of what you would like to do or be."

After sufficient practice, a conditioned reflex is established and deep relaxation is attained by merely closing the eyelids, by-passing the need for the progressive-relaxation techniques. The purpose of this meditative and self-reflective state, somewhat like communion or deep prayer, is to repeat the autosuggestions or affirmations long enough, strong enough, and often enough. Eventually the adverse stimuli responsible for the over-eating are inhibited. This is direct symptom removal, but yet permissive and patient-centered. The patient is now taught dehypnotization. In well over 50,000 inductions, all promptly terminated hypnosis. In fact, often it is difficult to maintain the hypnosis.

I explain that the patient should learn autohypnosis for the following reasons: a) You will have a feeling of pride and self-esteem that you were able to remove the symptom; b) you will *not* be dependent upon me or any other physician or drugs; c) that if any excess poundage returns, you will be able to utilize the never-to-be-forgotten affirmations that once removed the overeating; d) should a substitute symptom replace the removed one, such as excessive smoking (and this is highly equivocal), you can also remove it in the same way as the overeating.

Recent data indicate that a new symptom does not replace a removed symptom, especially if it is the patient himself who eliminated the original symptom. Eysenck[12] states, "Behavior therapists consider it a trifle odd that they should be criticized for only curing 'symptoms' by those who cannot even cure 'symptoms.'"

After making certain that the four premises mentioned above are understood, I teach the patient the following affirmations.

If you really wish to lose weight, roll the food from the front of the tongue to the back of the tongue and from side to side in order to obtain the last ounce of satisfaction and the "most mileage" out of each morsel and each drop. This satisfies the thousands of taste cells on the tongue which are connected to the appetite center located in your brain. As a result your caloric intake will be immeasurably curtailed. (This is the old "Fletcherization" treatment popular at the turn of the last century.)

Try to "think thin," that is, keep an image uppermost in your mind of how you once looked when your weight was normal. Pick your own good points (smile, eyes, hands, hair, complexion, etc.) and concentrate on how these will be enhanced by weight loss. Also, place a picture of yourself when you weighed less in a prominent position so it continually reminds you of the way you once looked.

Think of the most horrible, nauseating, and repugnant smell you have ever experienced; maybe the vile odor of rotten eggs. Whenever you eat something *not on your diet,* immediately associate this disagreeable smell with it.

You cannot "will" yourself to lose weight. The harder you try, the less you will accomplish. So relax, don't press. Purchase the most beautiful dress (or suit) that you can afford. Hang it in your bedroom where you can see it every morning and night. Then imagine yourself getting into it. Speculate how soon and the date this will be. Now this is important! The garment should be at least one or two sizes too small for you!

Following dehypnotization, the rationale for these affirmations can be discussed on the following bases: There is a sensory pathway connecting the thousands of taste buds and the impressions that they convey to the higher brain centers for interpretation. The "think thin" suggestion makes use to a degree of the alteration in body image secondary to strong emotional stimuli. That emotions can alter metabolic and endocrine activities to produce weight gain is vividly illustrated in phantom pregnancy or pseudocyesis; in this syndrome, the autonomic nervous system "tricks" endocrine activities and bodily processes into responding with a weight gain on the basis of expressed or unexpressed wishes for pregnancy. It also is conceivable that these neurohumoral pathways can produce weight loss with the proper inputs.

The fourth affirmation has a twofold meaning. First, it is highly motivating, as it stresses the value of a nice figure by indirection or extraverbal suggestion. This does not mobilize criticalness. I reiterate that not all the affirmations will become effective immediately, but that continuous repetition under autohypnosis leads to reinforcement learning and this can be of utmost benefit. If there has been some modicum of success with the first four, the following four affirmations are given.

If you wish to lose more weight, follow these suggestions. Do not lose more than six to eight pounds per month. Set a "deadline" date for this weight loss. One then tries much harder. Wonder if you will reach your objective before or after the deadline date!

The next affirmation might appeal to you, especially if you are interested in having a trim figure. Think of your ultimate goal in terms of the actual weight desired. Suppose you would like to get down to 130. I call this the "food stamp" suggestion. Every time you even think of eating something you are not supposed to, you will "see" the number 130 in blue *encircled by a blue ring,* just like the price of an item stamped on a can of food in a grocery store. Use this suggestion particularly at night if you get extremely hungry before retiring.

If you should eat something that is not on your diet, try to remember what you were doing and thinking at the time. Then discuss these situations with your doctor so that he can see whether there is a specific pattern to your eating.

If you get hungry before meals, especially before going to bed, try glove anesthesia. If you temporarily wish to delay eating your next meal for several hours, induce glove anesthesia over the pit of the stomach to "knock out" the hunger contractions initiated in this area.

Posthypnotic suggestions can be given to reduce or eliminate "eating between meals," "nibbling," and "smoking." Some of the above PHS have a psychophysiologic basis. Hypothalamic centers mediate hunger and satiety, not only having separate anatomic locations but also different behavioral consequences. Appropriate lesions made in these brain areas in experimental animals result in bulimia, and/or ravenous eating or appetite loss. Either a decreased satiability or an increased hunger drive obviously accounts for overeating. One of the principal physiologic centers for initiating hunger contractions is in the epigastrium. Many obese are not hungry but eat because the hunger contractions are conditioned to a time schedule. Glove anesthesia only supports the old adage, "Tighten up your belt a notch."

The "deadline" affirmation increases motivation. This applies also to the "food stamp" one. The others are based upon the correlation between taste and the visual senses being stimulated. The tongue and the connecting brain centers are continually stimulated by reciprocal feedback connections. No wonder one unidentified wit said, "One tongue may have three times as many taste buds as another and the empire of taste also has its blind men and deaf mutes."

Group hypnosis is more beneficial than individual sessions for obesity. The group attendance is a form of behavior. The same factors described in group training apply for behavioral conditioning of alcoholism or painless childbirth.[22] There is the emotional contagion inherently present in any group, the desire to please the leader (the physician) and the competitiveness. The increased socialization during and after the sessions is rewarding. The eating behavior becomes incompatible with their overeating and weight gain; no longer do they require food as a catalyst for talk-fests, the group discussions replace eating alone.

The author sees four to five patients for one hour, at first weekly and then biweekly. Gradually, they learn to replace high-caloric, low-bulk foods with the recommended foods. Autohypnotic affirmations are helpful in maintaining the optimal weight after it is reached. About 50 per cent of the patients relapse and require periodic reinforcement to prevent further weight gain.

It is recommended that the affirmations be used at least eight to ten times a day. As reinforcement learning increases, weight loss becomes a reward and the weight gain acts as a punishment. Thus far, treatment has been directed strictly toward the symptomatic level. A noncondemnatory attitude when failure occurs, combined with encouragement, facilitates the incorporation of the aforementioned affirmations into the total personality structure. I have successfully used a similar approach for treatment of the tobaccomaniac.[33]

The next phase is directed to the characterological level. The dictum is to treat the patient who has the obesity rather than the symptom *per se*. Otherwise, as Rynearson[39] suggests, "We will have a fat personality crying to get out of a thin man." As mentioned, I am interested in the significance of the overeating in the *here* and *now* more than its relationship to the longitudinal life development of the personality structure. Free association, interpretations and dream analysis are not used. I concur with Rado:[38] "Fishing into the past only yields diminishing returns."

Briefly, the therapeutic design is structured around the following: a) "How much of this overeating do you really need to keep?"; or, perhaps, "Could you *overeat* just enough to lose one and one-half pounds a week?" b) "What are you trying to prove by overeating?" c) "How rapidly can you divest yourself of the behavioral needs for the excessive eating?"

To expedite therapy, over 75 per cent of the patients are given an interview-in-depth and a complete psychometric evaluation by a clinical psychologist. This is time-saving and also brings many hidden problems into focus. Behavioral conditioning under hypnosis nearly always requires treatment of the associated anxieties with slow desensitization (exposure to small amounts of anxiety-laden material at each session).

There are only three therapeutic avenues open to the anxiety-ridden patient: a) He can "develop a thicker skin" and learn to live with his problems; b) he can walk away or retreat from his life situations to fight another day when stronger; c) he can come to grips with his difficulties, provided, and if, the therapist gives him the necessary coping mechanisms.

There are needs inherent in all emotionally disturbed persons, *i.e.* the need to talk, the need to be told what to do, the need to be accepted, the need to be one's real self, and the need to emancipate oneself from any undue dependency on the therapist.

Each patient is asked to bring a list of his urgent problems with the most vexing ones at the top and the minor ones at the bottom. We discuss this hierarchy of symptoms under hypnosis as described by Wolpe.[41] The relaxed patient senses the physician's interest and warmth. Who can deny that the strength of the interpersonal relationship is the important vector in any therapy, and that it is up to the therapist to mobilize the patient's desires to achieve self-mastery over his eating behavior? This best can be achieved by the best co-pilot any healer can have—faith in the therapist's methods. Successful behavioral conditioning is a collaborative and reciprocal effort between therapist and patient, each learning from the other. One salient fact stands out; namely, a high percentage of my patients are able to maintain their weight loss effectively for years. Though I have no statistical data to support my contentions, empirically the approach is more effective than conventional psychotherapy.

The hypnotic procedures are not dangerous as some psychiatrists contend. Their suppositions are all open to question and the burden of proof is on them. In an article,[23] "It Is Indeed a Wise Hypnotist Who Knows Who Is Hypnotizing Whom," I quote Pierre Janet who stated: "The only danger to hypnosis is that it is not dangerous enough!" Behavioral conditioning and hypnosis are both derivatives of ancient therapies. The fact that they have survived as meaningful therapeutic adjuncts indicates these will not be the "treatments of the year." There are drawbacks: not all patients are amenable, it is a time-consuming process for the therapist, and by no means are the methods a panacea. I have had dramatic successes as well as dramatic failures.

In the proper hands, used wisely and judiciously, the all-out attack consisting of behavioral modification by hypnotic conditioning can have a salutary effect for the "fat of the land who live off the fat of the land."

REFERENCES

1. American Medical Association Council on Drugs: *New Drugs*, Chicago, 1966, p. 413.
2. Berman, M. I. and Anderson, I. R.: Obesity: Manifestation of a behavioral deficit. *Clin Med*, 1966, April, 59-61.
3. Bruch, H.: Psychologic aspects of reducing. *Psychosom Med*, 14:327-332, 1952.
4. Bruch, H.: Role of emotions in hunger and appetite. *Ann NY Acad Sci*, 1955, 63. 1955, 63.
5. Bruch, H.: *The Importance of Overweight*. New York, W. W. Norton, 1957.
6. Bruch, H.: Conceptual confusion in eating disorders. *J Ner Ment Dis*, 133:46-56, 1961.
7. Bruch, H.: Psychological aspects of obesity. Symposium on Overnutrition, Folsterbo, Sweden, Aug. 1963.
8. Bruch, H.: Prognosis and treatment of obesity from a psychiatrist's point of view. *JAMA*, 19:748, 1964.
9. Bruch, H.: Neuro-psychological disturbances in obesity. *Psychiatric Digest*, 1966, 38.
10. Cooper, L. F. and Erickson, M. H.: *Time Distortion in Hypnosis*. Baltimore, Williams & Wilkins, 1954.

11. Erickson, M. H.: Special techniques of brief hypnotherapy. *Journal of Clinical and Experimental Hypnosis*, 2:109-129, 1954.
12. Eysenck, H. J.: Behavior therapy and techniques. Evaluation. *Medical Opinion and Review*, Feb. 1967.
13. Frank, B. W.: Gonadotrophin therapy in obesity. *Am J of Clin Nut*, 14:133-136, 1964.
14. Frank, J. D.: *Persuasion and Healing: A Comparative Study of Psychotherapy.* Baltimore, Johns Hopkins Press, 1961.
15. Garrison, O.: *Tantra: The Yoga of Sex.* New York, Julian Press, 1964.
16. Huxley, A.: *Psychology Today*, 1:69-78, 1967.
17. Kroger, W. S.: Psychologic factors in obesity and anorexic drugs. *American Practitioner*, 10:2169-2175, 1959. (a)
18. Kroger, W. S.: An integrated approach to obesity. *International Record of Medicine*, 172:212-222, 1959. (b)
19. Kroger, W. S.: Techniques of hypnosis. *JAMA*, 172:675-680, 1960. (a)
20. Kroger, W. S.: Hypnosis for relief of pelvic pain. *Clin Obst Gynecol*, 6:763-775, 1960. (b)
21. Kroger, W. S.: And psychotherapy is indicated. *Western Journal of Surgical Obstetrics and Gynecology*, 68:138-140, 1960. (c)
22. Kroger, W. S.: *Childbirth with Hypnosis.* New York, Doubleday, 1961.
23. Kroger, W. S.: An analysis of valid and invalid objections to hypnosis. *American Journal of Clinical Hypnosis*, 6:120-131, 1962. (a)
24. Kroger, W. S.: A comparison of anorexigenic drugs in the treatment of the resistant obese patient. *Psychosomatics*, 8:1-4, 1962. (b)
25. Kroger, W. S.: *Clinical and experimental hypnosis.* Philadelphia, Lippincott, 1963. (a)
26. Kroger, W. S.: Hypnotherapeutic management of headache. *Headache*, 3:50-62, 1963. (b)
27. Kroger, W. S.: Hypnotic pseudoorientation in time as a means of determining the psychological effects of surgical sterilization in the male and female. *Fertil Steril*, 14:535-538, 1963. (c)
28. Kroger, W. S.: Comparative evaluation of zen and yoga, with conditioning techniques and psychotherapy. *Excerpta Medica*, 119:175-180, 1966.
29. Kroger, W. S.: Hypnoanesthesia in surgery. *Western Journal of Surgical Obstetrics and Gynecology*, 68:138-140.
30. Kroger, W. S.: It is indeed a wise hypnotist who knows who is hypnotizing whom. *Western Journal of Surgical Obstetrics and Gynecology.*
31. Kroger, W. S. and Freed, S. C.: *Psychosomatic Gynecology.* Philadelphia, W. B. Saunders, 1951, Ch. 16.
32. Kroger, W. S. and DeLee, S. T.: Use of hypoanesthesia for caesarean section and hysterectomy. *JAMA*, 1957, 163, 442.
33. Kroger, W. S. and Libbott, R.: *Thanks, doctor, I've stopped smoking.* Springfield, Thomas, 1967.
34. Kroger, W. S.: *Symposium on biomedical engineering.* Chapter on Sensory Processing and Control, Milwaukee, Wis., Marquette University Press (in press).
35. Lindner, P. G.: *Mind over Platter.* Los Angeles, Wilshire Book Co., 1966.
36. Paterson, A. S., *et al.*: Acquisition of cortical control over autonomic malfunction in psychosomatic medicine through hypnosis. Read at International Congress for Psychosomatic Medicine and Hypnosis, Kyoto, June 13, 1967.

37. Platonov, K. I.: *The Word as a Physiological and Therapeutic Factor.* Moscow, Foreign Language Publishing House, 1955.
38. Rado, S.: Recent advances of psychoanalytical therapy in psychiatric treatment. *Proceedings of the Association for Research in Nervous and Mental Disease,* 31:57, 1953.
39. Rynearson, E. H.: In Kroger, W. S.: *Psychosomatic Aspects of Obstetrics, Gynecology and Endocrinology, Including Diseases of Metabolism.* Springfield, Thomas, 1962.
40. Stunkard, A.: Obesity and the denial of hunger. *Psychosom Med,* 21:281-290, 1959.
41. Wolpe, J.: *Psychotherapy by Reciprocal Inhibition.* Stanford, California, Stanford University Press, 1958.

21

The Utilization of Patient
Behavior in the Hypnotherapy
of Obesity

Milton H. Erikson

R EQUISITE to effective hypnotherapy and experimental hypnosis is the
  adequate communication of ideas and understandings to the hypno-
tized person. Since the object of hypnotherapy is not the intellectual clarification of understandings but the attainment by the patient of personal
goals, this cannot be achieved by a simple reliance upon the inherent values
of the ideas and understandings to be presented. Rather, communications
need to be presented in terms of the patient's personal and subjective needs,
learnings, and experiences, whether reasonable or unreasonable, recognized or unrecognized, so that there can be an acceptance and a response
and a feeling of personal fulfillment.

To illustrate this need to center the therapeutic use of hypnosis about
the individual personality needs and attitudes of the patient, three instances of obesity previously unsuccessfully treated by other procedures
will be cited.

CASE 1

A physician's wife in her late forties entered the office and explained that
she wished a single interview during which hypnosis was to be employed
to correct her obesity. She added that her normal weight was 120 lb, but
that her present weight was 240, and that for many years she had weighed
over 200 lb despite repeated futile attempts to reduce under medical supervision. She stated that in recent years she had been slowly gaining to her
present weight, and that she was distressed about her future because, "I
enjoy eating, I could spend all the time in the world just eating." Additional history was secured, but the only thing of particular note was her somewhat anxious unnecessary repeated assertions that she enjoyed eating and
liked to while away time by eating for purely gustatory pleasure.

Since she was insistent upon a single interview and hypnosis, an effort
was made to meet her wishes. She was found to be an unusually responsive
subject, developing a profound trance almost immediately. In this trance
state an understanding of time distortion as a subjective experience, particularly time expansion, was systematically taught to her. She was then instructed to have her physician husband prescribe the proper diet for her

and to supervise her weight loss. She was henceforth to eat each meal in a state of time distortion, with time so expanded and lengthened that, as she finished each portion of food her sense of taste and feeling of hunger for that item would both be completely satiated as if she had been eating for "hours on end with complete satisfaction." All of this instruction was given repetitiously until it seemed certain she understood fully, where-upon she was aroused and dismissed.

The patient, together with her husband, was seen nine months later. Her weight had been 120 lb for the past month, and her husband de-clared that her weight loss had occurred easily and without any medical complication. Both she and her husband spoke at length about their im-proved personal, social, and recreational activities, and she commented that, even though she ate much less, her eating pleasures had been inten-sified, that her sense of taste and smell were more discerning, and that a simple sandwich could be experienced with as much subjective pleasure as a two-hour dinner.

CASE 2

A patient weighing 180 lb explained half-laughingly, half-sobbingly, that her normal weight was about 125 lb, but that for over fifteen years she had weighed 170 or more "most of the time."

During these years she had been under medical supervision many times for weight reduction. She had always cooperated with the physician, ad-hering to the recommended diets, obeying every instruction, always losing at least the prescribed poundage each week, usually more. Each time she re-duced, she established a goal-weight which varied from 120 to 130 lb. As she approached this predetermined weight she invariably experienced much disturbing behavior of an obsessive-compulsive character.

When within 5 or 10 lb of her goal she would weigh herself repetitiously throughout the day, and the nearer she came the more frequent became the weighings with increasing anxiety. When the scales showed exactly the chosen weight, and not until then, she would rush precipitously to the kitchen and "gorge frantically," usually regaining at least 10 lb the first week. Thereupon the reduction program would cease and there would oc-cur a progressive systematic restoration of the lost weight accompanied by a feeling of despair mingled with a profound determination to engage upon another weight reduction program soon after she had completed re-gaining her lost weight. She had, in the past, reduced to the goal weight as many as three times within a year, but always under the direction of a dif-ferent physician.

She now sought reduction to 125 lb, stating frankly and with some amuse-ment, "I suppose I'll do exactly the same with you, even though you are a psychiatrist, as I do with every other doctor. I'll cooperate and I'll lose and then I'll gain it back and then I'll go to someone else and repeat the same old silly behavior." Here she burst briefly into tears. Recovering her poise she continued, "Maybe if you use hypnosis that will help, but I don't think it will even if you do hypnotize me. I'll just do the same darned old thing again and again, and I'm so tired of reducing and gaining. It's just a horrible obsession with me. But I don't want any psychiatry used on me."

Further explanation on the patient's part served only to emphasize more clearly what she had already related.

In accord with her wishes hypnosis was attempted, and by the end of the hour a medium trance characterized by a considerable tendency toward spontaneous post-trance amnesia was induced. She was given a second appointment, at which time her history was taken a second time. The details were essentially the same, and she reiterated her firm belief that she would again follow her pattern of losing and gaining weight, and again she sobbed briefly. She also reaffirmed her unwillingness to accept psychiatric help and restricted emphatically any help given her to the problem of her weight. She also declared her intention of terminating her treatment if any attempt were made to deal with her psychiatrically. Repetitiously she promised her full cooperation in all other regards.

A medium trance state was readily induced and she was asked to reiterate her promise of full cooperation. She was also induced to restate repetitiously that in the past her problems had centered around "gaining, losing, gaining, losing, gaining, gaining, gaining, losing, losing, losing," and to agree that throughout the proposed course of treatment she would keep this sequence of behavior constantly in mind.

As soon as it was felt that she had accepted these peculiarly but carefully worded statements, the assertion was offered that her treatment this time, "will be the same, yet completely different, *all of your behavior will be used,* your cooperation has been promised and will be given, and all of your behavior that you have shown so many times in the past will be used, but this time used to make you happy, used in a different way."

When it was certain that the patient knew what had been said to her, even though she did not understand what was meant or implied, she was reminded of the firmness of her resolve to cooperate completely, even as she had in the past, but this time, she was told, "things" would be "done differently" and therefore successfully and to her entire happiness and satisfaction.

Thereupon, while she was still in a medium trance, it was explained that always in the past she had approached her problem of obesity by setting a goal weight, by losing and gaining weight, by a performance of obsessional weighing, and then setting a second goal of her original overweight. These same items of behavior, it was emphasized, would again be employed but in another fashion and effectively for the medical purposes desired.

The explanation was continued to the effect that instead of letting her terminate her reducing by a process of gaining, the procedure would be reversed. Therefore, she was under obligation, as a part of her cooperation, to proceed at once, and at a reasonable rate, to gain between 15 and 25 lb. When this gain had been made, she could then begin reducing.

The patient protested vehemently that she did not want to gain but to lose weight, but it was patiently and insistently pointed out that her reducing programs had always included obsessive weighing, losing weight, gaining weight, the setting of goal weights, and full cooperation with the physicians. No more and no less was now asked. Finally the patient agreed to abide by the instructions. She was then aroused, and the instructions were explained again. She protested vigorously but slightly less so than in the trance state, and finally she reluctantly agreed to the proposed program.

Most unwillingly she began to increase her weight. When she had gained 10 lb she pleaded to be allowed to begin reducing. She was reminded that an increase of 15 to 25 lb had been prescribed and this would be insisted upon. As she approached the gain of 15 lb, she began weighing herself in a repetitive obsessive manner and demanded an appointment immediately when the scales showed the 15 lb increase. At that appointment it was carefully explained to her in both the trance and the waking states that the prescribed gain had been for a weight *between* 15 and 25 lb.

Less than a week later, after much obsessive weighing and eating, which was done with great reluctance, she reported for an interview and hesitantly stated that she had gained 20 lb and that this figure was exactly between 15 and 25. She pleaded to be allowed to reduce. Consent was given with the admonition that the *loss of weight must not exceed the average of 3 lb a week.*

The patient's progress was most satisfactory. She showed none of her previous obsessive weighing as she approached the weight of 125. She had almost at once calculated the date of her goal weight when she had first begun to reduce, but she had been admonished that weight reduction was on a weekly average. Hence, she could only set the week but not the day of achieving the goal weight.

She was seen only at intervals of three to six weeks. She was always adequately praised for her cooperation in both the trance and waking states, and each time the hope was expressed that no intervening problem would develop to alter the expected week of final achievement.

She forgot her appointment for the final week, but made one for the next week. At that time she weighed 123 lb instead of 125. She explained that she had failed to weigh herself regularly and hence did not know exactly when she had reached 125 lb. She declared her intention to remain approximately at that weight.

In the nine months that have passed since then, the patient has succeeded comfortably in this resolve. In addition she has developed recreational and vocational interests, particularly golf and a book review club, and she has for the first time in her life participated in social and community affairs.

CASE 3

A physician's wife in her middle thirties sought aid for her obesity in an amused, half-hearted manner. This had begun in her junior year in high school, at which time she weighed 110 lb, and each succeeding year of life had been marked by a progressive increase to the current weight of 270 lb.

During the past thirteen years she had sought help from one physician after another, but each time failed to secure results. Her explanation was, "Oh, I always cooperate with the diet they put me on. I always eat that and everything else I can lay my hands on. I always overeat, and I suppose I always will. As a forlorn hope, I'm trying you to see if hypnosis will work. I know it won't, but my husband will feel better if I do try it. But I warn you not to expect too much because if I know me, and I think I do, I'll overeat as usual."

Hypnosis was attempted. She developed a medium to deep trance readily, but it was difficult to maintain that depth of trance. She would repeatedly arouse, laugh, and explain that she was curious why the writer would be willing to waste his time on her in view of her "unfavorable prognosis" of her own behavior. The explanation was offered to her that neither time nor effort would be wasted since it was intended to utilize her own behavior to effect therapeutic results. Her reply was, "But how can there be therapeutic results when you and I both know that I'll eat any diet you recommend and everything else even if I have to make extra shopping trips? I've had too many years of overeating to give it up, and I'm here only because my husband wants me to come. I've always tried to cooperate but it's no use. I know the exact caloric value of any serving of food, but all my knowledge does not keep me from overeating. Even my teen-age daughter's embarrassment about my obesity doesn't keep me from overeating. But I'll play along with you, at least for a while, but nothing will work."

Again she was assured that her own behavior would be employed to produce effective results, and she was asked to redevelop a trance state so that hypnosis could be employed. She declared that she would only awaken herself from the trance state if this were done. Even as she completed her statement she developed a medium to deep trance but almost immediately aroused herself by laughing.

She was then asked to develop and to maintain a light trance and to listen carefully to what was said to her, to understand completely what was said, to go into a deeper trance whenever she wished, or to lighten her trance if she felt so impelled, but, at all events to listen to the entire explanation about to be offered her without interrupting it by arousing from the trance. She agreed to cooperate on this basis.

Slowly, systematically, she was instructed:

1. Your weight is 270 lb.
2. You know the caloric values of any food serving.
3. You always have and always will overeat.
4. Your own behavior has always defeated you in the past.
5. Your own behavior will be used this time to effect therapeutic results. This you do not understand.
6. You will cooperate as you always do and you will also overeat. (The patient first shook her head vigorously at this, then sighed and slowly nodded her head affirmatively.)

When it was felt that she understood these instructions adequately, she was given the further instructions:

1. You now weigh 270 lb, not 150 or 140, but 270 lb. You not only will overeat but you need to eat excessively in order to support that poundage.
2. Now bear this in mind and cooperate fully: During this next week overeat, *doing so carefully and willingly,* and overeat enough to support 260 lb. That is all you need to do, overeat sufficiently to support 260 lb. Now I am going to arouse you and dismiss you with no further discussion or even comments. You are to return at this same hour one week from today.

She was seen again a week later. Her opening remark was, "Well, for the first time in my life I enjoyed overeating, and I checked on my husband's office scales today, because I don't trust our bathroom scales. I weighed 260 lb too, a few ounces less in fact, but I call it 260 lb."

A trance was induced again, light in character, and she was again similarly instructed, but this time to overeat sufficiently to support 255 lb and to report in another week's time. On that occasion, a new goal was established at 250 lb.

On the next visit she hesitantly explained that she and her husband were going on their annual two weeks' visit at her parental home, and that "I always gain on my mother's cooking, and I hesitate to go this year, but I see no way out of it."

In the trance state she was asked what weight she ought to overeat sufficiently to support on this two-week holiday. She answered, "Well, we'll really be gone 16 days so I think I ought to eat enough to weigh a good fat 238."

She was emphatically told that she was *to overeat sufficiently to support 238 lb, and also sufficiently to gain 3, 4, or even 5 lb.*

She returned from the trip jubilant, weighing 242 lb, and stated happily, "I did just as you said. I gained 4 lb. This is a silly game we are playing, but

I don't care. It works. I like to overeat and I'm so grateful that I don't overeat as much as I used to."

A variation was introduced into the procedure by insisting that she maintain her weight unchanged on two occasions for a two-week period. Both
times she reacted with impatience, declaring "That's too long a time to
overeat that much."

In six months' time she has reached the weight of 190 lb, is enthusiastic
about continuing, and is in the process of window-shopping for "something
that will look good on a chubby 130 or 140."

SUMMARY

The medical problem for each of these patients was the same, a matter
of weight reduction, and each had failed in numerous previous attempts.
By employing hypnosis a communication of special ideas and understandings ordinarily not possible of presentation was achieved in relation to personality needs and subjective attitudes toward weight reduction. Each was
enabled to undertake the problem of weight loss in accord with long-es-
tablished patterns of behavior but utilized in a new fashion. Thus, one
patient's pleasure in eating was intensified at the expense of quantity, a
change of sequence of behavioral reactions led to success for the second,
and a certain willfullness of desire to defeat the self was employed to frustrate the self doubly and thus to achieve the desired goal.

22

The Treatment of Obesity by Individual and Group Hypnosis

FREDERICK W. HANLEY

OBESITY is a disfiguring psychosomatic disorder with many causes. Regardless of etiology, any individual patient, with his specific genetic, metabolic, and emotional make-up, gains weight because, in the last analysis, he is taking in more food than he actually needs for energy and maintenance. For the obese, overeating is not simply an occasional practice but has become a habit, a learned pattern of behavior involving long-standing attitudes to food and eating. Added to this are self-dislike generated by the disfigurement and discouragement due to the frequent failure to reverse the process of weight gain or even to control it adequately by dieting. The obese person gradually comes to build up rationalizations and other defenses about his condition but these do not resolve the underlying feelings of guilt and self-dislike, which he very often assuages by further eating. Thus the corpulent are caught in the familiar vicious circle.

The basic problem with obesity is to help the patient to learn new, more satisfactory eating habits and to have these become so firmly implanted that they will last indefinitely. It is true that in many cases eating is an emotional outlet for other problems, but psychotherapy directed solely toward these and the maturation of the personality is very seldom successful without, in addition, direct attention to the habits themselves. The situation is similar to that of the alcoholic in whom the drinking has become a major part of the disease, causing its own repercussions and ravages to the personality. In the obese person the very acquisition of better eating habits and the loss of weight bring a feeling of encouragement and control which can lead to significant development and maturation of the personality and hence less and less need to use the primitive gratification of eating. A positive cycle is established to replace the former *impasse*.

To achieve the goal of relearning, hypnosis can be of great value as a method of communication to increase rapport, to motivate learning and to facilitate the acquisition of new eating patterns. It is not used to deprive the patient of satisfaction, i.e. to remove a symptom, but to alter the eating behavior on the basis of the patient's needs.

The first step is to define clearly the patient's goals and motivations. How much weight does the patient want to lose? What would he like to weigh and how long does he think it will require to reach this weight? Discussion

291

of these concrete matters helps the patient to adjust to a realistic expectation and at the same time communicates the physician's understanding that
he is prepared to work with him on a relatively long-term, consistent program which he expects the patient to maintain after the termination of
treatment. The motivations for losing weight are brought out and explored
and all positive aspects are strongly supported. The eating habits are then
carefully examined to learn how the patient overeats and his lifelong as
well as his present attitudes to food are looked into. At this point some
tentative agreements are reached, e.g. that it would be best to eliminate
eating between meals or perhaps that a mid-morning snack should replace
the usual mid-day meal. Individual variations must be taken into account.
In this whole process a good rapport is being established and the patient is
committing himself to a definite program.

At this stage the patient is trained to enter a hypnotic trance, which
usually requires only one or two sessions. Acting on the knowledge that
has been gained the physician then formulates positive suggestions. The
patient is told that he will derive a great deal of pleasure from eating, that
he will enjoy even more the taste of his food and the satisfaction of
chewing it and that when he swallows the first mouthful he will begin to
feel satisfied and full. It is suggested that by the time he has eaten a very
small portion of food he will feel so satisfied and full that he will have no
desire to eat anything more until the time of the next meal. Increased feeling of confidence and self-esteem are suggested. He is also asked to visualize
himself at the size and weight he would like to be, doing the things he cannot do now, wearing the clothes he would like to wear, enjoying additional
energy and so on. As one learns more about the individual patient, one can
formulate various suggestions to suit the specific case. The unconscious is
reeducated so that the satisfactions of achievement come to outweigh
the primitive gratifications of eating, and food loses its central place in the
patient's life. Practice and repetition are essential until the new eating
habits are thoroughly learned.

An important feature of the learning process which is often overlooked
is the relapse and discouragement following the initial enthusiasm and ac-
complishment. It is at this point that the patient has often given up in the
past but it is precisely at this stage in the learning process that there is a
potential for basic change. The initial success is always superficial and
deeper change does not occur until at least one recrudescence of the old
habits. When the relapse comes it is carefully explained to the patient that
this was expected and that it is part of the learning process. In fact he is con-
gratulated on having relapsed so quickly and so well. At this juncture the
patient will often bring out some of his deeper attitudes and problems
and the rapport will be greatly strengthened. It is sometimes useful in

the hypnosis sessions at this time to give the patient permission to fail at any time he feels he really needs to. This is not only supportive but subtly transfers the responsibility to the patient. Depending on the degree of personality problem present, a considerable amount of psychotherapy may have to be done at this time. This may be usefully combined with hypnotherapy. After passing this phase, the patient often settles down to more or less steady progress in acquiring his new eating habits, but in many cases the relapse may have to be repeated several times.

Recently the author began group treatment of six to eight females aged 21 to 44. The first forty minutes of the hour are used for group discussion, which at first centers around the problem of obesity, but later extends into areas of other personal difficulties. It has been found that this group therapy has been most valuable for the ventilation of feelings of guilt, discouragement, and hostility associated with eating and obesity. Patients express their feelings and their attitudes more freely when they find that others feel the same way. There is a great deal of mutual support and an interchange of helpful ideas. Motivation is maintained and friendly competition may develop. When a patient announces that she has lost seven pounds in the previous week, the motivation of the others is increased. On the other hand, when patients relapse others come to their support, thereby increasing their own motivation. In fact, several of the patients have worked out a procedure similar to that of Alcoholics Anonymous—if one is feeling depressed or otherwise tempted to overeat, she will call another member of the group to be "talked out of it." The group has been found to be especially useful for the withdrawn patient.

Following the group discussion, twenty or thirty minutes are spent on group hypnosis. When everyone is in a satisfactory trance state, general suggestions outlined above are given and then specific suggestions are offered to individual patients by referring to them by name and by telling other patients that they may disregard these remarks. It has been interesting to note that sometimes a specific suggestion was rejected by the patient to whom it was offered but has been picked up and used effectively by some other member of the group. The fundamental fact holds true here that patients accept those suggestions and only those suggestions which are meaningful and useful to them.

Each member of the group loses weight at her own individual rate, the average loss being around two to three lb a week. The greatest weight loss has been seventy lb in six months. Invariably, patients report that their outlook on life changes and that they find themselves improving in many ways they had not expected. This is contrasted with their previous experience in losing weight by dieting, where the effect was limited to the one specific matter of weight and there was little or no effect on other aspects of their lives. Although it is too soon yet for meaningful follow-up, most patients feel that they will be able to maintain their new weight because their attitudes to food have changed, their new eating habits are firmly established and their accomplishments and satisfactions in life preclude the necessity of using food for emotional relief. Patients with a poor prognosis are the very immature who expect hypnosis to accomplish magic with no effort on their part.

REFERENCES

1. Brodie, Earl I.: A hypnotherapeutic approach to obesity. *Am J Clin Hypnosis,* 6: No. 3, 1964, p. 211.
2. Erickson, Milton H.: The utilization of patient behavior in the hypnotherapy of obesity: Three Case Reports. *Am J Clin Hypnosis,* 3:No. 2, 1960, p. 112.
3. Wollman, Leo: Hypnosis in weight control. *Am J Clin Hypnosis,* 4:No. 3, 1962, p. 177.

VIII

DIET

23

The Social Psychology of Dieting

Johanna T. Dwyer
Jacob J. Feldman
AND
Jean Mayer

THE prevalence of excess weight in the American population as a whole is high—so high, in fact, that in some segments of the population it has reached epidemic proportions. Excess weight is a serious health problem because it is associated with respiratory, arthritic, gall bladder, and cardiovascular diseases.[46] Certain types of coronary heart disease, namely angina pectoris and myocardial infarctions, are more common in obese persons and frequently lead to sudden death.[36] The significance of excess weight on the public's health may therefore be considerable.

Dieting is a popular American avocation. Because the reduction to or maintenance of weight at normal levels can result in decreased risk and severity of certain chronic diseases, successful weight control has great medical significance, and health reasons cause many persons to diet. However, since social factors are equally, if not more, important in motivating weight control behavior, one must understand the social psychology of dieting.

DEFINITIONS

Overweight

It is important at the outset to define what health professionals mean when they speak of overweight and obesity. Overweight is defined as body weight in excess of an ideal weight, based on height-specific and sex-specific standards. Overweight can result from excesses of bone, muscle, fat, or, more rarely, fluid. Almost everyone who is more than 20 per cent overweight is also overfat, or obese. However, not all people who are heavy are excessively fat. The relative contributions to overweight of bone, muscle, and fat vary from person to person, and it is often hard to recognize these differences. The component that actually causes weight in excess of normal is less than clear when overweight is in the more moderate range (i.e. less than 20 per cent over ideal weight), and this brings diagnostic difficulties if weight alone serves as the criteria for overfatness. This brings us to the definition of a second term: obesity.

297

Obesity

Obesity is defined as body fatness in excess of an age and sex specific standard. Body weights grossly in excess of standards are indicative of obesity. Moderate overweight sometimes, but not always, is due to obesity. Some people whose weights are normal are also obese. Thus, overweight (heaviness) and obesity (excessive fatness) are not necessarily synonymous, and weight deviations give only imprecise estimates of obesity. Football players, for example, may be overweight because of their massive bone and muscle structure, yet not be overfat at all.

Body Type

Body types, or somatotypes, which describe differences in physical conformation and structure between persons, are important in the study of weight deviations. These variations in outward appearance are due, at least in part, to underlying anatomical differences in the amount, distribution, or conformation of fat, muscle, and bony tissue, which are reflected in body form. These variations have been precisely defined and described systematically by Sheldon *et al.*;[41] his system contains three major components: a) endomorphy, which is characterized by softness and roundness of appearance; b) mesomorphy, characterized by a combination of bone and muscle development; and c) ectomorphy, characterized by linearity, fragility, and attenuation of body build. The most common somatotypes in the population combine all three of these components to varying degrees.

Most obese persons are not simply thin persons with an excessive body burden of fat; their body types have been found to differ in other aspects as well. The majority of the obese tend to be somewhat larger in their bone and muscle components as well as fatter than their nonobese counterparts.[37, 39] Different weight goals are thus necessary for persons of different body types to allow for the fact that they vary in relative contribution of the nonfat components to their weights.

Dieting

The word "dieting" covers a multitude of different types of eating behavior. Some persons believe that they are dieting when they substitute noncaloric sweetners for sugar, while others consider they are doing so only when they are subjecting themselves to a total fast. In most of the studies reviewed in this article, few attempts were made to identify the types of changes in eating habits that were categorized as dieting. Thus, all that can be inferred from statements that respondents were "on diets" is that these persons reported changing their usual food intake in some way in order to lose weight, however effective or ineffective, extensive or limited, their efforts may have been.

PREVALENCE OF OBESITY

Obesity is the major health factor that motivates people to diet; therefore, the epidemiology of obesity in this country needs scrutiny. The prevalence of obesity varies with age, sex, probably socioeconomic class, and perhaps ethnic variables such as race. The percentage of persons who are obese (that is, 20 per cent or more above ideal weight) generally rises with age from early childhood until late in life, so that far more adults than children or adolescents are obese.[33] Sex differences in the prevalence of obesity do not appear until adulthood. Men gain more weight with age during their early 20's than do women, and by the end of their 20's and 30's more men are obese or overweight than women.[21, 46] Women achieve their maximum weights about two decades later than men and have a greater relative gain with age, however, so that by early middle age the proportion of obese women exceeds that of men. By late middle age many more women are obese than men. This may be due in part to obese men dying in proportionally greater numbers than obese women or nonobese men.

The prevalence of obesity also apparently varies somewhat by socioeconomic class. In their study of whites in midtown Manhattan, Moore et al.[32] found that as social class rose, the prevalence of obesity decreased, particularly among women. In adolescents, associations between obesity and social class appear to be weaker: Huenemann et al.[23] found that higher mean income of the home census tracts of California adolescent subjects was associated with deceased prevalence of obesity, but Canning and Mayer,[6] working in New England, found no relationship between the educational levels or occupations of the adolescents' fathers and the prevalence of obesity in their sample.

Occasionally racial differences in the prevalence of obesity have been mentioned,[21] suggesting that the prevalence of obesity among Negro women is higher than among white women. Differences among men are not as pronounced and suggest a slightly higher prevalence among white men. However, racial differences are usually confounded with socioeconomic class variations, so that it is difficult to say from presently available evidence whether racial differences would exist if class were held constant.

PREVALENCE OF CONCERN ABOUT WEIGHT
AND DIETING BEHAVIOR

Age

Excessive weight deviations tend to be more common and severe among adults than adolescents, yet adults are much less concerned about their weights and less apt to take remedial measures than teen-agers. An opinion poll conducted in 1964 on a national stratified sample[47] revealed that over 30 per cent of those adults who had a weight problem were not even concerned about their weights. Only about 10 per cent of the adults with weight problems were dieting to lose weight, about 20 per cent were watching their weights so that they would stop gaining, and the rest were concerned but took no action against overweight. Another poll done in the early 1960's showed that concern with weight in adults rarely led to dieting; if any action was taken, it was more likely to cut out food regarded as "fattening" to prevent future gains, rather than to attempt to remove excess weight which had already accumulated. The "wishful dieters," as those adults who were concerned about their weights but doing nothing to lower them were called, gave as their main reasons for failure to diet lack of will power, enjoyment of eating, and procrastination.

In contrast, the studies of Huenemann *et al.*[23, 24] and Dwyer *et al.*[12] indicate that almost all obese and many nonobese adolescents are concerned about weight, and that they engage in remedial efforts more often than adults.

Sex

Sex differences in the prevalence of concern about weight clearly favor females, although the prevalence of obesity is not always higher and, in some age groups, may be lower than in males.

Dwyer and Mayer's[16] analysis of several national public opinion polls revealed that concerns about weight and dieting behavior were much more common among adult women than among men. Polls taken in 1956 found that 45 per cent of the women and 22 per cent of the men wanted to lose weight, and that 14 per cent of the women and 7 per cent of the men were currently on diets to do so. Polls in 1966 showed that 42 per cent of the women and 35 per cent of the men interviewed felt that they were over their best weights, and 14 per cent of the women and 6 per cent of the men claimed that they were doing something to lose weight. While concern with weight appeared to be rising among the men over time, dieting behavior was not.

Weight was perceived as much more of a problem by teen-age girls than by boys in the surveys of health concerns of adolescents done by Deisher and Mills[10] and Adams.[1] Huenemann *et al.*[23, 24] investigated concerns about weight in senior high school students. On the basis of physical measurements, about 25 per cent of both the boys and the girls were classified as being obese or somewhat obese. Almost 50 per cent of the girls and somewhat less than 25 per cent of the boys expressed concern about their overweight and described themselves as being too fat. Concerns about overweight and obesity were present in many nonobese girls. A large proportion of the girls and a much smaller proportion of the boys were trying to lose weight or change their body proportions. Dieting was the most popular method of doing this.

Dwyer *et al.*[12] studied attitudes of high school seniors toward their weights. Sixteen per cent of the girls and 19 per cent of the boys had triceps skinfolds that would be classified as obese. Over 80 per cent of the girls but less than 20 per cent of the boys wanted to weigh less than they did. Among the twelfth-grade, upper-middle-class New England girls they studied, over 60 per cent of all the girls had dieted by the time they were seniors in high school. Thirty per cent were on reducing diets on the day they were questioned. Only 16 per cent of all the girls were obese, and virtually all these girls had dieted, and many leaner girls as well. Of the boys in the same high schools, only 24 per cent of all the boys had ever dieted, and only 6 per cent were on reducing diets on the day they were questioned. Nineteen per cent of these boys were obese, but only a small proportion even of this group was on a reducing diet.

Weight Status

Heavier people in general tend to be more concerned about weight than lighter people. Almost all of the studies relevant to this point have been done on adolescents, however; little work has been done on adults. Hinton *et al.*,[22] Dwyer *et al.*,[12] and Huenemann *et al.*[23, 24] found that overweight or obese adolescents were more likely to be concerned about their weights and dieting to change them than nonobese adolescents.

Social Class and Ethnicity

Dieting and concern with overweight seem to be somewhat more prevalent among upper-class than lower-class adults, although there are fewer obese persons in the upper classes than in the rest of the population. Only 11 per cent of the population falls in the upper-class or upper-middle-class brackets, but they contain 24 per cent of all dieters.[47] Dwyer and Mayer's analyses[16] of opinion polls showed that concern with weight and dieting behavior increased slightly with occupational status but not educational level in men, and with both education and occupation in women. Newman[34] found that a greater proportion of overweight upper-class women saw themselves as overweight and attempted to lose than did lower-class women.

The associations between obesity and social class are not as strong in adolescents as they are in adults. No data are available on the relationship of dieting to social class in adolescents. Little information also is available to indicate whether the prevalence of dieting varies by ethnic variables such as race, religion, or national origin.

THE CHAIN OF DECISIONS LEADING TO DIETING

Regarding dieting as the logical terminal behavior resulting from a step-wise choice of a certain set of options makes it easier to understand the social psychology of dieting. The sequence of events that may result in dieting are the following: a) recognition of a weight problem; b) decision to remedy it; c) choice of source of treatment; and d) choice of method of treatment. Each of these steps offers several options, so that the decisions and actions of the people involved may vary considerably at each step in the process. Let us turn now to a closer examination of the factors which come into play at each step.

Before he is likely to engage in dieting behavior, the potential *dieter must realize that he has a weight problem.* Equally obese people often differ in their opinions as to their body weights. Some are convinced that they are too fat, others are not, and still others have no opinion at all. One reason for the diversity of opinions is their salience. Membership in social and cultural groups may cause people to vary the attention and importance they place on body weight. Individuals within a particular sociocultural group differ in their exposure to various professional and lay persons and other sources of information that might make them perceive that they are too fat. In addition, individuals vary in their own inherent interest and concern about fatness and appearance.

Differences in opinion may also evolve from the type of prevailing standards or norms that are used. Various types of standards are used as criteria for diagnosing obesity; health professionals and laymen often differ in their assessments of fatness status, since their standards are based on different considerations.

The standards most universally used by physicians, other health workers, and many laymen to diagnose obesity are the tables of ideal or desirable weights for each height, frame, and sex. These have been derived by insurance companies[30] from actuarial studies and are based on health considerations. However, these tables have rather severe shortcomings.[35, 37] The problem most germane to the current discussion is the fact that no clear specifications are given of what is meant by frame.

If overweight that may be due to large amounts of bone and muscle is mistaken for obesity—which is due to overfat alone—this may lead to misdirected and fruitless dieting efforts or unrealistic goals for body weight. While diets and exercises make it possible to reduce the weight due to extra fat, it is impossible to reduce the bone and muscle components of weight by these measures. Conversely, if overweight due to excessive fatness is wrongly identified as being due to a large build, no action may be taken against obesity. Thus, the distinctions of build are important ones to make.

Moreover, ideal weights for persons of certain builds, particularly for those with large muscle and bone, may be unrealistically low as weight goals for the general population.[35] Norms of obesity more valid and precise than weight alone are available.

One simple way of assessing body fatness is to measure the size of the triceps skinfold, the subcutaneous fat depot over the triceps muscle on the back of the upper arm. This measurement allows a reasonably satisfactory estimate of the total body burden of fat to be made, and standards for obesity based on this measurement have been established.[37] A slightly more complicated method of estimating body fatness is the "body envelope method" of Behnke,[3] which is based on a number of physical measurements, including several fat depots. Many of the studies reported here use one of these two measurements for the objective assessment of obesity.

Many laymen rely on standards based on appearance or social acceptability as well as weight tables to evaluate their weight or fatness status. But is there any regularity or consistency in aspects of physical appearance related to weight that are aspired to? If so, how stable are they? Obviously, if ideas of what is "too fat" or "too thin" change either as the individual progresses through the life cycle or from year to year like fashions in dress, judgments about what is "too fat" or "too thin" may also change.

Fairly uniform, implicit norms for the appearance of the body do appear to exist in this country. While they vary somewhat from person to person because of their strong roots in individual opinions and attitudes, these norms are on the whole quite consistent. They are probably based on collective observation by the population of what is common in the community or in society in general, coupled with an unconscious judgment about what is to be regarded as normal. Norms for certain aspects of appearance are regarded as unattainable for some; for example, if the norm is that American women should be about 5 ft 6 in tall, a 5 ft 1 in woman can never attain the norm and will always be regarded as short. Other norms for physical appearance, such as lack of obesity, are generally regarded as attainable by all. While aberrations or striking deviations from these norms may not be regarded as abnormal or pathological from a medical standpoint, society's judgment or the opinion of influential members of society that they are not "normal," or deviant, may generate concern and discomfort in the unfortunate individuals who happen to possess these characteristics.

Homogeneous ideals for these aspects of physical appearance also exist within this country. Ideals arise from man's attempts to visualize and classify not what is common or normal, as is true in the case of standards or norms, but what is perfect, that which is uncommon and desirable for that reason.

Just as fashions in clothes vary, norms and ideals for bodily appearance change from culture to culture and over time. Arabs, for example, esteem different, plumper body types than do Americans. During the late Renaissance, a young woman who had wide hips and an ample expanse of abdomen regarded herself as beautiful, while her twentieth-century American counterpart abhors these very characteristics in herself. Thus, since norms and ideals do change, there is no reason to assume that the current ones will last forever. Slimness may remain in vogue, or it may be replaced by a more amply padded figure. Such shifts could have striking effects on the prevalence of concern over weight and on dieting efforts.

Almost no work has been done on adult norms or ideals for weight, although a few studies have been done on adolescents. Their weight aspirations appear to vary with sex, body fatness, weight, and perhaps race. Dwyer *et al.*[12] explored weight goals among high school seniors in a New England suburb. Among the girls, means for the weights they thought were the best for themselves on the basis of health decreased with decreasing body fatness and were always lower than their actual weights, except for the leanest girls, who felt that they should weigh a few pounds more than they did. When the same girls were asked what they wished to weigh, taking all considerations (health, appearance, etc.) into account, weights were even lower. The situation was quite different for the boys: Both weight goals were higher than actual weights. Huenemann *et al.*[23, 24] reported racial as well as sex differences in desires for body weights for high school sophomores. Caucasian girls wanted to lose more weight than Negroes or Orientals, although Negro girls were heavier. In contrast to the girls, boys of all races wanted to weigh more than they actually did and also wanted to be taller. Oriental boys were the lightest and shortest and also those who wished the greatest increases in weight and height.

Within each sex adolescents have fairly uniform ideals for the relative size of body parts, and these may influence their weight goals. Many adolescents appear to believe that appearances closer to their ideals in body parts can be brought about by a change in body weight. The studies of Huenemann *et al.* and Dwyer *et al.* suggest that boys wish to gain weight and to be larger in almost all dimensions, especially in those that might signify strength or athletic prowess, such as the upper torso or arms. Girls, on the other hand, want to be smaller in almost all dimensions and to lose weight, although they are content about their heights. Girls also have very different concerns about their bodies; they wish to be smaller, especially in their torsos (with the exception of the busts) and thighs. Huenemann *et al.* suggested that while adolescent girls attribute their overweight to overfatness and regard it as undesirable, boys attribute their overweight to build components other than fat and regard it as desirable.

Uniform ideals of body type that may affect weight aspirations also exist. In Dwyer *et al.*'s[12] study, adolescents were asked to choose among six female silhouettes (ranging from extreme ectomorphs to extreme endomorphs), first, the silhouette they considered to be their ideal, and second, that which was regarded by them as the most feminine. A majority of both sexes picked the female silhouette representing a mesomorphic ectomorph as being their ideal and also the most feminine figure. A substantial portion of the girls chose the extreme ectomorph, while the boys did not, suggesting that the girls' ideals were more ectomorphic than those of the boys. When male silhouettes were rated, the silhouette representing the extreme mesomorph was chosen by an overwhelming majority of the boys and a majority of the girls as their ideal and as the most masculine. Girls showed a wider range of responses, suggesting that the boys' ideals for masculinity were more mesomorphic than those of the girls.

A great deal of confusion seems to exist between what are attainable norms or realistic expectations and what are virtually unattainable ideals and unrealistic with regard to physical appearance. Time spent attempting to alter aspects of appearance that cannot be changed is wasted, while that spent striving toward attainable norms is time well spent. It is thus of crucial importance to ascertain how realistic weight-related norms are and how much hope of fulfillment they offer before people are urged to aspire to attain them. Clearly, both the feminine ideal of a slender, full-bosomed fashion model's build and the masculine ideal of the barrel-chested, muscle-bound football player are only realizable for a small percentage of the population, since such body builds occur only rarely in actuality.

Even after the potential dieter has realized that he is too fat, he must be *motivated to undertake a weight control program*. It is abundantly clear that the factors encouraging people to follow through involve more than health motivations, even among those with the greatest health risk from their obesity.

Among adults, fear of poor health is the primary, but not the only, reason given by men who undertake reducing diets.[47] Other reasons such as appearance appear to be equally if not more important in motivating women to lose weight. In adolescent girls, the desire to change certain aspects of appearance or become more attractive is almost universally the primary reason for dieting behavior.[13, 14] On the other hand, Dwyer *et al.*[12] found that boys embarked on reducing diets primarily to improve their physical fitness and sports ability. Huenemann *et al.*[24] also found that the adolescent boys and girls they studied undertook diets for appearance rather than for health reasons most of the time.

Many Americans decide to lose weight because of the pervasive negative attitudes toward obesity that permeate the social climate. Obesity is regarded as more than solely a health issue, not only by the afflicted individuals themselves, but even by physicians and other members of society. Obesity evokes negative stereotypes about behavior and personality traits as well as appearance, although these generalizations may not correspond to actuality. Maddox *et al.*[26] recently showed that most Americans regard obesity as a socially deviant form of physical disability. The subjects in their study blamed the obese for being fat, but felt that persons with other physical handicaps should not be blamed because they were not responsible for their conditions. The authors of the study expected certain groups, notably low-income subjects, Negro males, and elderly persons to be indifferent to the standard American preference for leanness and to value fatness instead. However, the negative attitudes toward obesity ran so deep that even members of these groups considered fat persons less likeable than nonfat ones. Some members of society are even more extreme and look upon obesity as downright immoral. They apparently base such judgments on the belief that it arises from either or both of the sins of gluttony and sloth.

An obese appearance evokes negative and stereotyped attitudes as early as childhood. Staffieri[42] asked boys from four to ten years of age to assign various behavior or personality traits to silhouettes representing extremely endomorphic, mesomorphic, and ectomorphic body types. He found that stereotyped responses began to appear between the ages of four and five, and that differences had become apparent by the age of seven. At age seven, all adjectives assigned to the endomorph with a significantly greater frequency than to the other silhouettes were socially unfavorable (for example, fights, cheats, mean, and lazy). All of those assigned to the mesomorphic silhouette were favorable (for example, strong, best friend, and clean), and those assigned to the ectomorph were personally unfavorable or indicative of social submissiveness (for example, sneaky, afraid, and quiet). The children liked the mesomorph better consistently after the age of seven, and after this age they were also able to classify their own body types fairly accurately. Hassan[20] also noted that stereotyped ideas of the character traits and behavior of persons with different body types existed in grade-school children of both sexes, and that those whose body types were less favored had less self-regard and less accurate self-concepts.

Professional persons such as physicians, who are trained to regard all sorts of physical problems dispassionately, might be expected to be free from such stereotyped beliefs about the obese. However, a study by Maddox and Liederman[27] revealed that a negative evaluation and characterization of obese persons extended to doctors' attitudes as well. Obese patients were described by their doctors as being more weak-willed, ugly, and awkward than their other patients. The obese have also been noted to appear to accept more blame and feel more guilt about their condition than those with other types of physical disabilities. Perhaps this is due in part to physicians' attitudes toward them.

Obesity may affect interpersonal relationships even in childhood. Matthews and Westie[28] reported that grade-school children indicated the greatest social distance from overweight children in their classes. Among the children he studied, Staffieri[42] found that mesomorphic boys received the highest number of "best friend" choices, and endomorphs the fewest, from their peers.

Obese children, especially girls, have particular social problems when they reach adolescence and heterosexual interest picks up. Bullen *et al.*[5] found that extremely obese girls had significantly fewer dates than nonobese girls. The obese were in fewer nonsport clubs, organizations, and groups in and outside of school than the nonobese. They did not participate as actively in those groups of which they were members as did the nonobese.

Canning and Mayer[6] presented evidence that unconscious prejudices of high-school teachers in writing recommendations or among college interviewers against obese adolescents may hinder their chances of being accepted by the colleges of their choice. Application rates and academic qualifications among the obese were equal to those among nonobese twelfth graders in the schools they studied, yet acceptance rates into high-ranking colleges were lower for obese students, especially for girls. Canning and Mayer[7] also found that obesity did not have any effect on high school performance as measured by IQ scores, PSAT or SAT scores (achievement tests), absences, or enrollment in extracurricular activities. Thus it appears that the extreme concern of the obese with weight and their own and teachers' negative evaluations of obese adolescents do not prevent them from performing well or even excelling in many areas.

Our own self-regard largely reflects what others think of us. Other factors being equal, persons with an attractive appearance tend to develop high self-regard, while those whose appearance is regarded as unattractive tend to have lower self-regard, and may strive to change this appearance. Therefore, it is not surprising to find that obese children and adolescents have extremely negative self-images. In a study of high-school girls at a summer camp in New England, Monello and Mayer[31] found that the obese girls showed personality characteristics such as passivity, obsessive concern with self-image, expectation of rejection, and progressive withdrawal—all strikingly similar to the traits of ethnic and racial minority groups due to their status as victims of prejudice. They also accepted the dominant negative values toward obesity prevalent in our society. Canning and Mayer[8] demonstrated that the obsession with their weights was so great that nonrelated areas became involved in the issue. In sentence-completion tests dealing with interpersonal situations, obese girls were more apt to give responses indicating concern about weight, while the responses of normal-weight controls were related to other normal concerns and reactions of adolescents. The obese girls persisted in interjecting concern with wishes or things in their lives that generated anxiety. Direct questions about weight and appearance also brought significantly higher response from the obese than the nonobese.

Alexander,[2] in working with female college freshmen, found that endomorphs were significantly less accepting of themselves than were ectomorphs or mesomorphs. Maddox *et al.*[26] found that the disvaluation of fatness and denial of identification with the obese extended not only to the general public but to people who were themselves obese. When obese subjects were asked to compare themselves to their ideal selves and to fat people for various characteristics, their answers revealed that they felt they were less like their ideal selves but also less like obese people than did normal-weight subjects.

The early and prolonged exposure to negative sociocultural attitudes toward obesity encountered by those whose obesity begins in childhood appears more detrimental to self-image than does obesity of adult onset. Stunkard and Mendelson's[44] study indicates that adults afflicted with obesity of the latter type do not approve of their overweight, but do not loathe their bodies or hate themselves because of it. Tarini[45] has shown that many of them deny their fatness. In contrast, the Stunkard and Mendelson[44] study found that certain obese adults, most of whom had been obese since childhood or adolescence, looked upon themselves as grotesque and ugly; they tended to blame their weights for far-removed troubles, to divide the world into fat and nonfat, and to disregard factors such as talent, intelligence, and wealth in favor of appearance in judging others. Stunkard and Burt[43] confirmed these findings on another sample of obese adults and again found that disturbances in body image clustered in persons obese since childhood or adolescence. Bruch[4] observed that many persons obese since early life who later successfully reduced their weights still felt that they were ugly and fat.

Thus, from many standpoints—conformity to current standards and ideals for appearance, self-regard, social acceptability, and health—obesity is detrimental. Many obese persons undoubtedly undertake weight control behavior to escape some of this social and moral opprobrium as well as to decrease health risks.

The potential dieter must now decide whom to consult for help in losing weight. He may seek advice from a health professional, a lay practitioner, or he may choose to treat himself. This choice is probably largely determined by the individual's perceptions and opinions on the cause and severity of his condition. If he believes that his obesity is connected to a pathological, physical, or psychological condition, he is likely to seek medical or psychiatric help; if he believes that he is well and that his obesity is uncomplicated from the medical standpoint, he will probably treat himself or engage the services of a lay practitioner such as the leader of a diet club. However, other variables may also influence his decision. In terms of the economy of money, time, and effort involved in arranging for treatment and access to treatment, the self-administered methods rate the highest. However, if we examine the adequacy of medical supervision and the amount of psychological support they provide, some of the methods employed by lay practitioners and health professionals are superior. Further, persons whose obesity is severe (or who regard it as such, even if it is not) are more likely to choose these sources. Those whose obesity is complicated by some other physical or emotional problem often seek medical help. In addition, many other related variables that involve the perception of illness and of health-motivated behavior may determine the source of treatment.

The next decision confronting the individual who wishes to lose weight is the method. There are *three basic popular methods* that can be used either alone or in combination to bring about weight loss: a) dietary modifications, b) increased physical activity, and c) medications. Dietary modifications accomplish the objective by decreasing caloric intake, increased physical activity by raising caloric output. Medications vary in their action; some act as appetite depressants, others as laxatives or diuretics, and a few, such as thyroid extract, increase metabolic rate and therefore energy expenditure. Psychiatric treatment for obesity is based on the premise that solving the patient's emotional problems will motivate him to lose weight. These last two treatments are usually coupled with or result in changes in food intake or energy expenditure as well.

The source of treatment chosen to some extent dictates the methods and techniques available for losing weight. For example, lay practitioners are usually involved in managing diet clubs and health spas, while health professionals are the only ones who can prescribe most medications or refer patients to dietitians for diet therapy. However, choice of method is also influenced by several other interrelated factors: a) the individual's views on the cause of his obesity, b) cost and availability of the method, and c) compatability of the method with the individual's life style.

Views on the Causation and Proper Treatment for Obesity

Mayer[29] has recently reviewed and summarized current scientific opinion on the etiology and pathogenesis of obesity. The most common type of obesity in this country today is generally agreed to be environmental in origin, arising from inactivity rather than from excessively large food intakes on the part of the obese versus the nonobese. Only a small percentage of cases appears caused by preexisting pathological conditions, either physical or psychiatric. Thus, most competent physicians treat most of their obese patients through reducing diets or increased physical activity, and they are extremely conservative in using medications. The more potent medications such as thyroid extract or "rainbow diet pills" (consisting of thyroid extract, diuretics, digitalis, and amphetamines) in combination with extremely rigid diets have in the past few years been misused by some disreputable "diet doctors." Their patients have paid dearly in money and may also have jeopardized their health by their patronage.

Lay and medical opinion on the cause and proper treatment for obesity vary. Lay opinion stresses overeating rather than inactivity as the major cause of obesity, and perhaps these views lead to the high value placed on the efficacy of dieting. For example, in Huenemann et al.'s[23] study of knowledge in high school students of the causes of obesity, over half of the freshman boys and even more of the girls believed that fatness was due chiefly to overeating. Modifications in diet greatly overshadowed changes in activity levels among both boys and girls. Less than half of both sexes realized that the obese did not exercise as much as the nonobese. By the time these students had reached the twelfth grade, boys had begun to adopt the opinion that obesity was due to underactivity, while girls remained committed to their earlier beliefs. Boys had also become more partial to exercise than girls. Dwyer et al.[11] also found that twelfth-grade boys were more likely to incorporate greater physical activity into their weight control efforts than were girls. Bullen et al.[5] similarly found that the obese adolescent girls they interviewed thought they were fat primarily because they ate more, had greater appetites, and snacked more than their nonobese friends.

Unfortunately, no work has been reported on the opinions of adults on the causes of obesity, but it is likely that their beliefs are similar to those of adolescents. Given the public's general conviction that food and overeating are the major cause factors operating in obesity, it is easy to understand why reducing diets are so popular.

Cost and Availability

Self-administered methods are the easiest to employ. Dietary modifications and increased physical activity can be undertaken by anyone who chooses to do so without any contact with a physician, although they are often more effective under a physician or dietitian's direction. Psychiatric treatment with some weight-loss technique is available only from physicians. The more potent medications are available only by prescription, and access to them therefore entails seeing a physician. Some of the less powerful drugs such as certain appetite-depressants, weak diuretics, bulk producers, laxatives, and other nostrums can be obtained over-the-counter in drugstores without prescription, but these are usually used in conjunction with dieting.

Compatability of Method with Life Style

The ease with which weight loss can be fitted into one's normal life is vitally important in determining choice of reducing method. Most people acknowledge the value and stress the beneficial effects of exercise and activity, and they may be partial to reducing drugs in controlling weight when discussing it or advising others, but when it comes down to their actual weight-control efforts, in practice they rely chiefly, if not exclusively, on dietary methods. The difficulty of obtaining diet pills and the inconvenience involved in taking them probably account for their rather limited use.

However, the unpopularity of physical activity has a more complex explanation. People seem to think that dieting is an easier method of curing obesity than burning off calories by increasing exercise and physical activity. Considering the relative amounts of disruption to established habits and life style in general that go along with each type of modification, they are probably right. The constraints imposed by life style on activity levels seem to be even greater than those on eating habits. Patterns of inactivity probably have an even stronger hold and are more difficult to overcome than habits of overeating. In addition, increased physical activity usually requires a greater rather than a lesser time input, which busy people are loathe to make, while the skipped meals and eating less that are often involved in dieting patterns require no time expenditures and may even save time. Special facilities, such as swimming pools, are required for many of the types of exercise people like best; other sports require several teammates or other players for a game. Further, many simple activities such as walking, which seem to face none of the above obstacles, are difficult in many areas where streets are unsafe. Finally, the disinclination to increase activity as a means of controlling weight is due partly to the widely held but mistaken belief of most Americans that they are not inactive or sedentary. The great majority of Americans do lead sedentary lives; they do not perform much physical labor that involves substantial energy expenditures. Inactivity and the sedentary life are apparently confused in many people's minds with sloth—laziness, sluggishness, idleness, or indolence. To say that a person is sedentary has no moral overtones. Americans are sedentary, but this does not mean that they do not engage in a great deal of tiring activity; it simply means that most of this activity does not involve large caloric outputs.

Another widespread belief that works against the adoption of activity as a means of losing weight is that exercise must be violent and unpleasant, such as calisthenics, jogging, or weight lifting, in order to contribute substantially to weight loss. While this is not true, it undoubtedly discourages many persons from engaging in greater physical activity. In terms of all of these variables that affect life style, the easiest, most pleasant, and most popular method of losing weight seems to be dieting.

At last the potential dieter has become an actual dieter and has embarked on his diet. This, of course, gives no assurance that he will actually lose weight. The efficacy of the dietary treatment will depend on the soundness of the regimen itself, the zeal with which it is followed, and its duration. Unfortunately, very little has been written on the psychological factors that influence these variables, and more intense study is needed in this area.

POSSIBLE EXPLANATIONS OF THE GREATER RATE OF DIETING AMONG FEMALES THAN MALES

On the basis of evidence that has been presented, several plausible reasons can be suggested for the greater rate of dieting among females than among males.

First, weight deviations are more of a social liability for females than for males. If their weights are excessive, females are at a greater social disadvantage both in their relationships with other females and in their relationships with males. Their social mobility is also inhibited to a greater extent. Successful men are often overweight or obese; successful career women and the wives of famous men rarely are.

Second, weight-related aspects of appearance are more intertwined with the self-concept in females than in males. The sensitivity of the self-images of females to weight problems may encourage them to undertake corrective efforts. It is little wonder that, since women know the importance of their physical appearance particularly in determining how the male half of the human race will regard them as well as in influencing other females' opinions of them, appearance becomes so tightly bound up with self-image. Men have always desired physical attractiveness in their mates and have valued it highly. Although appearance is certainly an important factor in how females assess the eligibility of their male partners, other considerations such as the prospective husband's potential as protector and provider tend to rank higher among the criteria important to their selection. Extra pounds pose a powerful threat to a female's appearance, and hence generate greater concern and ego involvement in females than in males. Men's concerns with respect to their bodies seem largely tied to functional aspects of appearance that suggest physical or sexual prowess. Obesity and leanness must be severe before they become real detriments or imply deficits in the area of physical performance to others. The self-concepts of females, on the other hand, are more intimately involved with myriad aspects of body appearance other than those suggesting physical prowess, and their body images are adversely affected by much smaller deviations. As soon as many women gain a few pounds they feel obese, even though the level of fatness is not sufficient to be noticed by others, and certainly not enough to affect physical performance. Thus, similar deviations in pounds of excess weight above normal that might be merely annoying to a male are devastating to a female's concept of herself.

These differences in the salience of weight status to the individual are illustrated in the accuracy of self-reporting of weight. Huenemann *et al.*[24] found that sixteen-year-old girls reported their weights much more accurately than did boys of the same age. They attributed this to the boys' lack of awareness of their weights. Dwyer *et al.*[12] found that boys weighed themselves less frequently than girls, which might indicate that they were less interested in their weights. Girls, particularly the fatter girls, showed a striking tendency to report weights on questionnaires that were markedly less than their actual weights, while boys reported their weights quite accurately. Perhaps girls knew what they weighed but were embarrassed and sensitive about reporting it, resorting to intentional underreporting.

A third reason for the heightened concern of females about weight is rooted in physiology: obesity is more visible in females than in males. Normal, young, mature females have almost twice as much fat on their bodies as do males. Furthermore, fat on females is distributed more conspicuously; women tend to have more fat on the extremities, hips, and chest, while men have most of their fat on their torsos and are leaner in the extremities. Females thus add extra fat at highly visible or interesting points, and attention is called to it automatically.

A fourth reason that may explain the zeal of females to lose weight and the relative torpor of males to do so may be due to differences between the sexes in the prevalent mistaken notions about body composition and weight loss. Males tend to overestimate the contributions of build to weight and consequently are often uninterested in lowering their weights. Many males seem to believe that reducing diets will result in muscle as well as fat loss. For example, Glucksman and Hirsch[17] observed men who were undergoing weight reduction and found that they were obsessed with the thought that their loss of weight was causing the physical disintegration by affecting their strength and virility. Some adolescent boys believe that dieting will stunt their growth. Loss of strength and size is very threatening to males, and perhaps because of these beliefs they shy away from dieting. When males do diet, they seem partial to high-protein diets in combination with increased physical activity similar to the types used by athletes in training. This form of dieting, which might be labeled the "training-table mystique," appeals to them for several reasons. It has a virile aura about it, is in line with males' convictions that underactivity is an important cause of obesity, and conforms to cultural beliefs that males should be physically active. Unfortunately, the physical activity aspect often degenerates into only perfunctory efforts to do push ups, or, in the case of adult men, an occasional sauna bath and massage to ease the conscience and provide the illusion of fitness. Thus, the relative disinclination of males to lose weight by dieting and their propensity to do so only if it is coupled with physical activity are probably rooted in their aspirations to appear larger and more mesomorphic.

Underestimation of the contribution to weight of build components other than fat is common in girls and women and can lead to dieting or other weight-loss behavior when it is not called for. For example, Dwyer *et al.*[18] found that a large number of adolescent girls were dieting because they mistakenly attributed their relative largeness and heaviness to fatness rather than to the other components of build that were truly responsible. They were on diets because they thought they were obese, although they were really below average in body fatness as measured by the triceps skinfold. Similarly, Goldman *et al.*[19] found several girls at a special summer camp for treatment of obesity who, although far from obese, believed that they were. Casual observation of the members of "Weight Watchers" and similar dieting clubs suggests that many adult women labor under similar misconceptions. Cultural stereotypes that females should be dainty eaters and less physically active than males also encourage dieting. The desire of girls to lose weight probably reflects their desires to be smaller and more ectomorphic as well.

A fifth reason for the predominance of female dieting is fashion. Since the dawn of history, clothes designs have been influenced by three principles: seduction, the attraction of persons of the opposite sex; hierarchy, the expression of personal or social superiority through clothing; and utility, the protection of the body. Male fashions in dress have generally been dominated by hierarchy and modified by utility, with very little emphasis on the seduction principle. Thus, most men's clothes are shapeless enough to conceal large amounts of fat and all but the most deviant body conformations. What little male fashion is present is found largely among young unmarried men. Female fashions, on the other hand, have been largely under control of the seduction principle, modified by utility and hierarchy. They are designed to call attention to the erotic potential of the body. Until modern times, modish dress was the prerogative of the unmarried young girl and the not-quite-respectable older woman of the world. Traditionally the married female had very little concern for her attractiveness, and her seclusion in the home and devotion to her family gave little incentive and few opportunities for the display of attire. However, over the past fifty years fashion has become important for almost all American women, and today, women of all ages and matrimonial states follow it to some extent. It has been theorized that female fashions change periodically to direct attention to a new area of the body that has remained hidden in the recent past and thus become erotically interesting. For some reason, at any rate, areas given particular emphasis do change; the breasts are emphasized during one decade, the legs in another.

Clothes tend to be designed with an ideal female body type in mind. These ideals change, as do fashions and hemlines, but more slowly. Since early in this century the somewhat ample, mature figure favored by the Victorians and Edwardians has been out of fashion. The slight frame has been the ideal, although emphasis has shifted from the legs to the bosom and back again. For the past several decades, fashions have been tailored for the very tall and slim, or, alternatively, for the tall, narrow-hipped, rather wide-shouldered female figure. Women who are short, stout, or wide hipped with narrow shoulders have difficulty dressing à la mode. Women with more ample endowments are at a disadvantage and often take steps to bring their figures more in line with current ideals. Male body ideals, like male fashions, are relatively static and do not change so dramatically.

POSSIBLE EXPLANATIONS FOR DIFFERENCES IN DIETING PREVALENCE BETWEEN ADOLESCENTS AND ADULTS

Adolescence is a period that is particularly favorable for dieting and other weight reduction efforts for several reasons.

First, adolescents are more self-conscious about their bodies than are adults. This may be due in part to their recent experience with the dramatic physical changes brought about by the accelerated growth of puberty, which confer a virtually new appearance. The heterogeneous nature of adolescent growth patterns accentuates physical differences and makes them extremely noticeable. Adolescent girls mature about two years sooner than boys, so that by late high school they have reached their fully-mature size and are likely to become concerned if the weights at which they have stabilized seem to be too high. On the other hand, many boys of the same age are still growing. Even obese boys may convince themselves that their weight problems are only temporary and that they will grow out of them, although this is unlikely to actually be the case. Concerns about underweight are extremely common among adolescents who are late maturers and who, because of this, are shorter and lighter than their peers. Asynchronism, or lack of coordination in development, is also often present during adolescent growth. A common asynchronism is rapid weight gain with height gain lagging behind. It may cause embarrassment and generate weight-control efforts in afflicted adolescents. All of these physical changes occur at the very time in life when social and cultural pressures are the strongest for homogeneity and conformity in matters of appearance as well as in many other aspects of life. Dwyer and Mayer[13-15] have shown that failure to attain appearance ideals can cause a great deal of discontent and unhappiness among adolescents, especially among those more noticeably deviant from them. These wounds may still smart among some adults.

Adults, whose adolescent growth is far behind them, have had more or less constant physiques for years, and have had time to become accustomed to and accept their bodies, imperfections and all. Accordingly, obesity of adult onset usually has less severe and detrimental effects on self-image than does obesity of juvenile onset and is less likely to impel the afflicted individual to diet.

Second, recent experience with extensive body alterations during the adolescent growth spurt may make teen-agers receptive to the idea that changes in weight are possible and encourage their optimism about the probable success of their weight-control efforts. By comparison, adults are used to their bodies as they are and know from experience that weight changes are difficult to achieve.

Third, adolescents are more physically active than adults. Thus, their physical performance is more hindered by the effects of extreme obesity. However, there are some sports in which sheer crushing power is important, and for these a slight degree of overweight may be an advantage.

Fourth, the desire to conform to others and to ideals in weight, appearance, and many other aspects of life is particularly strong during adolescence, probably stronger than it is in adult life. Teen-agers tend to regard being different from their peers as tantamount to being inferior. These feelings often lead to attempts to change body weight and to bring it back into line with the norms for the group. Adults are less likely to feel the need to conform in these respects.

Fifth, adolescent desires to demonstrate their independence or to rebel against their parents may sometimes lead them to alter their eating habits, especially if their parents are opposed to the idea or manner in which they do it.

A final factor is that weight deviations among adolescents are more likely to be diagnosed and treated early. Teen-agers are almost universally given yearly school medical exams, and those who are obese are urged to take action against it. School health personnel are usually advocates of preventive medicine and encourage adolescent weight-control efforts. Conversely, adults often go for years without any physical examination, and their weight deviations are thus likely to be more severe, established, and difficult to reverse by the time they are finally diagnosed. Even then, as Maddox *et al.*[25] have revealed, many obese adults are not urged to take action against it because of their physicians' disinterest in preventive medicine or dismal experience in past efforts to treat obese adults.

VARIATIONS IN DIETING PREVALENCE BETWEEN DIFFERENT SOCIOECONOMIC GROUPS

Little evidence is available on variations in the perception of obesity by socioeconomic status, race, or ethnicity. Goldblatt *et al.*[18] have suggested that perhaps lower-class persons do not regard obesity as culturally undesirable as do those of higher social status, because their experiences with deprivation may have led them to connect obesity with well-being and prosperity. With respect to this, it would not be surprising to find that variations by social class existed in views toward obesity. People in different social classes vary in the types of lives they lead and in their behavior toward many problems, particularly health problems. Therefore, they would not be expected to exhibit homogeneous behavior in dealing with obesity. On the whole, however, the similarities between social classes are more impressive than class differences with regard to concern about weight and dieting. Every social class contains many persons who are obese, concerned about their weights, and dieting to correct them. Perhaps this is due to the fact that all are exposed to the same mass media, schools, and other factors that might generate homogeneous attitudes toward obesity.

APPROACHES FOR MORE EFFECTIVE PREVENTION AND TREATMENT OF OBESITY

Left alone, obese children and adolescents do not outgrow their condition; they become obese adults. Since the cure of obesity is rare once it is well established, with few exceptions they remain obese adults. Other persons, nonobese until adulthood, are afflicted with obesity at maturity and are never cured. Therefore, prevention or early treatment is vital if prevalence rates of obesity are to be substantially decreased.

Moderately successful methods of weight reduction already exist, but no appreciable inroads have yet been made into the high prevalence of obesity. Weight reduction efforts by persons acting by themselves or under the direction of their physicians have been widespread in this country for many years. These measures alone do not seem to reach enough people, are often expensive, and consume a great deal of the time of health professionals who are involved in treatment, although they should certainly not be abandoned.

Group rather than individually organized efforts might have more hope of success in reaching the millions of persons who require some kind of expert support and guidance, yet whose obesity does not require highly-specialized medical supervision because it is uncomplicated by other medical problems. Such group efforts have the added attraction of being less expensive to the patient in terms of medical manpower and cost. The more successful group programs mentioned below deal with persons who are obese or at high risk of becoming so. They might be organized on a broader scale in order to test their adaptability as weight-control programs on a public health basis.

Many health agencies have begun anti-coronary clubs for middle-aged persons, particularly men, which combine calorie restriction with low-cholesterol, highly unsaturated fat diets. These are designed to decrease weight as well as serum cholesterol and consequently, to reduce the risk of coronary heart disease. Most of these groups encourage their members to exercise, and some provide sports facilities and organized classes as well. Others also try to attack the smoking problem, another risk factor involved not only in heart disease but in various lung conditions. Such clubs have been quite popular in many cities, and their methods do indeed seem to substantially decrease risks of heart attacks.

The past few years have also marked the epidemic spread of "Weight Watchers" and similar clubs for reducing among women. Most of these groups are private, profit-making organizations. The reducing diets prescribed by such clubs are usually a standardized low-calorie diet of roughly 1200 calories. Strict adherence to the rather limited choice of foods and weighing of portions is required. Many people are losing weight through such clubs, whose techniques contain many useful elements of group support and group therapy that might be adopted more widely by health professionals. Members are usually friends or acquaintances. This lends a social nature to meetings, and the fact that the members know each other apparently generates social pressure to succeed in dieting by developing a spirit of camaraderie and good-natured competition among the members of the group. Meetings are held in a neighborhood church or school at times convenient to members. The format is partly social, partly business; the members are weighed, exhorted to follow the club's particular diet, and given helpful hints and low-calorie recipes.

From the large membership lists of such clubs and the substantial, if temporary, weight-loss records of members, it appears that many American women are amenable to this type of weight reduction program. However, the clubs have two failings. First, in some states they are outside the realm of supervision by knowledgable physicians or health agencies so that they are difficult to monitor. Second, the major qualifications for the instructors is that they have themselves reduced successfully and are good leaders, but they are given no training in the science of nutrition or the other health sciences. Consequently, they have often given fallacious information on nutrition and weight control to members who regard it as authoritative knowledge. Unfortunately, the instructors' well-intentioned effort to explain why their diet works are usually derived from the pseudoscientific theories presented in the mass of books and articles written by prolific quacks who find the topic of weight control so profitable.

There is an urgent need to educate these instructors in the rudiments of scientific nutrition, with particular emphasis on energy balance, energy metabolism, and weight control, so that such misconceptions will not be disseminated further. However, the deficits in these programs with respect to nutrition education should not discourage nutritionists and other health professionals from adopting the more positive aspects for designing weight-control programs tailored to fit the needs of the community.

Unfortunately, the implementation of weight-control programs on a wide-scale basis at present seems far off. One shortcoming of such efforts, in any case, is that many of them possess the inherent disadvantage of being curative rather than truly preventive programs. Attempts to organize weight-control programs among adults run into the problem that adults are difficult to assemble on a regular, frequent basis, even if motivation is high. Children are more accessible. Schools have captive populations of youngsters who are easy to reach. Moreover, working with persons early in life often makes it possible to prevent obesity, or to arrest its progress. Therefore, school-based group approaches to preventing obesity in children in order to decrease the potential reservoir of obese adults offer great promise.

The first objective of such school programs should be the improvement of nutrition education with regard to obesity. Strong in-service courses in nutrition for teachers, with special emphasis on weight control in the context of adolescent development, as well as more coordination between different teachers whose subjects touch nutrition, are desperately needed to improve the quality and presentation of weight-control-related topics in the classroom.

A second objective should be to increase the efforts of school health personnel in combating overweight. Periodic screening procedures should be instituted to enable early diagnosis of weight problems. Because they lack the time, only a few school health nurses and physicians can give students direct assistance in initiating weight-control measures and supervising their dieting efforts. This service gap could be filled by augmenting the staff with a part-time nutritionist who could prescribe therapeutic diets and assist students. At the least, there should be an adequate referral system to alert parents and family physicians to the problem. Although direct intervention in altering food habits is beyond the scope of the school, the school cafeteria manager could cooperate by serving special low-calorie lunches to those who wished them, to demonstrate and encourage sensible dieting.

The third objective should be to improve physical education programs. Schools can intervene directly in matters relating to the activity component of overweight, since most of them have compulsory physical education classes, as well as a variety of extracurricular athletic programs. Presently most school physical education programs cater to the physically fit rather than to the unfit. Obese youngsters are inactive and sensitive about their clumsiness and lack of skill. Needed here are in-service instruction of physical education teachers about the special needs of the obese and an extension or redirection of departmental programs to refurnish intensive, frequently-scheduled special classes in physical education adapted to the handicaps of the obese.

Two projects have demonstrated the feasibility and success of a combination nutrition education-physical fitness program for controlling adolescent obesity. Christakis *et al.*[9] used nutrition lectures, individual dietary consultations, and extra biweekly programs of physical fitness in addition to regular classes to attack obesity in high school boys. A larger and more intensive program carried out among junior-high-school boys and girls by Seltzer and Mayer[40] concentrated on special before-school and after-school physical education classes several times a week. Some nutrition advice was given, but no supervised dieting was attempted.

Certainly, even if well-organized programs to control obesity were instituted in every elementary and secondary school in the land today, we would still be far from solving the obesity problem, since we still would not have reached the millions of obese adults. However, this would be a good beginning and an excellent investment in the health of the adults of tomorrow. A "spin-off" effect of such programs might be to excite interest in weight reduction in the children's parents.

Another means to make dieting as painless as possible for large groups of people would be the expanded development of low-calorie, high-nutritive-value foods that are tasty, safe, and competitively priced. Such products of modern food technology would allow dieters to lose weight while maintaining satisfactory nutritional status in other respects and eating food that both looked and tasted good, without suffering the social stigma and lack of gustatory satisfaction that often accompany the eating of many of the bland, unexciting, and expensive diet foods now on the market.

A final approach to facilitating weight control that has hardly been begun yet in this country is the improvement of opportunities and facilities for exercise and the development of physical activity programs for adults. These programs might do much for the activity component of the energy balance equation.

In summary, this review has attempted to shed light on the epidemiology of weight-loss behavior and the processes that lead to it. Hopefully it will stimulate better teaching, more sympathetic counseling, and more effective treatment of those with real or imaginary weight problems, and help to identify points at which intervention might be effective in encouraging weight control or establishing preventive programs.

REFERENCES

1. Adams, J. F.: Adolescents' identification of personal and national problems. *Adolescence*, 1:240-250, 1966.
2. Alexander, W. R.: A study of body types, self image, and environmental adjustment in freshman college women. *Dissertation Abstracts*, 28:28A:3048, 1968.
3. Behnke, A. R.: Quantitative assessment of body build. *J Appl Physiol*, 16:960-968, 1961.
4. Bruch, H.: Psychological aspects of obesity. *Borden's Rev Nutr Res*, 19:57, 1958.
5. Bullen, B. A., Monello, L. F., Cohen, H. and Mayer, J.: Attitudes toward physical activity, food, and family in obese and nonobese adolescent girls. *Am J Clin Nutr*, 12:1-11, 1963.
6. Canning, H. and Mayer, J.: Obesity: Its possible effect on college acceptance. *New Engl J Med*, 275:1172-1174, 1966.
7. Canning, H. and Mayer, J.: Obesity: An influence on high school performance. *Am J Clin Nutr*, 20:352-354, 1967.
8. Canning, H. and Mayer, J.: Obesity: An analysis of attitudes, knowledge, and weight control in girls. *Res Quart*, 39:894-899, 1968.
9. Christakis, G., Sajeckie, S., Hillman, R. W., Miller, E., Blumenthal, S. and Archer, M.: Effect of a combined nutrition education-physical fitness program on weight status of obese high school boys. *Fed Proc*, 25:15-19, 1966.
10. Deischer, E. and Mills, M.: The adolescent looks at his health and medical care. *Am J Public Health*, 53:1928-1936, 1963.
11. Dwyer, J. T., Feldman, J. J. and Mayer, J.: Adolescent dieters: Who are they? Physical characteristics, attitudes, and dieting practices of adolescent girls. *Am J Clin Nutr*, 20:1045-1056, 1967.
12. Dwyer, J. T., Feldman, J. J., Seltzer, C. C. and Mayer, J.: Body image in adolescents: Attitudes toward weight and perception of appearance. *J Nutr Ed*, 1:14-19, 1969.
13. Dwyer, J. T. and Mayer, J.: Variations in physical appearance during adolescence: Part I. Boys. *Postgrad Med*, 41:99-107, 1967a.
14. Dwyer, J. T. and Mayer, J.: Variations in physical appearance during adolescence: Part 2. Girls. *Postgrad Med*, 41:91-97, 1967b.
15. Dwyer, J. T. and Mayer, J.: Psychological effects of variations in physical appearance during adolescence. *Adolescence*, 3:353-380, 1968.
16. Dwyer, J. T. and Mayer, J.: Potential dieters: Who are they? *J Am Diet Assoc*, 56:510-514, 1970.
17. Glucksman, M. L. and Hirsch, J.: The response of obese patients to weight reduction: A clinical evaluation of behavior. *Psychosom Med*, 30:1-11, 1968.
18. Goldblatt, P. B., Moore, M. C. and Stunkard, A. J.: Social factors in obesity. *JAMA*, 192:1039-1044, 1965.
19. Goldman, R. F., Bullen, B. A. and Seltzer, C. C.: Changes in specific gravity and body fat in overweight female adolescents as a result of weight reduction. *Ann N Y Acad Sci*, 110:913-917, 1963.

20. Hassan, I. N.: The body image and personality correlates of body type stereo-types. *Dissertation Abstracts,* 11A:4446, 1968.
21. Hathaway, M. L. and Foard, E. D.: *Heights and Weights for Adults in the United States.* Washington, D. C., Home Economics Research Report 10, Agricultural Research Service, U. S. Department of Agriculture, Government Printing Office, 1960.
22. Hinton, M. A., Eppright, E. S., Chadderdon, H. and Wolins, C.: Eating behavior and dietary intakes of girls 12-14 years old. *J Am Diet Assoc,* 43: 223-227, 1963.
23. Huenemann, R. L., Hampton, M. C., Shapiro, L. R. and Behnke, A. R.: Adolescent food practices associated with obesity. *Fed Proc,* 25:4-10, 1966a.
24. Huenemann, R. L., Shapiro, L. R., Hampton, M. C., Mitchell, B. W. and Behnke, A. R.: A longitudinal study of gross body conposition and body conformation and their association with food and activity in a teen-age population: Views of teen-age subjects on body conformation, food, and activity. *Am J Clin Nutr,* 18:325-338, 1966b.
25. Maddox, G. L., Anderson, C. F. and Bogdonoff, M. D.: Overweight as a problem of medical management in a public outpatient clinic. *Am J Med Sci,* 252: 394-403, 1966.
26. Maddox, G. L., Back, L. K. and Liederman, V.: Overweight as social deviance and disability. *J Health Soc Behav,* 9:287-298, 1968.
27. Maddox, G. L. and Liederman, V.: Overweight as a social disability with medical implications. *J Med Ed,* 44:214-220, 1969.
28. Matthews, V. and Westie, C.: A preferred method for obtaining rankings: Reactions to physical handicaps. *Am Soc Rev,* 31:851-854, 1966.
29. Mayer, J.: *Overweight: Causes, Costs, and Control.* Englewood Cliffs, N. J., Prentice-Hall, 1968.
30. Metropolitan Life Insurance Company of New York. New weight standards for males and females. *Statistical Bull,* 40:2-3, 1959.
31. Monello, L. F. and Mayer, J.: Obese adolescent girls: An unrecognized minority group. *Am J Clin Nutr,* 13:35-39, 1963.
32. Moore, M. C., Stunkard, A. J. and Srole, L.: Obesity, social class, and mental stress. *JAMA,* 181:962-966, 1962.
33. National Center for Health Statistics: *Weight by Age and Height of Adults: 1960-62.* Washington, D. C., Vital and Health Statistics, Public Health Service Publication No. 1000, Series 11, No. 14, Government Printing Office, 1966.
34. Newman, J.: *Motivation Research and Marketing Management.* Boston, Division of Research, Harvard Business School, 1957.
35. Seltzer, C. C.: Limitation of height-weight standards. *N Engl J Med,* 272:1132, 1965.
36. Seltzer, C. C.: Overweight and obesity: The associated cardiovascular risk. *Minn Med,* 52:1265-1270, 1969.
37. Seltzer, C. C. and Mayer, J.: Body build and obesity: Who are the obese? *JAMA,* 189:677-684, 1964.
38. Seltzer, C. C. and Mayer, J.: How representative are the weights of measured men and women? *JAMA,* 201:221-224, 1967.
39. Seltzer, C. C. and Mayer, J.: Body build (somatotype) distinctiveness in obese women. *J Am Diet Assoc,* 55:454-458, 1969.

40. Seltzer, C. C. and Mayer, J.: An effective weight control program in a public school system. *J Am Public Health Assoc*, 60:679-690, 1970.

41. Sheldon, W. H., Stevens, S. S. and Tucker, W. B.: *The Varieties of Human Physique*. New York, Hafner, 1963.

42. Staffieri, J. R.: A study of social stereotypes of body image in children. *J Pers Soc Psychol*, 7:101-104, 1967.

43. Stunkard, A. J. and Burt, V.: Obesity and body image II: Age at onset of disturbances in the body image. *Am J Psychiat*, 123:1443-1447, 1967.

44. Stunkard, A. J. and Mendelson, M.: Obesity and body image I: Characteristics of disturbances in body image of some obese persons. *J Am Diet Assoc*, 38: 328-331, 1961.

45. Tarini, J. A.: *Do Fat People Like to Be Fat?* Chicago, Weiss, 1962.

46. U. S. Public Health Service, Center for Chronic Disease Control: *Obesity and Health*. Washington, D. C., Government Printing Office, 1966.

47. Wyden, P.: *The Overweight Society*. New York, Morrow, 1965.

24

Therapeutic Starvation in Obesity

David W. Swanson

AND

Frank A. Dinello

SINCE ancient times people have gone without food for protracted periods. Such starvation was usually unintentional being due to economic deprivation or political abuse. Under such stressful circumstances one could logically expect evidence of psychological strain. This is illustrated in a thirteenth century Russian chronicle of a famine.[1] "A brother rose against his brother, a father had no pity for his son, mothers had no mercy for their daughters. . . . There was no charity left among us, only sadness; gloom and mourning dwelt constantly within and without our habitations." Suppression plus starvation produced extensive self-centeredness and depression.

Deliberate fasting has been used for religious or political reason or to highlight social protest. Under such circumstances psychological changes are again described. When the Old Testament prophet, Elijah, starved for forty days he developed great feelings of hopelessness for his nation and himself. He deprecated himself and at the same time was suspicious of his countrymen who, he thought, were seeking to harm him.

More recently the fasting person has undergone scientific study. In persons of normal weight this has revealed evidence of adverse psychological reactions. Schiele and Brozek[2] studied semi-starvation in thirty-six men and all of the subjects developed emotional difficulties, varying in intensity from mild to severe. These included borderline psychotic episodes, flight of ideas, suicidal threats, depression and compulsive behavior. Meerloo[3] described a psychological syndrome which he attributed to the combined effects of starvation and deprivation of oral gratification which consisted of irritability, suspicion, secretiveness, aggressive feelings, and general regression. Kollar, et al.[4] studied several healthy adult males who fasted only four to six days yet increased irritability, apathy, and depression were reported in all but one patient.

Keys, et al.[1] in their two volume work on the semi-starvation of thirty-two nonobese subjects also reported certain definite psychological reactions. The cumulative stresses resulted in a generalized emotional instability. The men experienced transitory and sometimes protracted periods of depression, and the threshold for such reactions diminished during the late stages of the project. Irritability increased until it became an individual and group problem. These authors defined a "starvation neurosis" consisting of indecisiveness, rumination, guilt feelings, and depression. In certain cases this was complicated by episodes of elation or urges toward violence. One subject had a definite psychotic episode.

Fasting is also used as a therapeutic technique, specifically in the treatment of obesity and associated medical complications. This has recently culminated in the use of total starvation of the severely obese person, a procedure usually done in the hospital with careful monitoring of the vital physiological functions. Some subjects have gone over one hundred days without caloric intake and even these lengthy periods have not produced serious physical complications; in fact, they are tolerated well. In comparison with the careful day-to-day observation of temperature, blood pressure, pulse, respiration, blood count, electrolytes, kidney function and liver function, psychological effects of starvation have received less attention. This paper reviews the psychological data which is available and the efficacy of total fasting in the production of sustained weight loss.

THE STARVATION TECHNIQUE

Starvation in the treatment of obesity is applied for varying periods of time dependent on the patient and the specific approach utilized at various centers. The motivated subject with confirmed exogenous obesity is evaluated to rule out significant physical disorder (e.g. cardiovascular, hepatic, or renal). Obvious psychiatric disorder also prompts exclusion under most circumstances. The subject is often given a reduced caloric intake for several days and then total starvation is begun. No caloric intake is provided; however, a defined fluid intake, vitamins, and electrolyte supplements as required are mandatory. Physical activity is not restricted but excessive perspiring is contraindicated. The usual subject experiences hunger cravings for 48 to 72 hours but then no longer has the physical discomfort of hunger. This is presumably due to the accumulation of ketones. Many subjects continue to have preoccupations with food manifested by recurrent thoughts, dreams, by collecting recipes, and talking about food.

Starvation subjects lose between one and two pounds daily. Physical complications such as hypotensive episodes and intestinal cramping are aggravating to some patients and starvation is terminated if hepatic dysfunction, infection, cardiac complications or very high levels of uric acid develop.

Total Starvation in the Obese Subject

There are three major fasting techniques: a) Short-term fasting up to two weeks; b) intermittent starvation using repeated periods of fasting interrupted by specific diets; c) prolonged fasting.

Short-Term Fasting

At least four attempts at short-term fasting are reported in the literature. In 1958 Bloom[5] fasted nine patients for four to nine days with an average per day weight loss of 2.7 pounds. He reported no adverse psychological symptoms and did a limited follow-up. Five of the nine patients maintained their moderate weight loss and continued to lose a small amount of weight; two patients maintained the weight loss during the fast but did not reduce further, and two patients did not maintain their fasting loss. Actually only two patients lost substantial amounts of weight (40 and 50 lb) from the time fasting began and the follow-up period for these two patients was three and nine months. Only one of the nine patients approached an ideal weight through the fasting and follow-up period. Schultz *et al.*[6] starved seventeen subjects for thirteen days. Their research dealt largely with adrenocortical function but observations were made on general effects. The authors made optimistic and encouraging statements regarding starvation as a tool for consistent and progressive loss of weight and felt that the technique was safe with no apparent or absolute contraindications. Seventeen subjects lost an average of 1.8 lb over thirteen days, ranging from 16 to 35 lb. No emotional disturbances were mentioned. In this study no follow-up was described and apparently if weight loss was maintained, it represented in most individuals, a moderate loss. No patient in the study reduced to his ideal weight. The authors decided that periods of starvation are not likely to change the long-term management of obesity since eating habits and attitudes are not altered during fasting.

Biggers[7] has made an effort to measure the affective changes produced by fasting. For ten days he starved thirty-four patients ranging in weight from 141 to 314 lb. He employed psychological testing which suggested that fasting under hospital conditions for the period tested was not a stressful situation and even results in affective improvement. The patients averaged a 15 to 20 lb weight loss but there was no follow-up. The author feels weight loss represents a return to a more natural state for the obese person and that the psychological gains parallel this correction of pathology. This conclusion seems to contradict the suggestion that obesity is psychological in origin and maintenance or that some obese individuals are made uncomfortable when forced to give up what to them is supposedly a defensive pattern. It is possible, however, that psychological disturbances were not triggered by short-term fasting.

In a similar study Fischer[8] evaluated twenty obese subjects who were starved for ten to fourteen days. Psychological testing was used and, as in the previous study, it suggested an affective improvement during the fasting period. For follow-up purposes a success criterion was the maintenance of the weight loss present at the end of the fasting period. At the end of one month six patients had maintained their weight loss. In a long term (1 to 2 years) follow-up, by personal letter, four subjects had gained weight and nine had lost weight. The weight loss in the nine "successes" ranged from 8 to 85 lb, but only four had lost more than 17 lb and only one had approached his ideal weight.

Research with short-term fasting apparently indicates that obese individuals can be starved with a minimum of psychological and physical discomfort. At least no overt psychiatric disorder was exposed. However, only a few patients were motivated to continue reducing to an ideal weight following the termination of starvation.

Intermittent Fasting

Duncan and his associates[9] have studied the effects of starvation on an intermittent schedule. The technique consists of a short-term fast of approximately fourteen days, then subsequent one or two day fasts per week until an ideal weight is achieved. In an initial study, fifty patients were observed during a 4 to 14 day in-patient fast, followed by a 1 or 2 day per week fast as an out-patient.[9] It appeared that the patients enjoyed the more liberal diets permitted by the one or two day per week fasting period. There were no details regarding long-term successes or follow-up. Duncan[10] expanded the number of cases studied to 107. A follow-up period up to 32 months showed 40 per cent maintained the moderate weight loss from the short-term fast but did not lose additional weight by intermittent starvation, and 17 per cent continued to lose weight during the more liberal 1 or 2 day fast per week period. In yet another paper[11] this author expanded the number of subjects studied to 683. He continued to utilize intermittent starvation since many hazards of long-term fasting were apparently prevented by using this technique; also, that the desired goal was a continued reduction in weight, not the immediate loss provided by more prolonged starvation. His figures for these subjects at a one year follow-up were, 60 per cent weighed less than they did at the end of the hospital fast, 40 per cent weighed more. However, there were no figures indicating how many subjects approached an ideal weight figure. The loss for all patients during the hospital fast was 20 to 32 lb which is a rather mild loss in the grossly obese individual. While intermittent fasting did not always lead to the desired goal of "continued reduction" Duncan was prompted to conclude: "Ultimate failures are frequent but this does not justify depriving others of the prompt and long-term advantages which short intermittent periods of total abstinence from food have to offer."

In a final paper Duncan[12] expanded the number of subjects studied to 890. In this paper he reports that approximately 50 per cent of patients were progressing favorably in their weight reduction program. A sampling of 118 of these patients indicated that 52 per cent continued to lose weight after their hospital fast but only 8 per cent were near an ideal weight, 19 per cent had remained unchanged since the two week hospital fast, and 29 per cent had gained weight. Those patients who were successful in reaching ideal weight were "subjects with obesity of the lesser degrees." As was the case with short-term fasting, no disturbing psychological reactions were reported in these four studies.

Prolonged Fasting

There have been several attempts at prolonged starvation in the hope that if a patient's weight could be reduced to near an ideal figure under hospital conditions that it would be maintained afterward. Drenick, *et al.*[13] in their initial report described eleven patients who were starved from twelve to a maximum, in one case, of 117 days. The average per day weight loss for these patients was 0.91 lb per day. The aim was to "accelerate weight loss to a maximum so that normal weight could be reestablished in a reasonable period of time." As usual in starvation studies hunger was virtually absent. Unfortunately, no detailed follow-up was provided concerning the patients' ability to maintain weight loss after leaving the hospital. The authors gave emphasis to medical observations rather than psychological reactions. However, cause of termination of starvation included three patients for personal reasons, three for noncooperation, and four for medical reasons (postural hypotension or gout). Only one was terminated because an ideal weight was reached.

Drenick,[14] in a second paper, reported on thirty-three patients. At this time the author made the following comment on prolonged starvation: "It is not known whether a period of starvation has a more permanent effect than conventional methods of weight reduction. It may be that starvation is merely a rather drastic method of securing for the patient a few months freedom from obesity." In this report Drenick concluded that a minimum of one month fasting is necessary "to break the habit of overeating" and "the period of total fasting should not exceed two months." Of the thirty-three patients studied in an eight month follow-up, nine were considered failures because of regaining weight or because they were lost to follow-up. The twenty-four remaining patients who were put on a low calorie diet (300-350 calories) following the period of starvation had various degrees of success. Approximately 30 per cent in this group had approached an ideal weight at the time of the follow-up. No comments are made regarding psychological reactions in the specific patients studied. However, Drenick warns that severe psychological disorders constitute a contraindication to prolonged starvation treatment. He also states that severe food addiction may make fasting impossible with aggravation of the underlying psychological disorder during weight loss or as the result of food deprivation. Drenick's success surpasses the results of most other investigators.

Three papers were published during 1966 reporting on prolonged starvation techniques. Crumpton, *et al.*[15] attempted to measure the psychological stresses of long-term starvation using observation and psychological tests. Twenty-one subjects were starved for 37 to 121 days. The authors discovered no impairment of intellect, psychomotor function, learning ability, immediate memory, hand steadiness, or strength of grip. As weight reduction continued, however, testing indicated that the patients were more tense and excitable. There were statistically significant increases in preoccupation with food, irritability, depression, and resistance to testing. Behavioral observations revealed more evidence of psychological stress than noted in the psychological tests. Typical reaction to fasting involved subjects becoming more immature, childlike, dependent, and even infantile. The longer the fast, the more self-centered the individual subject became. The authors concluded that these changes did not represent a significant threat to the psychological health of emotionally stable subjects; but less stable persons had difficulty remaining on the starvation regime and also created more management problems. Weight losses averaged over 100 lb for each individual during the prolonged starvation but there is no report on maintenance of the losses or information on those who dropped the program.

Rowland[16] studied six starvation patients from 10 to 50 days and provided each with individual psychotherapy. The patients lost weight at a typical rate during starvation but no follow-up detailing long-term success or failure is available. Marked psychological changes occurred in the patients during starvation including an increase in aggressiveness, depression, resentment and self-depreciation. Two subjects displayed psychotic features. One of the six patients had a relatively quiet course in the hospital, lost 100 lb, and left the hospital gratified by the change in himself. During starvation all six patients exhibited excessive control of their emotions, yet an obvious indirect expression of hostile feelings. None of the six had sufficiently well-marked emotional disturbance to justify a neurotic or psychotic diagnosis prior to fasting, but all did have some definite defects in character structure.

Kollar[17] did a pilot study of the psychological and physiological effects of fasting for 14 to 80 days. The goal was to reduce seven patients to normal weights, not to lose just a few pounds. During the fasting period patients were stubborn and expressed hostility more directly. Episodes of depression and anxiety occurred in all patients and there was a common problem of covert eating. One suicide attempt, an episode of withdrawal, and other ward management problems also occurred. The author related these psychological disturbances not to fasting but to problems in the doctor-patient relationship, in ward milieu and with family members. The conclusion by the authors was that starvation is not harmful psychologically or physiologically in the treatment of obesity. The hospital starvation period led to a major weight reduction (75 to 206 lb) in six of the seven patients. However, there is no follow-up clarifying whether these losses were maintained, although the authors stress the necessity of such a follow-up before the routine use of starvation in obesity can be recommended.

The authors have studied fifteen grossly obese patients undergoing starvation for periods from ten to eighty-six days. Many negative psychological reactions occurred during the study including resistance to the program, infantile behavior, paranoid reactions, and increased dependency. Follow-up investigation has revealed discouraging results as most patients regained the weight lost during hospitalization. Post-hospital group meetings with these patients revealed a good deal of bitterness and anger toward the medical profession because of the lack of success in maintaining weight losses. These meetings also suggested that the patients viewed the starvation program as a magical technique resulting in large, permanent weight losses.

Two studies have been done concentrating on a follow-up of patients treated for obesity by fasting. Hunscher[18] made a mail survey of the 709 patients starved by Duncan on an intermittent basis. These patients while hospitalized had lost 1 to 2 lb per day. After hospitalization they were expected to continue a fast one day per week and adhere to a moderately restricted diet until an ideal weight had been reached. Approximately 50 per cent responded to the questionnaire and the respondents tended to be those patients who were hospitalized most recently. Forty-six per cent of the respondents had continued to lose some weight, 21 per cent stayed the same, and 33 per cent had gained weight. A study of the findings of the respondents did not suggest any particular pattern. There were no statements regarding the number of patients actually reaching an ideal weight except that 5 per cent of those responding indicated they were now satisfied with their weight status. Thirty-three per cent of those who lost weight made the comment that success depends on an alteration of eating habits leading to a permanent change in the dietary pattern. During 1968, MacCuish, *et al.*[19] conducted a follow-up study of twenty-five patients who had fasted twenty-five days in a hospital. The authors found the results were not encouraging. Within some months of going home most had regained the weight lost in the hospital. Of the fifteen patients followed as out-patients for at least a year, only four weighed less than they did before fasting. The one patient who weighed substantially less was given special mention by the authors. This patient made strenuous and partially successful efforts to keep his weight down after hospitalization was completed through intermittent out-patient fasting but lost his job, and became so depressed that he eventually required psychiatric help.

DISCUSSION

These studies suggest that no starvation technique used to date is particularly successful in treating obesity. Short-term and intermittent starvation do not result in an appreciable weight loss nor is there continued reduction in most individuals on the subsequent low calorie diets advocated for continuing weight loss. However, as reported, these short-term techniques are not accompanied by notable psychological disorder in the obese patient.

Prolonged starvation techniques result in large weight losses but there is danger of disruptive psychological reactions during these periods. Under such circumstances the very obese person show some of the emotional complications previously noted in the nonobese person subjected to food deprivation. The fact that the very obese person shows this disturbance while still grossly overweight presumably reflects the stress of starvation, the loss of an addicting substance or the removal of a necessary psychological defense mechanism—that of excessive oral gratification. It is of research interest that an underlying psychological conflict in the obese patient possibly is exposed by food deprivation.

In prolonged starvation studies so far attempted, most individuals have regained their weight after leaving the hospital. Long-term efficacy is doubtful. Because of this, Mayer[20] expressed concern about the publicity given to this method of weight reduction, concluding it has greater potential as a research tool than as a therapeutic measure. It is dramatic in its immediate effect as a very obese person can lose 50 to 150 lb during a hospitalization. However, reduction to a less obese state is not alone sufficient motivation for continued restriction of food intake. It is not unusual for this same obese patient to regain weight at the rate of 20 lb per month after leaving the hospital, indicating that the encouragement of a more normal weight and appearance does not compete well with the food addiction.

Since the majority of subjects do not profit from starvation the present need is continued research study of this technique, particularly in the occasional successful subject. At present, starvation cannot be considered any more successful than the various other approaches to this difficult psychological and physiological problem.

REFERENCES

1. Keys, A., Brazek, J., Hanschel, A., Mickelson, O. and Taylor, H. L.: *The Biology of Human Starvation*. Univ of Minn Press, Vol. II, 1950.
2. Schiele, B. C. and Brozek, J.: Experimental neurosis resulting from semi-starvation in man. *Psychosom Med*, 10:31-50, 1948.
3. Merloo, J. A. M. and Klauber, L. D.: Clinical significance of starvation and oral deprivation. *Psychosom Med*, 14:491-497, 1952.
4. Kollar, E. J., Slater, G. R., Palmer, J. O., Docter, R. F. and Mandell, A. J.: Measurement of stress in fasting man. *Arch Gen Psychiat*, 11:113-125, 1964.
5. Bloom, W. L.: Fasting as an introduction to the treatment of obesity. *Metabolism*, 8:214-220, 1959.
6. Schultz, A. L., Werner, L. A. and Kerlow, A.: The use of total starvation in the management of chronic obesity. *Minn Med*, 48:441-447, 1965.
7. Biggers, W. H.: Obesity: Affecting changes in the fasting state. *Arch Gen Psychiat*, 14:218-221, 1966.
8. Fischer, N.: Obesity, affect and therapeutic starvation. *Arch Gen Psychiat*, 17:227-233, 1967.
9. Duncan, G. G., Jenson, W. K., Frazer, R. and Cristofori, F. C.: Correction and control of intractable obesity. *JAMA*, 181:301-312, 1962.
10. Duncan, G. G., Jenson, W. K., Cristofori, F. C., and Schless, G. L.: Intermittent fasts in the correction and control of intractable obesity. *Am J Med Sci*, 245:515-520, 1963.
11. Duncan, G. G., Cristofori, F. C., Yeu, J. K. and Murthy, M. S. J.: The control of obesity by intermittent fasts. *Med Clin N Am*, 48:1359-1372, 1964.
12. Duncan, G. G., Hunscher, M. A., Cristofori, F. C., Duncan, T. and Scheless, G. L.: Intermittent total fasts and obesity. *Postgrad Med*, 38:523-535, 1965.
13. Drenick, E. J., Swendseid, M. E., Blahd, W. H. and Tuttle, S. G.: Prolonged starvation as treatment for severe obesity. *JAMA*, 187:100-105, 1964.
14. Drenick, E. J. and Smith, R.: Weight reduction by prolonged starvation. *Postgrad Med*, 36:95-100, 1964.
15. Crumpton, E., Wine, D. B. and Drenick, E. J.: Starvation: Stress or satisfaction. *JAMA*, 394-396, 1966.
16. Rowland, C.: Psychotherapy of six hyperobese adults during total starvation. *Arch Gen Psychiat*, 18:541-548, 1966.
17. Kollar, E. J. and Atkinson, R. M.: Responses of extremely obese patients to starvation. *Psychosom Med*, 28:227-246, 1966.
18. Hunscher, M.: A post-hospitalization study of patients treated for obesity by a total fast regimen. *Metabolism*, 15:5, 383-393, 1966.
19. MacCuish, A. C., Munro, J. F. and Duncun, L. J. P.: Follow-up study of refractory obesity treated by fasting. *Br Med J*, 1:91-92, 1968.
20. Mayer, J.: Reducing by total fasting. *Postgrad Med*, 35:279-282, 1964.

25

A Comparison of a Self-control and a Contract Procedure for Weight Control

MARY B. HARRIS

AND

CAROL G. BRUNER

TRADITIONAL approaches to effecting lasting weight loss in over-weight people have generally achieved minimal success. Although a large number of medical treatments have been tried, ranging from psycho-therapy[1] to drugs[12] to fasting[3] to a wide assortment of varied diets, the long-term results of such programs have, with few exceptions, ranged from disappointing to dismal.[5, 17] Since it is universally accepted even by such proponents of exercise as Mayer[10] that a reduction in the caloric value of food eaten is both necessary and sufficient for weight loss to occur, it would appear that the control of obesity could be most effectively dealt with in terms of the control of eating behaviors. In recent years psychologists have finally become interested in the question of obesity and weight control, and a number of studies utilizing behavior modification techniques to control overeating have been undertaken. Several of these studies have involved aversive counter-conditioning of the smell, taste, and thought of food, using either electric shock,[11] nauseous odors,[7] or cognitively-produced nausea as aversive stimuli.[2] Although the reports of these studies have been encouraging, possibly due to the very small number of subjects involved, the fact that all but Cautela's technique involve the purchase and the use of equipment in a laboratory makes their practical value quite limited.

A second type of behavior modification approach to weight reduction and the approach used in this study has been that of contingency management, generally involving self-control procedures.[6, 8, 15, 18] Because such programs have actually taught the subjects how to use behavior modification techniques such as positive reinforcement for refraining from eating, punishment for eating, and stimulus control procedures, such an approach might be expected to have more lasting success that procedures which do not focus on producing permanent changes in the overweight person's knowledge or behaviors. On the other hand, it may not be the information given to the overweight person which is responsible for the apparent success of these programs but rather the increase in motivation caused by the personal relationship with and reinforcement from the experimenter. The importance of this relationship is generally stressed not only by psychiatrists but also by behaviorally oriented psychologists.[7, 8, 18] To assess the importance of increased motivation for losing weight without any specific information about techniques being given, the present research also utilized a contract procedure for weight control similar to that used by Elliott and Tighe[4] to reduce smoking.

Two separate projects are being reported in this paper, both of which were designed to assess the effectiveness of a self-control approach to weight reduction. The first project compared a group taught the principles of behavior modification for changing eating behaviors, an attention-placebo control group and a contract group, in which Ss signed a contract agreeing to make a monetary deposit which would be returned to them contingent upon weight loss. The second project compared a behavior modification group with an attention-placebo control group. These studies were designed to provide information about the relative short-term and long-term effectiveness of these three methods.

EXPERIMENT 1

This study attempted to assess the relative effectiveness of a self-control approach, a contract system and an educational attention-placebo control procedure on weight loss. It was also designed to assess long-term results of such programs, since the overwhelming majority of reported research studies on weight control report only short-term losses.

Subjects

Twenty-six female and six male subjects were recruited by means of notices placed in the campus newspaper. Ages ranged from eighteen to forty-eight years and weights from 130 lb to 300 lb. All Ss reported that they needed to lose at least twenty lb. Sixteen of them were students who worked part-time, eight were housewives, and eight were full-time professional or semi-professional workers. Pairs of friends or relatives and individual Ss were randomly assigned to the three groups, with twelve in the self-control group, twelve in the contract group and eight in the control group.

General Procedure

Evening meetings were held from July through September, with a female graduate student serving as E. During the first meeting with each group, E advised Ss of the experimental nature of the program and emphasized that research on obesity indicates that metabolic factors are extremely rare and that overeating is consistently the major factor for continuing overweight. Ss were told that each procedure had been demonstrated to be of some value for weight loss, but that direct comparisons of such techniques were lacking. They were told that the treatment period would consist of twelve weeks of regular weight checks using a commercial bathroom scale and that follow-up checks would be scheduled at infrequent intervals. Ss were asked to maintain a nutritionally sensible diet and to restrict their weight loss to not more than 2 lb per week. Instructions for maintaining daily diet records, computing caloric values, and noting circumstances surrounding their eating behaviors were given to all Ss. The format for the initial meeting was identical for each group with the exception of the description of the treatment specific to that group. In addition, all Ss were invited to a lecture given by an expert on diets and nutrition and were given handouts of low calorie recipes and calorie sheets for native New Mexican foods.

Self-Control

The program used to train Ss in the use of behavior modification techniques was almost identical to that used by Harris.[8] There were eight group meetings, during which the rudiments of behavior theory, particularly operant and respondent conditioning, were explained. Ss were asked to compile a list of their reasons for wishing to lose weight and of personal ultimate aversive consequences of eating.[6] They were instructed to read this list and any other negative consequences they selected as punishment for approaching food or overeating. The use of positive reinforcement for both long-term and short-term goals, such as not eating while studying for three consecutive nights, was also recommended. One lesson discussed the principle of chaining and made suggestions as to how the chain of specific acts involved in getting food to the stomach could be broken down or lengthened. Additional lessons discussed Schachter's external stimulus control hypothesis,[14] relevant research, and implications for weight control. Ss were then encouraged to examine specific techniques which could be used to limit the range of stimuli to which they responded by eating. E attempted to stimulate group discussion and encouraged Ss to suggest possible solutions for both personal problems and those of others. Relaxation training techniques and Cautela's[2] covert nausea conditioning procedure were discussed but not included in this program.

Twelve Ss (eleven female, one male) attended the introductory meeting. Their $\overline{X}$ weight was 164.7 lb; the range was 132 to 300 lb. All but one S continued the twelve-week treatment and absences were infrequent.

Contract

Twelve Ss attended the introductory meeting ($\overline{X}$ weight was 172.8 lb; the range was 130 to 220 lb). At this time the contract procedures were explained and each S was given a copy of the agreement. The contract specified that S agreed to make a cash deposit of XN dollars and would receive

TABLE 25-I

DATA ON SUBJECTS FROM EXPERIMENT 1

S	Sex	Participation for 2 or More Weeks: Yes/No	Original Weight (lb)	12-week Weight (lb)	Weight Change (lb)	Percentage Change	10-mo. Weight (lb)	Weight Change (lb)	Percentage Change
Self-control:									
1	F	Yes	300	283	-17	-.057	297	-03	-.01
2	F	Yes	175	178	+03	+.017	155	-20	-.11
3	F	Yes	163	151	-12	-.074	147	-16	-.10
4	F	Yes	161	158	-03	-.019	157	-04	-.02
5	F	Yes	139	139	00	.000	154	+15	+.11
6	F	Yes	137	134	-03	-.022	139	+02	+.01
7	F	Yes	134	130	-04	-.030	140	+06	+.04
8	F	Yes	132	118	-14	-.106	124	-08	-.06
9	M	Yes	189	174	-15	-.079	—	—	—
10	F	Yes	161	156	-05	-.031	—	—	—
11	F	Yes	151	139.5	-11.5	-.076	—	—	—
12	F	No	134	—	—	—	—	—	—
Mean*			164.7	160.0	-07.4	-.035	164.1	-03.5	-.018
Contract participants									
1	M	Yes	190	175	-15	-.079	187	-03	-.02
2	F	Yes	180	165	-15	-.083	188	+08	+.04
3	F	Yes	174	161	-13	-.075	182	+08	+.05
4	F	Yes	147	132	-15	-.102	145	-02	-.01
5	F	Yes	130	122	-08	-.061	—	—	—

	Sex	Participated	164.2	151.0	-13.4	-.080	175.5	+02.75	+.015
Mean									
Contract nonparticipants									
1	M	No	220	—	—	—	212	-08	-.04
2	M	No	210	—	—	—	193	-17	-.08
3	F	No	181	178	-03	-.016	—	—	—
4	F	No	169	—	—	—	175.5	+06.5	+.04
5	F	No	165	—	—	—	166	+01	+.01
6	F	No	156	—	—	—	148	-08	-.05
7	F	No	152	—	—	—	—	—	—
Mean			179	—	-03	-.016	178.9	-05.1	-.024
Control group nonparticipants									
1	F	Yes	168	170	+02	+.010	162	-06	-04
2	M	No	175	176	+01	+.005	—	—	—
3	F	No	150	—	—	—	150	00	.00
4	M	No	255	—	—	—	252	-03	-.01
5	F	No	207	—	—	—	—	—	—
6	F	No	178	—	—	—	—	—	—
7	F	No	163	—	—	—	—	—	—
8	F	No	133	—	—	—	—	—	—
Mean			178.6	—	+01.5	+.008	188	-03	.02

* Means are based on all Ss weighed at that time: therefore, the post-test means are based on smaller Ns.

it back at the rate of X dollars per pound ($1.00 or 50¢ in all cases) to be paid the week after each pound's loss was recorded, until N pounds had been lost and all XN dollars had been refunded. The contract also provided for forfeiture of the remaining dollars if an S did not appear at his weekly weight check or notify E that he would not be present, with the money forfeited to be divided equally among the remaining participants at the end of the twelve-week period. Ss were advised to consider the terms of the contract one week before making a commitment.

At the second meeting only five Ss attended. This meeting focused on determining how much weight each S wished to lose over the twelve-week period and how much each pound was worth. The remainder of the second meeting discussed Ss' personal dieting problems. No further group meetings were held. When Ss reported to E for weekly weight checks, E refunded the appropriate amount of the deposit. E offered no suggestions for altering eating habits aside from counting calories conscientiously. The $\overline{X}$ weight for the five Ss (four females, one male) who participated in the contract group was 164 pounds, while the $\overline{X}$ initial weight of the seven drop-outs (five females, two males) was 179 lb.

Eight Ss with a $\overline{X}$ weight of 178.6 lb and range from 133 to 255 lb attended the first meeting, at which time they were told that treatment would consist of individual counseling and weekly weight checks. At the second meeting, which was conducted as a group discussion of dieting problems, only four Ss (two males, two females) reported ($\overline{X}$ weight was 201.3 lb). Ss were encouraged to keep accurate daily diet records and to report for weekly weight checks, but no suggestions were made for alteration of specific eating habits. Pseudocounseling consisted of the E passively listening to S describe his personal dieting problems, weight history, and related problems. Only two Ss reported after the second week of meetings ($\overline{X}$ weight was 171.5 lb). As subject number 1 could not be considered a naive S (she was currently conducting a behavior modification smoking study), there was essentially no control group for this study. The $\overline{X}$ initial weight for the six drop-outs was 181 lb with a range of 133 to 255 lb.

Follow-up

Ten months after initiation of treatment, all Ss were asked to report for follow-up weight checks, including those Ss who dropped out after the first or second meeting. A very determined effort to contact all Ss was made, requiring a large number of phone calls. Although those Ss who dropped out do not constitute a true control group, it was felt that a comparison of their scores with those of participating Ss would be of value.

Results

Data from the Ss including original weights and short-term and long-term changes are presented in Table 25-I. T-tests for correlated means were performed, comparing original weights with twelve-week and ten-month weights for the contract and self-control groups. Both the contract ($t = 9.73$, $p < .01$, 4 df.) and self-control ($t = 3.66$, $p < .01$, 10 df.) groups lost a significant proportion of body weight between weeks one and twelve. In addition, after twelve weeks, the contract group had lost a significantly larger proportion of initial weight than the self-control group ($t = 2.96$, $p < .02$, 14 df.). As twelve-week weights were not available for the nonparticipating Ss, comparisons with treatment groups could not be made.

To evaluate the permanence of weight loss, t-tests for correlated means were done comparing initial with ten-month weights for the contract, self-control, contract nonparticipant and control nonparticipant groups. No significant differences were obtained. Additional t-tests revealed that the contract group had not maintained a significantly greater loss than the self-control Ss and that at the end of ten months the experimental groups did not differ significantly from the nonparticipating groups.

EXPERIMENT 2

Subjects

Eighteen female Ss were recruited by means of advertisements and posters. No males responded to these requests for Ss. Originally, Ss were randomly assigned to self-control, contract, or attention placebo control groups; however, all Ss assigned to the contract condition declined to participate. The typical reason given for refusal was lack of money. These Ss were then randomly reassigned to the self-control or control groups. Three Ss were deleted on the basis that they did not need to lose twenty lb.

Of the eight Ss assigned to the self-control condition, two did not attend sessions after the introductory meeting. The $\overline{X}$ weight for the remaining six Ss was 143.7 lb; the range was 131 to 160 lb. Of the seven Ss assigned to the counseling control group, three did not attend either the introductory or further sessions. The $\overline{X}$ weight for the remaining four Ss was 144.3 lb; the range was 132 to 164 lb.

Procedure

The procedure was essentially the same as that employed in Experiment 1, with the exception that there was no contract group. Meetings were held in a classroom on campus from 5:30 to 6:30 PM. As subject attendance was extremely sporadic, the sequence of lessons was extended over a sixteen-week period. Because no Ss came to meetings for the weeks immediately preceding and following the two-week Christmas vacation, a four-week no-meeting period was interspersed between the first four and last eight meetings. At each session E attempted to inform each S of what she had missed in preceding sessions. Follow-up weight checks were obtained at the end of sixteen weeks. At this time one S in the control group was unavailable.

TABLE 25-II

DATA ON SUBJECTS FROM EXPERIMENT 2

Treatment Group	Original Weight	16-Week Weight	Number of lb Lost or Gained	Proportion of Body Weight Lost or Gained
Self-control				
1	160	158	−02	−.01
2	155	156	+01	+.01
3	141	138	−03	−.02
4	140	142	+02	+.01
5	135	131.5	−03.5	−.03
6	131	126	−05	−.04
Means	143.7	141.9	−01.75	−.013
Control group				
1	164	162	−02	−.01
2	141	—	—	—
3	140	140.5	+00.5	+.003
4	132	128	−04	−.03
Means	144.3	143.5	−01.83	−.012

Results

At the end of treatment, the mean weight loss was 1.75 lb, or 1.3 per cent of initial body weight for the self-control group and 1.83 lb or 1.5 per cent of initial body weight, for the counseling control group. A Mann-Whitney U-Test revealed no significant difference between the two groups for proportion of body weight lost. These data are presented in Table 25-II.

DISCUSSION

The results of this study illustrate clearly the problems typical of most attempts to get people to lose weight, problems which are generally lumped under the nonexplanatory label of "lack of motivation." Most obese people do not seek treatment of their obesity, do not continue with treatment once begun, and do not keep off weight which has been lost.[17] The present study was unfortunately no exception. In Experiment 1, thirteen of thirty-two Ss did not return after the first two weeks of treatment; in Experiment 2, five of fifteen Ss were lost. The attrition rate was particularly high in the contract conditions, as only five of twelve Ss in Experiment 1 and none of those in Experiment 2 who were requested to do so would sign contracts and put up cash deposits. Since all of those who participated in the contract group did lose weight during the period of the contract but not when the contract was no longer in effect, it appears that the contract system serves a dual role: it screens out those who are less "motivated" or eager to lose and also provides extra incentives for weight loss during the period that the contract is in effect. As a short-term procedure for weight control, a contract system might be expected to be successful for those who are willing to participate; however, it is suggested that a contract be continued indefinitely if the weight loss is also to be continued indefinitely.

The self-control behavior modification program produced a lower rate of attrition and also more favorable comments from the participants on the value of the techniques they were learning. As previous studies[8, 13, 15, 18] had shown such techniques to be effective, it was expected that they would indeed produce a short-term weight loss, as they did in Experiment 1. The fact that these techniques could be used to control eating behaviors indefinitely and that the focus was on the production and maintenance of permanent changes in eating habits led to the mistaken prediction that such permanent changes would indeed occur. Although Stuart[16] has found a weight loss persisting for almost a year after the beginning of treatment with six Ss, this result is almost unique. Certainly, there is strong evidence that knowledge of how to change behavior is insufficient to assure that such a change will be attained or maintained. For instance, in a recent questionnaire, Harris[9] found that over 80 per cent of a group of professionals interested in weight control reported that they had a personal weight problem. The experience of the two authors ($\overline{X} = 120$ lb, range 120-120) would definitely confirm the above finding.

An ideal program for achieving weight control would accomplish three things: attract and retain participants, assist them in losing weight and enable them to keep weight off once lost. An attention-placebo control group condition involving information about nutrition, sympathetic listing, and a request for record-keeping did not accomplish any of the objectives in either study. The contract system attracted few participants and did not produce a long-term weight loss but did produce a significantly greater short-term loss than the other two procedures. The self-control procedure had a low attrition rate, was liked by the subjects and produced a significant short-term loss in the first but not the second experiment. All of the procedures, as is true for all other techniques for weight control, were inadequate in some respects. It may be that the best approach would be to offer a wide variety of alternatives in order to attract and maintain the participation of a large percentage of those people who need to lose weight. A combination of instruction in techniques of behavior control and powerful incentives for changing one's eating habits, such as a contract system might provide, may prove to be more effective than any single approach.

REFERENCES

1. Bruch, H.: *The Importance of Overweight.* New York, W. W. Norton and Co., 1957.
2. Cautela, J. R.: Treatment of compulsive behavior by covert sensitization. *Psychol Rec,* 16:33-41, 1966.

3. Drenick, E. J.: Starvation in the management of obesity. In Wilson, Nancy (Ed.): *Obesity*. Philadelphia, F. A. Davis Co., 1969.

4. Elliott, R. and Tighe, T.: Breaking the cigarette habit: Effects of a technique involving threatened loss of money. *Psychol Rec,* 18:503-513, 1968.

5. Feinstein, A. R.: The treatment of obesity: An analysis of methods, results and factors which influence success. *J Chron Dis,* 11:349-393, 1960.

6. Ferster, C. B., Nurnberger, J. and Levitt, E. B.: The control of eating. *J Math,* 1: 87-109, 1962.

7. Foreyt, J. P. and Kennedy, W. A.: Treatment of overweight by aversion therapy. *Behav Res Ther,* 9:29-34, 1971.

8. Harris, M. B.: Self-directed program for weight control: A pilot study. *J Abnorm Psychol,* 74:263-270, 1969.

9. Harris, M. B.: The portly psychologist, or on the perils of using a control group. *Psychol Rep,* 29:557-558, 1971.

10. Mayer, J.: *Overweight: Causes, Cost and Control.* Englewood Cliffs, New Jersey, Prentice Hall, Inc., 1968.

11. Meyer, V. and Crisp, A. H.: Aversion therapy in two cases of obesity. *Behav Res Ther,* 2:143-147, 1964.

12. Penick, S. B.: The use of amphetamines in obesity. *Psychiat Opin,* 1:27-30, 1970.

13. Penick, S. B., Filion, R., Fox, S. and Stunkard, A. J.: Behavior modification in the treatment of obesity. *Psychosom Med,* 33:49-55, 1971.

14. Schachter, S.: Some extraordinary facts about obese humans and rats. *Am Psychol,* 26:129-144, 1971.

15. Stuart, R. B.: Behavioral control of overeating. *Behav Res Ther,* 5:357-365, 1967.

16. Stuart, R. B.: A three dimensional program for the treatment of obesity. *Behav Res Ther,* 9:177-186, 1971.

17. Stunkard, A. J. and McLaren-Hume, M.: The results of treatment for obesity. *Arch Intern Med,* 103:79-85, 1959.

18. Wollersheim, J. P.: Effectiveness of group therapy based upon learning principles in the treatment of overweight women. *J Abnorm Psychol,* 76:462-474, 1970.

IX

TESTS

26

Nutrition Imagery in the Rorschach Materials of Food-Deprived, Obese Patients

ROBERT S. McCULLY
MYRON L. GLUCKSMAN
AND
JULES HIRSCH

THOSE factors which may underlie the emergence of specific types or classes of Rorschach imagery are poorly understood. An understanding of the processes which promote certain varieties of responses would improve our grasp of Rorschach theory and our knowledge about the relation between psychic structure and perception. Particular interest in food responses and their bearing on theory goes back to Brozek's[2] study of perception and association in Ss who experienced experimental semistarvation. Brozek reported only a small nonsignificant increase in Rorschach food imagery among his Ss during starvation, and an almost identical increase during a rehabilitation period when food intake was not under control. This finding led Brozek to point out that a "wish-fulfillment" explanation for the presence of certain kinds of classes of Rorschach imagery was untenable. Our study of hospitalized obese patients whose weight reduction was carefully controlled enabled us to observe aspects of food and body perception in a group who were food-deprived. Hirsch[6] and others have reported that there is a decrease in the size of adipose cells rather than a decrease in the number of adipose cells in both obese and average weight individuals following weight loss. Since our patients were studied over a considerable period of time during food deprivation (they subsisted on a liquid formula) and physiologically may have approached a state similar to that of starvation in nonobese subjects, it seemed worthwhile to isolate and analyze projective imagery related to nutrition in this population. This chapter represents a particular focus within a larger investigation of the behavioral response of obese patients to weight reduction. Glucksman and co-workers[5] have presented the first of a series of quantitative reports on the behavioral responses of our population.

Recently, Masling and co-workers[8] analyzed Rorschach images in obese patients. Unfortunately their data is not comparable with ours because food images per se were excluded. Epstein and Levitt[4] reported that hungry

345

Ss learned paired associates more rapidly when the stimulus word was a food noun. Spence and Ehrenberg[10] observed that overweight Ss were equally responsive to both subliminal and supraliminal food stimuli, provided they were deprived. The Rorschach does not provide subliminal stimulus qualities for food any more than any number of other entities. In fact, food in our culture is not a common Rorschach image. At the same time, one can introduce a variable that offers at least some degree of combining Rorschach conditions with supra and subliminal food stimuli. This can be done by using suggestion to look for food after the initial Rorschach is completed (limit testing). This may be introduced at a crucial stage and later repeated to check for its effects over time. Thus, direct suggestion may serve as a supraliminal stimulus for a repeated Rorschach at a later time. A food image in a hungry patient should have greater probability of being repeated upon retest with the same stimulus material. Our patients were studied in depth over a comparatively long period of time. They were starved to a considerable degree, and were deprived of the gustatory sensation process. Their environment was controlled in a systematic fashion as much as possible. A focus on nutrition imagery in the projective materials of our Ss offered the opportunity to check certain observations reported by others,[11] since our conditions were less simulated and more intensively controlled. It also provided another methodologic approach to a further understanding of obesity and the theory of Rorschach perception.

SUBJECTS AND METHOD

A group of six severely obese adult patients seeking weight reduction were hospitalized in the Behavioral-Metabolic Unit of the Rockefeller University Hospital. All the patients were of at least normal intelligence, and had been obese since childhold. (Obesity was defined as a body weight of more than 20% fat tissue.) Table 26-I shows age, IQ range, and other aspects of the group. Three of the patients were hospitalized and studied during an eight-month period, and the other three were studied for an additional year. The experimental program of weight reduction for the patients consisted of an initial six-week period of weight maintenance (Period I), followed by a fifteen-week period of weight loss (Period II), and a final six-week period of weight maintenance (Period III). A second period of weight loss (Period IV) lasted fifty-two weeks for three patients. Caloric intake during the final period of weight maintenance enabled the patients to remain at their admission weight. Weight loss was accomplished by the administration of 600 calories per day. Caloric intake during the final period of weight maintenance allowed the patients to remain at the lowest weight achieved during weight reduction. The total daily caloric intake was provided by feeding composed of orally administered liquid formulas with known amounts of carbohydrate, protein, fat, minerals, and vita-

TABLE 26-I

DISTRIBUTION OF AGE, SEX, INTELLIGENCE, AND WEIGHT CHANGES FOR THE GROUP

Patient	Age	Sex	Full Scale IQ	Weight on Admission[a] (lb)	Weight at Period II[a] (lb)	Weight at Period III[a] (lb)	Weight Loss at 8 Months (lb)	Weight at Period IV* (lb)	Weight Loss at 20 Months (lb)
(1)	23	M	128	407.0	330.5	300.7	106.3	189.8	217.2
(2)	20	M	97	396.0	325.6	300.0	96.0	175.1	220.9
(3)	20	F	90	213.4	179.9	170.9	42.5	124.0	89.4
(4)	36	F	134	358.6	290.4	263.7	94.9		
(5)	21	M	111	304.7	229.3	211.6	93.1		
(6)	27	F	112	325.6	245.6	238.5	87.1		

* Weight on date of testing.

mins.[1] Solid food was not allowed except for a brief period before discharge from the hospital.

The Rorschach was administered individually along with several other projective devices. It was administered first at the beginning of Period I, then at the termination of Period II, and at the end of Period III, prior to the return to solid food. For the three patients who remained in the hospital for another year, a fourth set of data was obtained at the end of Period IV, just prior to the time of their discharge. Table 26-I shows weight changes coinciding with the time of Rorschach administration. After a complete Rorschach was obtained at Period II, the examiner returned the Rorschach plates to the patient and requested: "Please look back through all the cards and see if you can find anything that looks like food." All remarks and images were recorded. This limits testing procedure was not repeated at testing Period III. However, for three patients, limits testing for food was repeated at the end of testing during Period IV. Table 26-III shows the effects this request had on the total number of nutrition images produced.

Those Rorschach images which fell under a category termed *nutrition* were analyzed. This category was defined by seven classes of images whose combined components represented a generic composite designated *nutrition*. It seemed important not to use certain common theoretical terms whose definition is seldom precise. For this reason, such descriptive terms as orality, oral dependence, oral sadism, and symbolic material that could be unconscious substitutes for any aspect of so-called oral experience were avoided. In the same fashion, scoring unequivocal food responses alone seemed to do violence to certain images in the data that were not food per se, but which had obvious relevance to the physical condition being studied. In addition to the senior author, an independent examiner was asked to designate a list of all Rorschach images in the groups' materials which appeared to him to pertain to the nutrition process. Responses so grouped were combined and classes or categories were given the following designations: a) organs or products of digestion (total of 15), b) food per se (total of 78), c) mouth activity (total of 7), d) nonpopular animals commonly used for food (total of 12), e) effects of nutrition (total of 3), f) food utensils (total of 6), g) carrion (total of 3). From the total shown above, it may be seen at once that food itself was by far the most frequent of these subcategories. Examples of each category were the following: a) "stomach," "intestines"; b) "lettuce," "steak on charcoal"; c) "person eating from bowl that's not there," "faces with bubbles coming out of the mouths"; d) "frog" on Plate VIII, "ducks" on Plate II; e) "fat man sitting on stool," "Jolly Green Giant who fell back and squashed a cow"; f) "picnic basket," "garbage pail"; g) "vultures with a carcass," "hyenas ripping on a dead animal." Our aim was to do no violence to the range and nuances of images associated with nutrition and, at the same time, to avoid ambiguity. (The bulk of the images were food, and there was no ambiguity there.) Although category four might seem ambiguous, it was decided that the images included had direct relevance to our analysis. There were only a dozen of these images, but in every case the patient himself authenticated the nonpopular animal as being associated with food. For example, the popular crabs on Plate X were never included, but "King Crab" for an unusual area on Plate VIII was included (reported by the patient as food). Animals absent from the common diet were not included (as deer). "Duck" on Plate II was counted because it is a highly uncommon association as an animal for this card; the patient associated it with food at some time during limits testing, and duck is a common food. Even though certain images could easily be classified as "orally aggressive" (i.e., "cannibals ripping a carcass"), such a classification was avoided because it was difficult to be precise about what this aggressive act entailed for the particular individual who produced the image. The data might have been analyzed in any number of other ways, but it was our intention to avoid the ambiguity of certain psychoanalytic definitions in this context.

FINDINGS

Table 26-I shows the extent of weight loss for the group and at the times of Rorschach examination. At the end of Period III, the mean length of hospitalization for the six patients was eight months, and the mean weight loss for the group was 86.7 pounds. The three patients who stayed a year longer were reduced to normal weight for their age and height. None received any formal psychotherapy during their hospitalization.

Table 26-II shows the individual distribution of nutrition responses and

TABLE 26-II

NUMBER AND PERCENTAGES OF NUTRITION RESPONSES
COMPARED WITH TOTAL NUMBER OF RESPONSES

Patient	Period I			Period II			Period III			Period IV		
	R	NR	% NR	R	NR	% NR	R	NR	% NR	R	NR	% NR
(1)	28	6	23.0	38	8	21.0	42	7	16.6	45	8	17.7
(2)	24	6	23.3	23	3	13.0	22	3	13.6	23	4	17.3
(3)	16	1	6.2	15	1	6.6	18	1	5.5	16	2	12.5
(4)	23	5	21.7	36	9	25.0	30	5	16.6			
(5)	32	4	12.1	38	5	13.1	39	5	15.1			
(6)	33	6	18.1	34	6	11.1	32	6	18.7			
Totals	156	28	17.9	184	32	17.3	183	27	14.7	84	14	16.6

R = Total Responses
NR = Nutritional Responses

their relation to the total number of Rorschach responses produced at any one examination. For the group as a whole ($N = 6$), the percentage of nutrition responses decreased even though the total number of Rorschach responses increased. At the end of the first weight loss period (Period II), the raw number of nutrition responses increased slightly for the group, but the greater number of responses in general reduced the percentage of nutrition responses at that period. At Period III there was a small decrease in the percentage of food responses, while the total number of responses was essentially the same as at Period II. When Period IV is considered ($N = 3$), two patients showed a small decrease in the percentage of food responses (after a year and eight months, and a return to a normal body size), while the third patient showed an increase. However, when the percentage of nutrition responses of the three patients who remained for Period IV are compared with their percentage of nutrition responses at Period III, all three showed a percentage increase in food responses when the total number of responses they produced is considered. When percentages at Period I are compared with those at the end of Period III, four of the patients showed some decrease in percentage of nutrition responses, while two showed an increase. The findings at Period IV tend to reverse the group trend at Period III.

Even though inspection suggested that statistical tests would lack utility with our data, several types of tests were applied. These included forms of chi square and rank order techniques. None proved useful primarily because the number of raw-score food images tended to remain constant or vary against a much larger change in the total number of responses at successive examinations. Raw scores, directional trends, and percentage changes have been utilized in evaluating the data.

Table 26-III shows the raw scores of the number of nutrition responses apart from percentages and total number of responses, and compares

TABLE 26-III

RAW SCORES, NUTRITION RESPONSES, AND IMPACT OF SUGGESTION ON NUMBER OF NUTRITION RESPONSES

Patient	Period I		Period II			Period III		Period IV		
	R	NR	R	NR	NL	R	NR	R	NR	NL
(1)	28	6	38	8	1	42	7	45	8	1
(2)	24	6	23	3	3	22	3	23	4	2
(3)	16	1	15	1	1	18	1	16	2	0
(4)	23	5	36	9	5	30	5			
(5)	32	4	38	5	3	39	5			
(6)	33	6	34	6	7	32	6			

R = Total Responses
NR = Nutrition Responses
NL = Nutrition Responses Reported in Limits Testing which did not occur in NR of the same period.

TABLE 26-IV
FREQUENCY DISTRIBUTION OF NUTRITION RESPONSES
FOR INDIVIDUAL RORSCHACH PLATES

Plate No.	Nutrition Resp.	Rank Order
I	8	7
II	18	2
III	15	4
IV	9	6
V	4	9
VI	2	10
VII	5	8
VIII	13	5
IX	16	3
X	27	1

them with the increase in number of nutrition responses obtained by suggestion in limits testing (Periods II and IV). We may see further the distribution of these responses and their relation to the total number of responses after limits testing was introduced during Period II.

Table 26-III indicates that our supraliminal stimulus (that of directing the patient to look actively for food in the Rorschach plates at Period II) produced no effect whatever on the number or kind of nutrition responses which appeared at Period III. No limits testing for food was done at Period III. However, at Period IV, of the three patients who remained, all showed an increase of one nutrition response when they were tested approximately a year later. For *one* patient, this added nutrition response (a food utensil) was the same image given during limits testing at Period II. For most of the group, when food responses were asked for at limits testing (Period II), additional food images appeared easily. The three patients who remained for an additional year were the three who gave the fewest food responses on request. Table 26-III shows that these three gave even fewer additional images at the second testing of limits. Further, no entirely new food image emerged for anyone at final testing (all were reported at some earlier time).

Table 26-IV shows the frequency distribution of nutrition responses in relation to individual Rorschach plates. Plates X and II elicited the greatest number of these responses, while V and VI produced the least (all in that order). The ten cards were divided equally, in that the colored plates ranked serially as producing the most nutrition responses, and the achromatic the least.

DISCUSSION

Given the conditions we have described, the data indicate that directions to find food images in Rorschach stimuli had little or no influence on subsequent Rorschach images. This result was independent of the total number of responses at any given time. A similar pattern was found in a seventh obese patient tested in the same setting, but one not included in the original group. Glucksman and co-workers[5] have reported that these same patients expressed frequent fantasies of food and eating during clinical interviews. None of the patients made any extensive effort to suppress thoughts about food. Most had colored magazine pictures of food decorating their rooms. *All* began with a remarkably elevated Rorschach food content. Even so, most found new food responses with ease when they were asked to do so. That form of testing the limits in a food-deprived group did not materially affect later Rorschach materials of the same patient.

This data supports the notion that a relationship exists between an individual and his imagery projected onto ink blots which may not be appreciably altered by outside interferences. Most Rorschach workers know that *conscious intent* on the part of the S to influence his images frequently has little effect on what actually ensues. McCully[9] has made particular note of this tendency before in discussing underlying processes in the Rorschach experience. It happens that a S who does not *consciously* believe he is sexually deprived may produce a flood of sexual responses. The meaning as to why these responses appear seems to transcend the outer state of the S. Failure to take this into account often interferes with interpretation of research data. We do not wish to imply that Rorschach imagery cannot be influenced, but we do emphasize that it is probably much less subject to influence than might be supposed. Our patients showed changes among Rorschach variables other than those described here. Qualities associated with anxiety and depression fluctuated. Glucksman's[5] paper describes them in detail. We merely wish to emphasize that the content of conscious preoccupations and Rorschach content may be quite disparate. Our subjects began with elevated food imagery, but it did not change significantly as the study evolved. Perhaps this has to do with the readiness for psychic experience to precipitate. Similarly, a particular dream may be a function of readiness for certain kinds of psychic experience to stimulate the visual cortex. When Rorschach images involve genuine symbol formation, there is doubtless a close kinship with dream imagery. Complex inner processes are mediated by the ink blots, and the images that appear may correspond with both inner and outer experiences as they play across the unique structure of a given individual. That some images vary in time and correspond with experiential changes, while others remain constant, corresponds to life and its fluctuation.

On initial examination, the group's mean percentage of food (per se) responses was 13.5 per cent. Using our definition of nutrition imagery, the group's mean percentage was almost 18.0 per cent. This is much above the percentage that might be expected for an average sample in our culture.

Brozek's[2] group of thirty-two patients had an initial Rorschach food count mean of 1.6%. A slight rise (mean of 2.4%) was found during semi-starvation. During a rehabilitation (no restriction of food) period, their mean food content rose to 3.1%, but none of the changes was significant. None of the changes in food imagery count was significant for our group either. In one S, whose number of Rorschach responses stayed relatively constant, there was a decrease in food count percentages at Periods I and III, but it rose over the longer period (IV). For the rest of the group, the food count fluctuation was small in relation to the change in total or non-food responses at every stage. Brozek's Ss were not prevented from eating solid food, and their Rorschachs were obtained by group methods. Further, they were not obese. Yet, both in his study and ours, food imagery was not significantly altered by the conditions of the experiment. It may be quite significant that our Ss began with a high nutrition imagery. Perhaps something in the nature of being obese over a long period of time increases the readiness of psychic processes to throw up nutrition imagery at a relatively constant rate. When first tested, no appreciable time had elapsed regards the effects of hospitalization, formula, or caloric deprivation. Hence, as Brozek *et al.*[2] observed, and Spence and Ehrenberg[10] have more recently repeated and emphasized, wish-fulfillment seems to have little to do with the content of Rorschach imagery. Perhaps such an assumption was naive, since much suggests that processes which contribute to the coming about of Rorschach images are complex and multi-determined.

It should be remembered that most food images on Rorschach are uncommon ones, and the majority of those given by our Ss were original responses. Hence, they were highly personal or individualistic. All had a dietary concern, and they could anticipate what would happen to them in the hospital. Elevated food responses was a group trend. Food certainly interested them, but the longer they were on a formula, and the longer their tastes were deprived, did not alter the state of Rorschach food content. Oddly, Brozek's Ss showed an increase in food imagery when there was no limitation about the Ss' diets.

We suggest that a perceptual readiness to construct nutrition imagery on Rorschach is related to the condition of being obese, or dietary concern. This does not simply mean that bakers tend to see bread on Rorschach. It may mean that their perception of bread on Rorschach may have a causal relationship to their occupation. We do not yet know how to identify the processes that underlie a group characteristic (elevated nutrition imagery).

We admit that our population was small indeed, but for some Ss, our measures occurred under controlled conditions for a year and a half. Brozek *et al.*[2] were unable to account for the rise in food responses after there was no restriction on food. The rise took place even though total responses decreased. He remarked he could safely say the rise was not a function of increased "food drive." Spence and Ehrenberg[10] have emphasized the drive state as being a more critical factor than the stimulus in influencing behavior. Neither our data nor Brozek's supports this per se. Spence and Ehrenberg[10] go on to state that a stimulus must resonate with an aroused and congruent drive in order to have a detectable influence on behavior. We suggest this is another way of saying that inner processes outside conscious awareness influence a precipitated pictograph or Rorschach perception. This would be in addition to the outer condition and the nature of the ink blot stimulus structure itself.

We found the same relationship between chromatic stimuli and their greater facility to elicit nutrition responses that Levine, Chein, and Murphy[7] found a quarter of a century ago. We expected Plate X might lend itself to nutrition imagery, but Plate II's second rank was more of a surprise. It emphasizes the relation between strong feeling (color) and food for our Ss. Yet, we found certain food or food-associated images in our Ss which would be disagreeable for humans to partake or ingest. This may be an important finding. All six patients produced at least one such image attended by strong, unsavory qualities. Examples were, "That card reminds me of having the 'runs' going to the bathroom"; "The contents of a garbage pail"; "Jackals eating remains." It may have been that something connected with this kind of negatively-toned quality or affect enabled them to agree to the rigors of dietary deprivation and experimentation. Those three patients who volunteered to spend an additional year in the hospital were those who gave the least amount of spontaneous food imagery at limits testing. We refer to what may be correlates with internal discipline. Perhaps an element of hostile feelings toward food or nourishment exists beside the need to ingest excessive food in the patient obese since childhood. Being willing to *do* something about obesity may be connected with a facility to inhibit food impulses. It would be interesting to discover whether obese individuals with an inertia about reducing have the negatively toned Rorschach images we found. Bruch[3] has reported that obese Ss frequently return to original weight levels after intensive reduction. The S in our study who produced the least negatively toned food images and who had the most food images was the one who least maintained her reduced weight status upon discharge. By the same token, at the end of two years, the only S who had maintained her weight-reduced status was the S who produced the highest number of unsavory nutrition images. Our population was too small to offer more than notation of these findings, but they may serve as tentative leads for later research.

REFERENCES

1. Ahrens, E. H., Jr., Dole, V. P. and Blankenhorn, D. H.: The use of orally fed liquid formulas in metabolic studies. *Am J Clin Nutr*, 2:336-342, 1954.
2. Brozek, J., Guetzkow, H., Vig Baldwin, M. and Dranston, R.: A quantitative study of perception and association in experimental semistarvation. *J Pers*, 19:245-263, 1951.
3. Bruch, H.: *The Importance of Overweight*. New York, Norton, 1957.
4. Epstein, S. and Levitt, H.: The influence of hunger on the learning and recall of food related words. *J Abnorm Soc Psychol*, 64:130-135, 1962.
5. Glucksman, M., Hirsch, J., McCully, R., Barron, B. and Knittle, J.: The response of obese patients to weight reduction: A quantitative evaluation of behavior. *Psychosom Med*, 30:359-373, 1968.
6. Hirsh, J., Knittle, J. and Salans, L.: Cell lipid content and cell number in obese and nonobese human adipose tissue. *J Clin Invest*, 45:1023, 1966.
7. Levine, R., Chein, I. and Murphy, G.: The relation of the intensity of a need to the amount of perceptual distortion. *J Pers*, 13:283-294, 1942.
8. Masling, J., Rabie, L., and Blondheim, S.: Obesity, level of aspiration, and Rorschach and TAT measures of oral dependence. *J Consult Psychol*, 31:233, 1967.
9. McCully, R. S.: Process analysis: A tool in understanding ambiguity in diagnostic problems in Rorschach. *J Project Tech Pers Assess*, 29:436-444, 1965.
10. Spence, D. and Ehrenberg, B.: Effects of oral deprivation on responses to subliminal and supraliminal verbal food stimuli. *J Abnorm Soc Psychol*, 69:10-18, 1964.
11. Stunkard, A. J. and McLaren-Hume, M.: Results of treatment for obesity: Review of literature and report of series. *Arch Int Med*, 103:79,1959.

27

Body and Self-cathexis of
Super-obese Patients

HARRY GOTTESFELD

THE Psychosomatic Division of the State University of New York, Down-state Medical Center has been investigating the physiological and psychological make-up and social functioning of "super-obese" patients. The following study is concerned with one aspect, the feelings the "super-obese" patients have about their own bodies and their personalities.

The mean weight of the subjects of this investigation was 269 lb with weights ranging up to 369 lb. While there are now in the literature a number of psychological studies of obese patients, there is little reported about people of such extreme obesity. One wonders about the psychological nature of people whose obesity is so marked that they flirt with death by overtaxing the heart and other vital organs, risk serious injury through falls, bar themselves from many occupational and social functions in which their weight handicaps them, often have difficulty in taking care of themselves, and subject themselves to ridicule and rejection. These super-obese individuals suffer all this rather than diminish their food intake. The immediate cause of their obesity seems to be overeating; the possibility of organic etiology such as endocrine dysfunctions, hypothalamic lesions, and pancreatic tumors was ruled out by careful medical workup, including laboratory studies.

To understand the super-obese patient one must understand how he feels about himself. Specifically, how does he feel about his ponderous, bloated body and how does he feel about himself as a person? Many investigators, including Machover,[3] Murphy,[6] Schilder,[7] and Secord and Jourard[8] believe that the individual's feelings about his body and feelings about himself as a person are related. Secord and Jourard have made systematic studies of feelings about the body and the self. These investigators have made use of the concept "body cathexis" which they define as the degree of satisfaction reported by an individual for the parts and processes of the body. They formulated a "body cathexis" questionnaire in which individuals rated various parts or aspects of the body on a five point scale ranging from "strong positive feeling" to "strong negative feeling." They also formulated a "self-cathexis" questionnaire, similar to the "body cathexis" questionnaire, in which the individual rated himself on such

356

qualities as "ability to express self," "conscience," "artistic talents," "personality." They found that the scores on the body cathexis questionnaire and the self-cathexis questionnaire were positively correlated.

METHODOLOGY

Subjects

The obese patients were referred to the Psychosomatic Division because they wished help with their obesity. To qualify as "super-obese" for our studies the patient had to be more than 50 per cent over ideal weight for age, height, and frame, according to the tables of the Metropolitan Life Insurance Company.[4, 5]

Thirty super-obese patients were equated with thirty patients who had applied for help at a Mental Hygiene Clinic and were diagnosed as "mixed psychoneurosis." The patients of the two groups were matched as to age, sex, socioeconomic background, education, and IQ.

Body Cathexis

To evaluate the body cathexis of the super-obese patients, their self-drawings were compared with the group of neurotics' self-drawings. Three methods were used to compare the drawings: global clinical judgment, omission of bodily parts, and degree of differentiation. Each patient of both groups was asked to draw a picture of himself, to include the whole body. It was assumed that the self-drawing would reveal feelings and attitudes, often unconscious, that the patient has toward his own body. Using Secord and Jourard's definition of "body cathexis" it was hypothesized that the super-obese group of patients would show a more negative "body cathexis" than the neurotic group.

Global Judgment

Five judges, all clinical psychologists, were given separately the sixty self-drawings of the super-obese and the neurotic patients without any identifying material or any knowledge of the purpose of the study. They were asked to sort the sixty drawings into two piles of thirty drawings each, one pile showing the most positive "body cathexis," the other pile the most negative "body cathexis," according to Secord and Jourard's definition of body cathexis.

Omission of Bodily Parts

It is generally believed among clinicians that when a patient draws a person and he omits a bodily part, this can be considered as negative feelings for that bodily part and/or what that part may symbolize for him. According to Secord and Jourard's definition of body cathexis as "degree of satis-

faction . . . for the parts . . . of the body" one indication of negative body
cathexis that could be evaluated is missing parts of the body in a drawing.

Two judges were given a list of major bodily parts and asked to go
through the sixty drawings and determine separately which drawings showed
any missing parts. The drawings of the super-obese patients and the neurotics could then be compared as to the number of missing parts.

Degree of Differentiation

It might be assumed, if intellectual factors are kept constant, that the
less differentiated a drawing of a body is, the less interest there is in the
body and the more negative the body cathexis.

Florence Goodenough,[1] the creator of the Draw-A-Man test, devised a
scale in which she was able to rate a drawing according to its complexity
and proportions. While Goodenough used her scale as a method of evaluating the mental age of children, in this investigation the scale was used
as a method for determining the degree of differentiation in the drawings
of the super-obese and the neurotics. Since the IQ's of the super-obese and
the neurotics were equated on another test, intelligence should not be a
factor in any difference obtained in the degree of differentiation between
the two groups. Each drawing was scored according to Goodenough's instructions and given a score.

Self Cathexis

Twenty-eight personal traits were compiled and listed on a sheet of paper. These traits were then rated on a five point scale by the patient according to the way he felt he was. The same group of traits was then rated
by the patient according to the way he would like to be. The trait lists for
self and ideal were given to both the neurotics and the super-obese. The
computation of the discrepancy between the self and the ideal self served
as a measure of the degree of dissatisfaction with the self. The neurotic and
super-obese patients could then be compared as to "self-cathexis."

Secord and Jourard[8] and Johnson[2] indicate that body cathexis and self-
cathexis are positively related. Accordingly it was hypothesized that if the
super-obese group showed a more negative body cathexis they would show
a more negative self-cathexis, i.e. show a greater discrepancy between ideal
and self ratings.

RESULTS

Body Cathexis

Global Judgment

Agreement among the judges as to whether a drawing belonged in the
most positive body cathexis pile or the most negative body cathexis pile was
high. For twenty drawings all five judges were unanimous, for thirty-

three drawings four of the five judges agreed, for seven drawings three judges agreed. The thirty drawings which the majority of judges agreed showed the most negative body cathexis were then identified. Twenty-five of these drawings were by super-obese patients, five by neurotic patients. According to the Chi-Square Test the difference is statistically significant at the 0.01 level of confidence.

Omission of Bodily Parts

The two judges who evaluated the drawings for missing parts agreed in every case, except one which they decided in a conference together, as to whether the drawing showed at least one major missing part of the body. Thirteen drawings demonstrated missing parts. Twelve of these drawings were by super-obese patients and only one by a neurotic patient. The Chi-square test indicated that the difference is statistically significant at the 0.01 level of confidence.

Degree of Differentiation

On the Goodenough Scale the super-obese patients obtained a mean of 19.7 with a standard deviation of 9.9. Neurotics obtained a mean of 42.6 with a standard deviation of 6.8. It was considered that the higher the score, the greater the degree of differentiation. A *t*-test indicated that the difference between the means of the two groups was significant at the 0.01 level of confidence.

Clinical Impression

Aside from the comparison with the neurotic patients, in more absolute terms the self-drawings of the super-obese show a negative body cathexis. After the experiment was over, the clinical psychologists who did the sorting of the drawings were shown the drawings of the super-obese patients. In general, the psychologists felt that the drawings showed more negative attitudes toward the body image than other groups of adult out-patients or adult "normals" whom they had examined. "Poorly executed," "childish," "crude," "amorphous," "unstable stance," "difficult to tell what sex the figure is," "little detailing" were some of the typical comments of these clinicians. When the other methods of analysis used in this study are considered in absolute terms the results are also quite striking. Clinical psychologists tend to view the omission of a major bodily part in human figure drawings as quite pathological; over one-third of the super-obese omitted such parts. The poorly differentiated drawings of the super-obese rated a mean IQ of 59 according to Goodenough's norms. However, the super-obese patients' mean IQ was 102 on a standardized intelligence test. The difference between means is statistically significant at the 0.01 level of confidence. If the IQ's are considered as indicating ability to differentiate, it would seem that the super-obese patients' general ability to differentiate is much better than their ability to differentiate on a task involving their body image.

Self-Cathexis

For all patients rating themselves on 28 personal traits on a five point scale there were a total of 520 traits in which the discrepancy between self and ideal ratings was two points or greater. These particular traits then resulted in relatively greater dissatisfaction than the others and may be considered as "dissatisfactions." The number of such "dissatisfactions" was totaled for each patient. The thirty patients who had the most "dissatisfactions" were then identified; eight were super-obese patients, twenty-two were neurotics. The hypothesis that the super-obese patients would be more dissatisfied with their personalities was not supported.* Had the opposite hypothesis been advanced, i.e. the super-obese patients would be more satisfied with their personalities, a Chi-square test indicates that this would be significant at the 0.05 level of confidence.

ADDITIONAL FINDINGS

If the super-obese patients are more satisfied with their personalities, one explanation of this may be that the super-obese may have "better" personalities and their satisfaction is based on realistic factors. To test this the following method was used.

Each of the super-obese patients was in the hospital for a two week evaluation. During this time, in addition to a psychological examination, psychiatric interviews, and a social history on each of these patients, there was an opportunity to observe his interaction with other patients and staff. Two psychiatrists and a psychologist, who had all this information, then acted as judges, each rating the patient on the same five point personal trait list as the patient had rated himself.

Reliability among the judges was high. Out of a total of 840 traits to be rated, on 264 traits there was perfect agreement among the judges, on 440 traits, a one point discrepancy existed, on 125 traits, there was a two point discrepancy and on 11 traits there was a three point discrepancy.

The super-obese patients' rating of themselves were then compared to their ideal rating of themselves and to the average rating of the three judges. It was assumed that if their self-ratings were closer to their ideal ratings than to the ratings of the observers (judges) of their behavior, their self-evaluations were relatively unrealistic.

---

* Chi-square tests do not indicate any differences between the super-obese and neurotics in their ratings of their ideal or between the two groups rating of their ideal and a cultural stereotype of ideal ratings.

A difference score between a self rating on a trait and the ideal rating was determined. Then a difference score between a self rating and the average ratings of the observers was determined for each trait and averaged for all trait ratings by a super-obese patient. The two total average difference scores were computed for all super-obese patients and then compared by means of a *t*-test. The difference scores between self ratings and average ratings of observers were greater than the difference scores between self ratings and ideal ratings, significant at the 0.01 level of confidence. Thus the super-obese patients tend to be unrealistic.

One explanation of the results obtained thus far may be in terms of techniques used. Human figure drawings are generally considered to elicit more unconscious material than by questionnaires utilizing self-evaluation of traits. Thus the more negative body cathexis and the more positive self-cathexis of the super-obese patients, as compared to the neurotics, may not be due to differences in these two areas but rather that it is easier to guard against a negative self-picture on a trait list than on the drawing. To test this first of all, items on the trait list were surveyed to see if any of them seemed to have any direct connection with body cathexis. The one item of the trait list which seemed to have relevance was "good-looking." Then the ratings for "good-looking" by the super-obese and the neurotics were compared. A Chi-square test was applied. No significant difference was found between the two groups. Twenty-six of the thirty super-obese patients gave themselves an average intermediate rating on "good-looking." Thus while the super-obese patients are more dissatisfied than neurotics with their bodies according to a drawing test, this difference does not hold up when rating themselves on a trait related to body cathexis.

DISCUSSION

Using three criteria for measuring body cathexis on a self-drawing, the super-obese patients on all three criteria showed a more negative body cathexis than the neurotic group. The super-obese drawings were judged as having more negative body cathexis by a group of clinicians; their drawings had more major parts of the body missing; the super-obese drawings were less differentiated. However, on a self-descriptive scale to measure self-cathexis, the super-obese group did not demonstrate a more negative self-cathexis.

These findings are not in accord with the findings of Secord and Jourard[8] and Johnson[2] that body and self-cathexis are related. However, it must be borne in mind that these investigators used self-descriptive scales for both body and self-cathexis, and were dealing with the same psychological level on both scales. Thus, an individual who expressed conscious dissatisfaction with his body tended to express conscious dissatisfaction with his self.

SELF-DESCRIPTIVE SCALE

I. "Here is a series of words which apply to most people to some extent and which describe you to some degree. Read each word and decide if it is always true of you, often true of you, sometimes true of you, rarely true of you, or never true of you, then put a check in the column under the correct heading. For example, the first word is affectionate. You decide if it is always true of you, often true, sometimes true, and so on. Put the check under the right column. Now continue with the rest."

II. "Here is the same list of words again. This time, instead of deciding to what extent the word applies to you, decide to what extent you would like it to apply to you. After you have decided put a check under the proper heading. Remember, this time you are to decide how you would like to be, not how you are."

Part I   I am
Part II   I would like to be

	Always	Often	Sometimes	Rarely	Never
1. affectionate	—	—	—	—	—
2. ambitious	—	—	—	—	—
3. angry	—	—	—	—	—
4. anxious	—	—	—	—	—
5. ashamed	—	—	—	—	—
6. bored	—	—	—	—	—
7. bossy	—	—	—	—	—
8. cheerful	—	—	—	—	—
9. complaining	—	—	—	—	—
10. confident	—	—	—	—	—
11. confused	—	—	—	—	—
12. easily-hurt	—	—	—	—	—
13. fearful	—	—	—	—	—
14. frank	—	—	—	—	—
15. friendly	—	—	—	—	—
16. good-looking	—	—	—	—	—
17. independent	—	—	—	—	—
18. intelligent	—	—	—	—	—
19. jealous	—	—	—	—	—
20. lonely	—	—	—	—	—
21. neat	—	—	—	—	—
22. optimistic	—	—	—	—	—
23. popular	—	—	—	—	—
24. practical	—	—	—	—	—
25. rebellious	—	—	—	—	—
26. reliable	—	—	—	—	—
27. showing-off	—	—	—	—	—
28. suspicious	—	—	—	—	—

Whatever psychological mechanisms of awareness or defense operated on one scale were likely to operate similarly on the other scale. In the present study two different types of techniques were used to measure body and self-cathexis. One was a projective technique, the other a questionnaire. One cannot fully guard against unconscious attitudes revealing themselves through projective drawings. The drawings of self reveal many unconscious aspects of attitudes toward the body; the self-descriptive scale apparently is on a more conscious level. Probably the super-obese patient is unable to accept a negative self-description of himself, and on the conscious level portrays himself as well satisfied. At a less conscious level the super-obese is more dissatisfied with himself, as in his self-drawings. It is likely that it is not a matter of whether feelings toward the body or personality of the super-obese are being studied but whether or not the technique of measurement permits the super-obese patient to guard against the unsatisfactory image he has of himself and allows him to present a facade of satisfaction. Two of the findings support this. While the drawings of the super-obese patients show greater dissatisfaction with their bodies than the neurotics, when asked on the questionnaire how good looking they felt they were, the super-obese patients rated themselves for the most part as average, with no difference in evidence that they rated themselves any worse than the neurotics. Also when observers rated the super-obese patients, it appears that the super-obese patients' ratings of themselves are closer to their ideal than it is to reality.

It is generally believed that personality factors underlie the overeating of the super-obese patients and that the most satisfactory manner of treatment would include some form of psychotherapy. The findings of this study imply that at best the super-obese patients would make difficult cases for psychological treatment. These patients tend to deny that there is anything wrong with their personalities and hence their motivation for psychotherapy is poor. Also, the strenuous use of so pathological a defense as denial in itself suggests a poor prognosis.

SUMMARY

Super-obese patients were compared with neurotic patients on "body cathexis" and "self-cathexis" through a self-drawing and a self-rating personality trait list. While the super-obese patients show a more negative "body cathexis" on the self-drawing they do not show a more negative "body cathexis" on the trait list. The results are explained in terms of the types of measures used and the defensive structure of the super-obese patient.

REFERENCES

1. Goodenough, F. L.: *Measurement of Intelligence by Drawings.* Yonkers-on-Hudson, New York, World Book Co., 1926.
2. Johnson, L. C.: Body cathexis as a factor in somatic complaints. *J Consult Psychol,* 20:145-9, 1956.
3. Machover, K.: *Personality Projection in the Drawing of the Human Figure.* Springfield, Illinois, Thomas, 1949.
4. Metropolitan Life Insurance Company: Ideal weights for women. *Statis Bull,* October, 1942.
5. Metropolitan Life Insurance Company: Ideal weights for men. *Statis Bull,* June, 1943.
6. Murphy, G.: *Personality: A Biosocial Approach to Origins and Structure.* New York and London, Harper and Bros., 1947.
7. Schilder, P.: *Psychotherapy.* New York, Norton, 1938.
8. Secord, P. F. and Jourard, S. M.: The appraisal of body cathexis: body cathexis and the self. *J Consult Psychol,* 17:323-7, 1953.

28

Extreme Obesity

RONALD S. REIVICH

RENE A. RUIZ

AND

RUTH M. LAPI

ALTHOUGH obesity has been the subject of innumerable psychiatric studies, few investigators have restricted themselves to examining only those persons whose corpulence has become excessive to the point of being almost a defining quality. We are speaking of people who are so greatly overweight they attract unfavorable attention to themselves, impair their ability to function in society, and seriously endanger their health. Recent progress in biochemistry,[8] medicine,[3] and surgery[5] has helped to spotlight these so-called "super-obese"[6] patients. For the past three years we have been studying a collection of such extraordinarily fat individuals in hopes of developing fresh hypotheses about the role of emotional factors in obesity. The following is a preliminary report of some of our findings.

METHOD

Since September, 1962, every extremely obese referral to the Department of Psychiatry of the University of Kansas Medical Center has been considered for inclusion in the study. Thus far a total of thirty-three patients, including three men, have qualified with respect to the sole criterion that their weight be at least four standard deviations above the expected weight calculated for height, sex and age from standard tables.[18] This represents an incidence of six per 10,000 referrals, inpatients and outpatients, to the University of Kansas Medical Center.[11]

The data reported here derives from a review of hospital records, formal psychiatric consultations, psychological testing, group psychotherapy process notes and weekly weight records.

Hospital records were scanned to exclude patients whose obesity could be demonstrated to be a result of a metabolic defect or organic illness and to establish if any heretofore unreported pattern of laboratory test abnormality was present. Formal psychiatric consultation reports were available on thirty of the thirty-three patients in the group. Of these, nineteen were seen personally by the senior author. Psychological testing included the Minnesota Multiphasic Personality Inventory (MMPI), Shipley Hartford Institute of Living Scale (SH), Draw-a-Person test (DAP), Food At-

364

titude Scale (FAS), and a Biographical Data Sheet (BDS). Ten patients participated in weekly psychodynamically oriented sixty-minute group psychotherapy sessions for periods ranging from three to twenty-seven months. Psychotherapy was not directed at accomplishing weight reduction but at helping the patients with their problems in living. Discussion of dieting and related matters was neither encouraged nor discouraged. Two of the authors served as co-therapists for the duration of the study and the third observed the sessions by closed circuit television in an adjacent room where she recorded process notes on the group interaction. The facilities and equipment required for this procedure have been described elsewhere.[16]

TABLE 28-I

CHRONOLOGICAL AGE (CA), SEX (S), HEIGHT (H), WEIGHT (W), MARITAL STATUS (MS), REFERRAL SOURCE (R), AND NUMBER OF POUNDS ABOVE EXPECTED MEAN WEIGHT FOR AGE, SEX AND HEIGHT (LB > ME), FOR 30 FEMALE AND 3 MALE SUPER-OBESE PATIENTS

No.	CA	S	H	W	MS	R*	Lb > Me
1	29	F	5'0"	262	M	OPC	149
2	23	F	5'4"	204	M	OPC	83
3	50	F	5'6"	275	M	MED	123
4	16	F	5'3"	278	S	MR	134
5	25	F	5'6"	365	M	MR	232
6	41	F	5'4"	241	D	OPC	101
7	14	F	5'6"	235	S	MR	110
8	29	F	5'2"	201	M	GYN	82
9	52	F	5'6"	285	M	MED	133
10	33	F	5'5"	280	M	ER	145
11	36	F	5'3"	242	M	ER	116
12	30	F	5'6"	334	M	OPC	195
13	61	F	5'2"	319	M	MR	182
14	45	F	5'4"	245	D	OPC	105
15	45	F	5'0"	313	M	MR	106
16	45	F	5'6"	230	M	MR	83
17	32	F	5'7½"	312	M	MR	168
18	34	F	5'6"	435	S	MR	296
19	52	F	5'7"	312	D	MED	156
20	30	F	5'2"	248	M	OPC	122
21	30	F	5'1"	227	M	MED	104
22	41	F	5'8"	320	M	MR	175
23	38	F	5'3"	245	M	OPC	116
24	29	F	5'5"	222	M	OPC	87
25	23	F	5'1"	248	S	GYN	136
26	42	F	5'2"	291	M	MR	158
27	15	F	5'5"	300	S	MED	179
28	18	F	5'2"	240	S	MR	129
29	20	F	5'9"	322	S	MED	182
30	50	F	5'5½"	309	M		159
31	40	M	6'2"	521	M	MR	329
32	19	M	5'10"	232	S	MED	75
33	36	M	5'10½"	454	M	MED	282

* Referral Source: OPC (Out-Patient Clinic), MED (Medicine), MR (Metabolic Research), GYN (Gynecology), ER (Emergency Room).

After each therapy session, the authors met for fifty minutes to discuss their observations and to prepare a summary of their proceedings. These summaries provided an on-going clinical impression of the salient themes and interactional styles during the therapy period. Follow-up psychological testing was administered to the five patients who remained in the group two years after its initiation in an attempt to substantiate further any psychological changes in the subjects. In addition, the patients were required to "weigh in" weekly at the psychiatric out-patient clinic on a special scale (most hospital scales are calibrated to only three hundred lb). This procedure provided a weight record for each member of the therapy group.

RESULTS AND DISCUSSION

For purposes of clarity and convenience of presentation, interpretative comments have been included in this section.

Table 28-I enumerates the thirty-three subjects according to age, sex, height, weight, marital status, referral source and number of pounds above expected weight.

As expected, a review of available hospital records of thirty patients failed to reveal either a definitive metabolic etiology of the obesity in any case or an unusual pattern of laboratory values overall. Although many of the subjects had abnormal glucose tolerance tests and some had specific pathological findings apparently unrelated to their obesity, in general the medical findings were consistent with what one would expect from the literature.[20] The major results in our study were abstracted from psychiatric consultations, psychological testing and the group therapy experience.

PSYCHIATRIC CONSULTATIONS

Formal consultations were available on thirty subjects. A compendium of the consultation data may be organized with respect to those features of the psychiatric (or "mental status") examination that were frequently considered abnormal. These categories include affect (or "mood"), mechanisms of defense, miscellaneous psychopathology, and psychiatric diagnosis.

Table 28-II summarizes the most frequently cited descriptions of affect. It is of note that fourteen patients appeared overtly *depressed* and that of the twelve who were either *cheerful* or *anxious,* six were thought to be *labile* in mood, perhaps an indication of underlying depression. The finding of emotional lability, a tendency to shift abruptly (but not so abruptly or unaccountably as patients with "pseudobulbar palsy") from one predominant mood to another, often with circumscribed outbursts of tearfulness, was noted in eighteen patients. Seven patients were considered *paranoid,* a term which in this case refers to interpersonal "style" in the interview, chiefly to an attitude of distrust, suspiciousness, uncooperativeness, or outright hostility. Four patients were considered *bland,* a term that refers to an inappropriate lack of concern or involvement. Only two of the thirty patients, both considered cheerful, were not felt to have any perturbation of affect.

Table 28-II also provides a frequency count of the defense mechanisms which were thought to be excessively utilized by the patients. As in the assessment of affect, these findings should be considered descriptive and subjective; at best, roughly quantitative. One can conservatively say that the utilization of denial (or repression) is a singular feature of the group as a whole. Since conflictual stimuli, both from the environment and the intrapsychic apparatus, are sealed off from consciousness, many patients in the group essentially were unaware, superficially, of the presence of emotional problems.

In evaluating psychopathology in a retrospective study of consultations, it is mandatory to reflect that what is reported by the examining psychiatrist is only a fractional, and sometimes inadequate, representation of what the patient's actual psychopathology may be; a list of psychopathologic findings is useful only insofar as it may demonstrate the breadth and quality of disordered mental functioning. The following list is distinguished both in terms of its variety and severity (the parenthetical figures refer to the number of times terms used more than once were listed): depression (4), somatization (4), anxiety (3), obsession (3), phobia (3), compulsion (3), withdrawal (2), concreteness (2), sexual promiscuity (2), circumstantiality, frigidity, impaired remote memory, impaired judgment, temper tantrums, poor concentration, untidiness, and cyclothymia. One patient had a history of a psychotic illness with both the primary and secondary (including auditory hallucinations and delusions of persecution) symptoms of schizophrenia. Another patient had been a severe alcoholic until, with the help of Alcoholics Anonymous, she went "on the wagon" and became, in her own words, "a foodoholic." Five patients mentioned serious inter-

TABLE 28-II

FREQUENCY COUNT OF DESCRIPTIONS OF AFFECT AND MECHANISMS OF DEFENSE IN PSYCHIATRIC CONSULTATIONS ON 30 SUPER-OBESE PATIENTS

Affect	*n**	*Mechanism of Defense*	*n*
Anxious	5	Denial (repression)	30
Bland	4	Conversion	5
Cheerful	7	Projection	8
Depressed	14	Reaction-formation	8
Labile	18	Regression	1
Paranoid	7	Withdrawal	1

* n = number of times mentioned.

personal difficulties with their mothers, which some examiners labeled "symbiosis" with mother. Two patients openly acknowledged serious marital difficulties. Although most of the patients, as a group, were considered to lack sufficient insight and motivation to be candidates for psychotherapy, nine patients recognized a relationship between eating and emotional, physical, or other events. They commented that they overate when depressed, anxious, angry, or rejected; before menstruation, after dieting, after masturbating, and at night; and for reward. Six patients mentioned numerous dietary failures. While only two patients admitted sexual promiscuity, two others reported that they feared dyscontrol of sexual impulses.

Nineteen patients in the consult group were labeled with a diagnosis of "personality disorder." Such a diagnosis connotes that the psychiatric difficulty is manifested by a lifelong pattern of behavior rather than by the acute onset of mental or emotional symptoms.[1] Twelve of the above were classified as "passive-aggressive," one as "emotionally immature," one as "emotionally unstable," and five were unspecified. The remaining patients were diagnosed as follows: depressive reaction (5), anxiety reaction (1), schizophrenic reaction, paranoid type (1), and no diagnosis (4). The preponderance of "character" diagnoses indicates that the consulting psychiatrists tended to see the patients so listed as chronically disturbed but not particularly in subjective distress. They saw most of these characterologically afflicted individuals as being either passive-dependent (helpless, indecisive, clinging), passive-aggressive (pouting, stubborn, inefficient, obstructionistic, procrastinating) or aggressive (irritable, destructive, impulsive, resentful). Probably because they seemed to lack both subjective discomfort (and therefore motivation) and insight, they were generally appraised as being poor candidates for psychotherapy. Moreover, the psychiatric consultant rarely made a specific recommendation that might have been helpful in the long range management of the case.

PSYCHOLOGICAL TESTING

To determine how personality factors relate to extreme obesity, the MMPI was administered to twenty-eight super-obese females. The MMPI[10] is a personality test questionnaire which includes 550 "true-false" type items of diverse content. On the basis of several decades of empirical research, groups of items have been organized into three "validity" scales and ten "personality" scales.[21] The validity scales indicate the extent to which the test results may be accepted as being an accurate description of the subject's actual personality. The personality scales measure either maladaptive behavior patterns (e.g. social introversion) or similarity of response-patterns to a criterion group of patients homogeneous for a particular psychiatric diagnosis or trait (e.g. depression, hysteria). In the most elementary scheme of MMPI interpretation, any scale score equal to or greater than two standard deviations above a mean obtained from normative data is considered "significant" or "pathological." Twenty-two of the twenty-eight MMPI's (79 per cent) obtained from the super-obese group revealed a significant elevation on one or more of the personality scales. Of the total group for whom MMPI profiles were available, eight were referred for testing from the Department of Psychiatry; of this psychiatric subgroup, all (100 per cent) had significant personality scale elevations. Fourteen of the 20 MMPI's (70 per cent) obtained from patients who were referred for testing from medical or surgical (nonpsychiatric) services showed significant elevations. Comparison data are available from Pearson *et al.* at the Mayo Clinic.[15] Pearson and co-workers found that 74 per cent of 709 psychiatric patients and 43 per cent of 10,000 nonpsychiatric patients obtained significant elevations on one or more of the personality scales of the MMPI. It therefore appears that extremely obese females are more likely to demonstrate psychopathology as manifested on the MMPI than a comparison population, regardless of referral source.

To facilitate interpretation of the MMPI results for the super-obese group, the twenty-eight MMPI profiles were merged to form a single, comprehensive profile based on means scale scores. This comprehensive, or mean, MMPI profile admits to three broad conclusions.

First, the validity scales, which are within normal limits, suggest that the elevations on the personality scales represent an accurate assessment of the MMPI psychopathology in this group of subjects. Secondly, the profile of significant elevations does not fit any of the known actuarial code types,[7, 13] indicating that no singular or definitive personality trait characterizes the super-obese group. Thus, super-obesity is probably not pathognomonic of a particular kind of psychiatric disturbance in terms of the present nomenclature. Finally, the mean MMPI profile was submitted to a computer analysis program of the Mayo Clinic type,[19] the system in operation in the Department of Psychiatry of the University of Kansas Medical Center. The following statements were "printed-out":

Slightly more than average number of physical complaints. Some concern about bodily function and physical health.

Mildly depressed or pessimistic.

Probably somewhat immature, egocentric, suggestible, and demanding.

Somewhat rebellious or nonconformist.

Avoids close personal ties.

Dissatisfied with family or social life.

Normal female interest pattern for work, hobbies, etc.

Sensitive. Alive to opinions of others.

Conscientious, orderly, and self-critical.

Tends toward abstract interests such as science, philosophy, and religion. Normal energy and activity level.

Probably reserved in unfamiliar and social situations.

The Shipley Hartford Institute of Living Scale[17] was utilized to measure intellectual functioning. The SH consists of two parts, one a "multiple-choice" vocabulary subtest with forty items and the other a "fill-in" problem subtest. The two subtests together assess general intellectual potential (IQ) and the ratio between the two subtests measures impairment in abstract thinking; the ratio index is known as the "conceptual quotient" (CQ). IQ scores from twenty-one super-obese females range from 103 to 132, with a mean of 114.8 and a standard deviation of 8.02. Because this mean score is clearly above average, a deficiency in intelligence cannot be postulated as an explanation for extreme obesity, at least in this group of subjects. The CQ scores from the same patients range from 62 to 119, with a mean of 90.5 and a standard deviation of 14.6. The mean CQ for the group falls within the normal range (i.e. between 90 and 110), indicating that extreme obesity and intellectual impairment are independent. The fact that the mean CQ is near the low end of the normal range tends to confirm the impression derived from psychiatric consultations that some extremely obese patients do have difficulty in abstract thinking.

The Food Attitude Scale[2] was utilized to quantify attitudes toward food and eating. The FAS consists of a pool of 221 "true-false" items concerning food preferences and feeding attitudes. FAS scores for twenty-six extremely obese females range from 28 to 55, with a mean of 45.4 and a standard deviation of 6.53. This may be compared with normative data derived from a group of 430 female college students at the University of Texas[2] whose mean score was 49.3 with a standard deviation of 5.9. The direction and magnitude of this difference in FAS scores between the super-obese group and the college student group indicates that extremely obese females hold relatively negative or unpleasant attitudes toward food as compared to a control population ($t = 2.93$ and $p < .01$).

Because disturbances in body image have frequently been described in obese patients,[14] the Draw-a-Person test[12] was administered to twenty extremely obese females. In the DAP, the subject is provided with a plain, unruled sheet of white paper of standard size and instructed to draw the picture of a person; when the drawing is completed, the subject is requested to draw a person of the opposite sex. A total of forty human figure drawings were obtained. Sixteen of the twenty subjects drew female figures first, a common and expected result often explained in terms of identification with one's own sex. Despite this, there were numerous indications of disturbances of sexual identity in the group of subjects. Specifically, twenty-six of the forty drawings were asexual (absence of secondary sexual characteristics) or sexually unattractive (anatomic distortions or omissions, stick figures). Six drawings depicted blatant secondary sexual characteristics displayed in an exaggerated fashion (e.g. a buxom female in a scanty bikini). These findings suggest that super-obese females tend to regard their own sexuality in extremely polarized terms; they see themselves as relatively sexless or as sexually overpowering. There is no middle ground *vis a vis* sexuality.

Certain features of the drawings tended to confirm previously related findings about immaturity and dependency. For example, eighteen of the forty drawings were of small, childish-looking, or youthfully garbed persons. On twelve drawings, hands were either hidden or absent, suggesting that the subjects were disinclined to "handle" or cope with the environment. Of the twenty-eight drawings in which hands appeared, eight showed hands extended, as if asking for help, or at the sides, as if grasping for balance. Facial expressions of the figure drawings suggested the emotional states of the subjects: three figures were obviously smiling, two seemed bland, and nine appeared to be clearly disturbed (angry, distorted, frowning).

Twenty-six subjects filled out a six page Biographical Data Sheet designed to elicit information concerning physical health, growth and development, educational level, sexual history, and other personal matters. Only a fragment of this BDS data can be presented here. As expected, most (20 of 26) subjects acknowledged "weight" as one of their major current difficulties. Of the six who did not mention weight as a problem, two said they were seeking help for reasons of physical health. The remaining four listed various emotional problems, including "nerves," "tension," "depression," and "anxiety." Two of these four super-obese subjects admitted suicidal ideation, and one admitted an overt attempt. The group as a whole was preoccupied with matters of physical health. In responding to a question about the presence of physical discomfort, only five subjects replied negatively; the median number of complaints cited was 1.5; one woman noted five specific somatic complaints. The frequency of hospital admission for the group was high; excluding admissions related to parturition, the median number was approximately two. One woman had been hospitalized nine times. We may infer from this data that super-obese females tend to have a high incidence of physical distress or discomfort.

A cluster of questions about earliest memories indicated that recall dated from between two and eight years with a mean of four years. Because seven of the twenty-six women failed to cite a specific age, special attention was focused on the content of recollections. Ten women left content unspecified, ten remembered distinctly unpleasant events (death, accident, injury, being lost) and only six reported memories that were not obviously unpleasant. If early memories condense general childhood feeling tones, then the above data suggests that many of the subjects experienced their early years as unpleasant or distressful.

Data from the BDS implies little, if any, relationship between formal educational level and excessive weight. Excluding one teen-age subject still attending school, educational level ranged from completion of the seventh grade to completion of requirements for graduate degrees, with the modal response being completion of high school. Being extremely corpulent does not result from lack of education *per se.*

GROUP PSYCHOTHERAPY

Since its inception, the psychotherapy group has met 112 hours, once weekly, for 27 months. To condense the voluminous clinical material that accumulated in that period requires that we focus on the most striking features of the total experience. These organize themselves in terms of developmental influences on the extremely obese patient, therapeutic problems, and progress in treatment.

A frequently mentioned influence in the emotional development of our super-obese patients was the dissolution of the family unit through death, divorce, or marital strife during childhood. The early environment was often perceived as threatening and chaotic; a consistent relationship with a loving maternal figure was commonly unavailable. Thus, the formative years were characterized by unstable object relationships. Many of the patients appeared to have an impaired sense of "self" or failed to establish a feeling of separateness from others (individuation). This deficiency in individuation may have been central in determining the patients' characteristic life style of dependency, diminished self-esteem and inhibited aggressivity, with deflection of hostile impulses inward. Failure to develop a sense of trust in a nurturant maternal figure and subsequent failure to develop autonomy antedate later problems of sexual identification,[4] a recurrent theme in the group.

Historical material reported in group sessions suggests that sociocultural factors also shaped feeding behavior. Most of the patients grew up in families from the lower socioeconomic classes; food was not always plentiful and tended to be, in the family ethos, a major source of gratification and reward. In the patients' otherwise unpredictable environment, food became a reliable transitional object.[23] As one patient said, "Food was the one thing I could depend on. It never let me down." Another factor may have been that at least one of the primary identity models within the family was likely to have been obese. Pathological patterns of food intake may have been emulated, assimilated, and fixed in childhood.

Many of the patients were already noticeably overweight by latency, and a few were involved with parents or parent surrogates in a power-struggle over food-intake regulation; this probably represents not only a prolongation of the combat so characteristic of the anal phase of psychosexual development but also a manifestation of their characteristic passive-aggressive personality style. Before or during puberty, some of the patients experienced or were threatened by some form of sexual molestation, not uncommonly incest. During this development phase, most of the patients engaged in sexual promiscuity, feared loss of sexual control, or developed a rigid, overcontrolled reaction-formation (e.g. puritanism) to sexual impulse. Overeating and consequent extreme obesity (i.e. unattractiveness) served the dual functions of substitute gratification of repressed sexuality and safeguard against sexual dyscontrol. On the other hand, the abnormal eating behavior may have been merely another expression of a generalized breakdown of emotional control. The atypical patient, who remained relatively svelte throughout adolescence, gained weight sharply at other times of developmental stress, such as marriage or childbirth.

The typical extremely obese referral arrives in the group as a primitively organized individual with a long-standing habit of dietary indiscretion. Her immense proportions have been welded into her defensive armor, providing a shield against competition or threat as well as an excuse with which she can rationalize her failures. Moreover, she can symbolically equate her girth with "bigness and power," another recurrent theme. Although she has been told that the purpose of group psychotherapy is to help her with her problems in living, her expressed motive for joining the group is to lose weight. She has highly unrealistic, even magical, fantasies about weight loss. Because of her exorbitant use of repression and denial, she is unable to recognize problems other than those directly related to her obesity and believes that becoming slender will somehow eliminate all her difficulties. In psychotherapy, her passivity makes it difficult for her to contribute to the group or she may chatter glibly and circumstantially to control the group, thereby preventing scrutiny of her underlying problems. The group itself is perceived as a threat to which the patient may react by overeating, by terminating treatment, or by becoming more severely disturbed for a time. In fact, all three possibilities have obtained in individual cases.

Most patients have gained weight during their first few months in the group. Eight of ten gained during the first month, six during the second and seven during the third. Of six patients who completed six months in the group, four gained weight during this period. After two years, only two of the five patients in the group had lost a significant amount of weight and both of these were still super-obese. Two years of group therapy, then, was less than successful in helping this small number of individuals maintain a diet.

That the super-obese female referred for group psychotherapy is tenously motivated for treatment can be attested by the fact that of the ten patients so far referred, five have terminated therapy prematurely. One patient left because she felt "insulted" by the group; one because she felt she was "getting nowhere"; and another because she felt she had gained so much insight about herself that she no longer required treatment (a "flight into health"). A therapeutic dilemma is how to chip away at the denial which obfuscates the patient's intrapsychic conflicts without evoking too much anxiety for the patient to tolerate.

Treatment not only mobilizes anxiety but also exacerbates those symptoms which bind anxiety. Thus, the patient in her first half year of therapy will probably gain weight and feel worse. Even so, she may recognize that she is making gains in other areas, such as in her marital adjustment; she may have faith in the doctors or the institution;[22] or she may be, as one patient commented, "at the end of the line" of unsuccessful attempts to lose weight and consolidate the loss. Obviously, whether she stays in treatment or quits is a kind of algebraic sum of the above, and other, factors. It is our feeling, after Hacker,[9] that the patient's motivation for treatment should be dealt with directly and if necessary, repeatedly, in the group sessions as another manifestation of resistance that needs to be systematically clarified, analyzed, and worked through.

It has been our observation that psychological change occurs excruciatingly slowly in the typical extremely obese patient. Between six and eighteen months, the patient's symptoms and anxiety tend to diminish. During this phase of treatment, as she becomes somewhat more committed to psychotherapy, she may become more cognizant of her interpersonal difficulties, more appropriate and comfortable in her interaction with therapists and other group members, and gain more insight about the development of her problems.

Change in the individual patient is gradually reflected in group process. Discussion becomes animated as the patients talk more to one another and less to the therapists, and as they become less inhibited in expressing anger.

As her reality testing improves, the super-obese patient may take action to ameliorate her troubles, such as by getting a job to solve a financial problem. Despite these signs of improvement, maintaining a diet does not appear to get much easier. The patient grudgingly accepts the notion that dieting is hard work. Her rationalizations about her food intake begin to give way to the recognition that she sheds pounds when she eats less; she is forced to consider, perhaps for the first time, whether she really wants (or is emotionally ready) to lose weight. Follow-up psychological testing (MMPI, DAP) tends to confirm the above clinical impression (e.g. personality scale elevations on the MMPI diminish, figure drawings become more differentiated).

In summary, progress in group psychotherapy with extremely obese females is not unlike group therapy generally, except that it is routinely jeopardized by inadequate motivation and that "movement" is greatly attenuated. Progress is signalled not by weight loss but by a diminution of psychic symptoms and an improvement in life adjustment.

CONCLUSIONS

Twenty-eight Minnesota Multiphasic Personality Inventories, twenty-one Shipley Hartford Institute of Living examinations, twenty-six Food Attitude Scales, twenty Draw-a-Person tests, and twenty-six Biographical Data Sheets were administered and scored. Although their mean MMPI profile fit no known actuarial code, super-obese females were more likely to demonstrate psychopathology as manifested by MMPI personality scale elevations than a control population. An analysis of the super-obese mean MMPI profile was performed by an automated technique and the computer "print-out" was presented. The Shipley IQ and CQ results indicated that neither a deficit in general intelligence nor an impairment in abstract thinking could account for the development of extreme obesity in the group as a whole. FAS results showed our subjects held negative or relatively unpleasant attitudes toward food. It was inferred from the DAP productions that many of the subjects demonstrated disturbances in body-image and sexual identification and that the drawings reflected immaturity and dependency. The BDS suggested that the subjects often experienced their early years as unpleasant and that level of formal education did not appear to be a significant factor in the development of corpulence. They also admitted a high incidence of physical complaints and hospital admissions.

Developmental histories accreted over twenty-seven months of group psychotherapy indicated that many of the subjects suffered as impairment of "individuation" as a result of perturbed early object relationships and that learning in the formative years played a role in the pathogenesis of food-intake dyscontrol. Group psychotherapy was jeopardized and not infrequently terminated because of inadequate treatment motivation. Progress in therapy was very slow and signalled not by weight loss but by an improvement in life adjustment.

REFERENCES

1. American Psychiatric Association: *Diagnostic and Statistical Manual: Mental Disorders.* Washington, D. C., 1952.
2. Byrne, D., Golightly, Carole and Capaldi, E. J.: Construction and validation of the food attitude scale. *J Consult Psychol*, 27:215-222, 1963.

3. Duncan, G. G., Cristofori, F. C., Yue, J. K. and Murthy, M. S. J.: The control of obesity by intermittent fasts. *Med Clin N Am*, 48:1359-1372, 1964.

4. Erikson, H.: *Identity and the Life Cycle*. N. Y., International Universities Press, 1959. (Psychological Issues, V. 1, no. 1, Monograph 1.)

5. Ferstenfeld, J.: Surgical treatment of obesity. *Minnesota Med*, 48:1057-1061, 1965.

6. Fink, Geraldine, Gottesfeld, H. and Glickman, L.: The "superobese" patient. *J Hillside Hosp*, 11:97-119, 1962.

7. Gilberstadt, H. and Duker, Jan: *A Handbook for Clinical and Actuarial MMPI Interpretation*. Philadelphia, Saunders, 1965.

8. Gordon, S.: New concepts of the biochemistry and physiology of obesity. *Med Clin N Am*, 48:1285-1305, 1964.

9. Hacker, F. J.: Treatment motivation. *Bull Menninger Clin*, 26:288-298, 1962.

10. Hathaway, S. R. and McKinley, J. C.: *The Minnesota Multiphasic Personality Inventory; Manual*. Rev. ed. New York, Psychological Corp., 1951.

11. Kansas University Medical Center: *Analysis of Hospital Service*. Kansas City, Kansas, 1964.

12. Machover, K. A.: *Personality Projection in the Drawings of the Human Figure: A Method of Personality Investigation*. Springfield, Ill., Thomas, 1949.

13. Marks, P. A. and Seeman, W.: *Actuarial Description of Abnormal Personality: An Atlas for Use with the MMPI*. Baltimore, Williams and Wilkins, 1963.

14. Mendelson, M. and Stunkard, A. J.: Obesity and the body image. Paper read at the 21st meeting of the Psychosomatic Society, San Francisco, April 5, 1964.

15. Pearson, J. S., Swenson, W. M., Rome, H. P., Mataya, P. and Brannick, T. L.: Further experience with the automated Minnesota Multiphasic Personality Inventory. *Proc Mayo Clin*, 39:823-829, 1964.

16. Schiff, S. B. and Reivich, R. S.: Use of television as aid to psychotherapy supervision. *Arch Gen Psychiat*, 10:84-88, 1964.

17. Shipley, W. C.: A self-administering scale for measuring intellectual impairment and deterioration. *J Psychol*, 9:371-377, 1940.

18. Society of Actuaries: Build and blood pressure study, Chicago, 1959. V. 1.

19. Swenson, W. M.: The test. In: Symposium on automation technics in personality assessment. *Proc Mayo Clin*, 37:65-72, 1962.

20. Thorn, G. W. and Bondy, P. K.: Gain and loss of weight. In: Harrison, T. R. *et al.* (Eds.), *Principles of Internal Medicine*, 4th ed. N. Y., McGraw-Hill, 1962, pp. 187-201.

21. Welsh, G. S. and Dahlstrom, W. G. (Eds.) *Basic Readings on the MMPI in Psychology and Medicine*. Minneapolis, U. Minn. Press, 1956.

22. Wilmer, A.: Transference to a medical center—a cultural dimension in healing. *Calif Med*, 96:173-180, 1962.

23. Winnicott, D. W.: Transitional objects and transitional phenomena. In: Winnicott, D. W., Collected papers. *Through Pediatrics to Psycho-analysis*. N. Y., Basic Books, 1958, pp. 229-242.

X
PSYCHOSES

29

Weight Changes with Schizophrenic Psychosis and Psychotropic Drug Therapy

J. M. C. Holden

AND

U. P. Holden

VARIATIONS in weight which occur during psychotic episodes and during the treatment of schizophrenic and manic-depressive psychosis are well recognized. Though there have been convincing studies to suggest that water and ion shifts are responsible for weight changes in the affective psychoses,[1, 2] there is still considerable speculation as to the mechanisms subserving weight changes in schizophrenia. One explanation is that weight variations are dependent on variations in food intake, motor activity, or agitation.[3, 4] Other studies suggest that weight gain in schizophrenic in-patients is also due to interaction effects of hospitalization or psychotropic drugs themselves.[3-6] It has been shown, however, that weight loss can precede overt signs of psychosis and occur before refusal of food intake, appetite change, or the development of increased motor activity or agitation.[7] Likewise, increases in weight may occur during treatment before psychotic symptoms themselves show improvement.[7-9] These observations suggest the possibility that factors other than variations in appetite, motor behavior, or drug therapy are involved, and that weight changes may be closely associated with basic pathological processes.[7, 10, 15] There have been few controlled studies in which weight and detailed clinical changes have been followed in groups of schizophrenic patients over long observation periods. In this study, weight and clinical changes were analyzed in a group of male schizophrenic patients who followed a pattern of on-drug and off-drug periods of eight weeks over fourteen months. The main objectives of the study were to compare the psychopathological, psychosomatic, physical, and electroencephalographical effects of chlordiazepoxide, thioridazine, and a combination of these drugs given in half-dosage to a chronic schizophrenic population. Full details of these studies are reported elsewhere.[16, 18]

MATERIAL AND METHODS

The findings of this study are based on observations of twenty-two male patients with a diagnosis of chronic schizophrenia. Their subtypes included hebephrenic (7), paranoid (6), catatonic (1), and chronic undifferentiated (8). Their mean age was thirty-three years (range 19 to 44 years), and average length of present hospitalization was 4.1 (range 1 to 10 years). The average length of illness for the group was eight years (range 5 to 16 years). Sixteen were white and six black. All were actively psychotic and none had improved sufficiently with previous treatments to be discharged from the hospital. All were free of any neurological or systemic disease, mental deficiency, or psychopathy.

The patients were randomly divided into three groups, each group following a different pattern of medication sequence (Table 29-I). Each medication period of eight weeks was separated by eight weeks of placebo, and the sequence of treatments was staggered so that each group began treatment in the study four weeks after the other.

The drugs and placebo were made up in identical capsules and the former were administered on a mg/kg body weight basis, each patient receiving 1 mg/kg chlordiazepoxide; 5 mg/kg thioridazine; or the combination of 0.5 mg/kg chlordiazepoxide and 2.5 mg/kg thioridazine. The daily dose ranges, therefore, were 60 to 100 mg chlordiazepoxide; 300 to 500 mg thioridazine and a combination of 30 to 50 mg chlordiazepoxide and 150 to 250 mg thioridazine. The study was structured on a double-blind crossover basis, with a physician from another ward arranging changes in medication. No other medications were used apart from paraldehyde or chloral hydrate, and these only when definitely indicated to cope with disabling agitation, restlessness, etc.

All patients remained on the same ward and under the supervision of the same medical and nursing staff during the fourteen-month study period. All were subject to the same environmental effects, and diets and dining facilities were the same for all. The whole Institute was air conditioned so that the temperature remained steady within a 2 to 10 F range.

All patients were rated globally at the end of each eight-week period on a 7-point scale (absence of symptoms = 1; severe psychosis = 7). Therefore, if a rating of 7 changed to 4 in the next period, this would indicate a change score of plus 3.

During placebo and drug periods, individual psychopathological items were scored every two weeks using the Missouri Institute of Psychiatry psychopathological and psychosomatic rating scales[19] of 132 single symptoms divided into eleven clusters. Three symptom clusters and eight single symptoms for each drug and placebo period were analyzed for this study. The symptom clusters were disturbance of thought content (covering ideas of influence, reference, and persecution, paranoid delusions, and dereistic thinking); disturbance of association (covering confusion, rigidity of thinking, thought paucity, thought blocking, ambivalence, and asyndesis); and disturbance of perception (covering auditory and visual hal-

TABLE 29-I

THIORIDAZINE-CHLORDIAZEPOXIDE ALONE AND COMBINED
SEQUENCE OF DRUG ADMINISTRATION

Consecutive Eight-Week Periods

Group I (N = 8)	Placebo	Chlordiazepoxide	Placebo	Combined T + C	Placebo	Thioridazine
Group II (N = 7)	Placebo	Combined T + C	Placebo	Thioridazine	Placebo	Chlordiazepoxide
Group III (N = 7)	Placebo	Thioridazine	Placebo	Chlordiazepoxide	Placebo	Combined T + C

Double-blind drug administration sequence of Latin square design for twenty-two chronic schizophrenic patients.

lucinations). The single symptoms included motor activity (increase and decrease), apathy, depression, agitation, emotional lability, drive, confusion, and appetite. A 5-point scale was used (0 = absent, 1 = suspicious or slight, 2 = present, 3 = marked, 4 = not applicable). Each rating was based on psychopathological and psychosomatic changes noted during the previous week as well as interview impressions. The BPRS scale[20] was also scored at the end of each eight-week period, and scoring was based on the clinical picture at that time. For analysis, four clusters of this scale were considered: thinking disturbance (including conceptual disorganization, hallucinatory behavior, and unusual thought content); paranoid reaction (including hostility, suspiciousness, and uncooperativeness); withdrawal reaction (including emotional withdrawal, motor retardation, and inappropriate affect); and depressive reaction (including anxiety, guilt feelings, tension, and depressive mood).

Clinical laboratory screening was performed every two weeks for hematology and serum chemistry. The mean hemoglobin values during the latter half of each drug period were calculated for each patient. Thus, at least two, and sometimes three, mean values were obtained for each patient for each period. The values for other laboratory items, including cholesterol, were calculated in a similar manner for each period.

Patients were weighed in indoor clothing before breakfast and after voiding. The same scales were used on each occasion and weights taken on the same morning of each week during the fourteen-month study period. Percentage weight changes for each drug and placebo period were then derived for each patient. Both absolute and percentage weight change values were used in analysis.

RESULTS

At the beginning of the study, average weight for the group was 165 lb, with a range of 114 to 252 lb (S.D. = 27). At the end of the study (fourteen months later), the average weight was 164 lb, with a range of 126 to 224 lb (S.D. = 22). Initial weights were compared with the Metropolitan Life Insurance Company tables of age, weight, and build.[21] Twelve patients were above the maximum of the desirable range, with an average weight excess of 18 lb. Ten patients were within the normal range, and the average group deviation was 9.5 lb overweight. There were no significant correlations between patient age and being overweight. Nor did length of illness and last hospitalization values show any significant relationships to weight. Fifteen of the group had previously received chlorpromazine and the others trifluoperazine, thioridazine, imipramine, and chlordiazepoxide. There were no correlations between previous drug treatment and initial weights.

Global Clinical Changes Versus Weight Changes During Placebo Treatment

There was an average loss of 5 lb for the total population during all the placebo periods, but weight losses were greatest during the first placebo period. The average loss for each period was 7½ lb (first period), 4½ lb (second period), and 1 lb (third period).

Only three patients showed clinical improvement during the placebo period according to global change scores, two following chlordiazepoxide (with weight gains of 3 and 9 lb) and one following combined therapy (with no change in weight). There were twenty-six instances of 0 to −2 change scores. The average weight loss with these scores was 2½ lb. There were thirty-two instances of −4 and −5 change scores, accompanied by an average weight loss of 7½ lb.

Thus, the tendency was to lose weight with overall clinical deterioration, and the more marked the deterioration, the greater the loss in weight. This was significant at the < .01 level of confidence.

During Drug Treatment

The global clinical changes were combined for all three drug treatment periods and plotted against percentage weight changes. The results were similar to those for the placebo periods. Greater degrees of improvement were usually accompanied by greater gains in weight, and this was significant at the < .01 level of confidence. Both clinical and weight changes with chlordiazepoxide were small and variable. The average weight change for nine patients with change scores of 0 to +2 during thioridazine treatment was +6 lb, and for thirteen patients with change scores of +3 to +5, 8½ lb. With combined treatment, nineteen patients who showed improvement on the basis of change scores had an average weight increase of 11 lb. Eight patients with 0 to +2 change scores had an average weight gain of 5 lb; thirteen patients who had change scores of +3 to +5 showed an average gain in weight of 11 lb.

Analyses of changes in weight and global clinical change scores for each drug individually showed no statistically significant correlations. This may well have been due to the small sample size and the relatively short treatment periods.

With thioridazine and combined treatment, weight tended to increase steadily over the eight-week period, though there were some instances of sharp increases during the first two weeks of drug administration. Likewise, weight losses on placebo tended to be gradual and steady, with a few instances of rapid loss.

Symptoms Changes Versus Weight Changes During Placebo Treatment

The relationship of weight changes to changes in psychopathology is shown in Table 29-II. When the values for all placebo periods were considered, two symptom clusters (associative and perceptual disturbances) showed significant inverse correlations with weight changes. Motor activity, apathy, and confusion also showed a significant inverse correlation with weight changes. There were no significant correlations between increase in scores and weight changes for any of the items in the placebo period following chlordiazepoxide. The only item showing a significant relationship between symptom and weight scores in the placebo period following thioridazine was agitation; increase in scores covering agitation was associated with decreases in weight ($P = < .03$: Sign Test). The clinical change scores of four items (associative disturbance, thought content disturbance, per-

TABLE 29-II

SYMPTOM CHANGE SCORES VERSUS PERCENTAGE WEIGHT CHANGES
(P VALUES) PEARSON SIMPLE CORRELATION ANALYSIS

Symptom	Placebo N = 44	Chlordiaze- poxide N = 22	Thioridazine N = 22	Chlordiazepoxide/ Thioridazine Combined N = 22	All Drugs N = 66
Associative Dist.	< .01(−)		< .05(−)		< .01(−)
Thought Content Dist.					< .01(−)
Perceptual Dist.	< .05(−)				< .01(−)
Motor Activity	< .05(−)				
Apathy	< .01(−)				< .05(−)
Depression					
Agitation			< .01(−)		
Emotional Lability					< .05(−)
Drive		< .01(+)	< .05(−)		
Confusion	< .01(−)		< .05(−)	< .01(−)	< .01(−)
Appetite					

(+) = Positive correlation
(−) = Negative correlation

Changes in individual symptoms and symptom clusters versus percentage weight changes with placebo, each drug alone, drugs in combination, and all drugs taken together. The significant negative correlations with weight changes are particularly noteworthy during placebo administration and when all drug therapies are combined.

ceptual disturbance, and motor activity) during placebo treatment following combined therapy showed a significant correlation with weight decrease ($P < .001$: Sign Test).

During Drug Treatment

The relationship of weight changes to the changes in symptom scores with each drug is also shown in Table 29-II. Apart from a positive correlation with drive, there were no significant relationships between changes in symptom scores and weight for any of the items during chlordiazepoxide treatment.

One cluster and three items (associative disturbance, agitation, drive, and confusion) showed a significant relationship between decrease in scores and increase in weight with thioridazine. Only one item (confusion) showed a significant inverse relationship between symptom and weight changes during combined treatment.

When the changes with all drugs were compared, there were significant inverse correlations in three clusters (associative, thought content, and perceptual disturbances) and three symptoms (apathy, emotional lability, and confusion).

When decreases only in symptom scores during drug therapy were compared with associated weight changes (Sign Test), associative, thought content, and perceptual disturbances showed a significant inverse association with weight increase ($P < .001$). Motor behavior ($P < .001$), apathy ($P < .01$), and depression ($P < .04$) were also related inversely.

BPRS Scores and Weight Changes

Comparative analyses of the four clusters of the BPRS were performed for placebo and drug periods. These are shown in Table 29-III. During

TABLE 29-III

PERCENTAGE WEIGHT CHANGES AND BPRS CHANGE SCORES
SPEARMAN RANK ORDER CORRELATIONS

	Thinking Disturbance Cluster	Paranoid Reaction Cluster	Withdrawal Reaction Cluster	Depressive Reaction Cluster
Placebo	Correl. −.291056 (P < .08)	Correl. −.312274 (P < .05)	N.S.	N.S.
Chlordiazepoxide	N.S.	N.S.	N.S.	N.S.
Thioridazine	N.S.	N.S.	N.S.	N.S.
Chlordiazepoxide/ Thioridazine Combined	Correl. −.564265 (P < .01)	Correl. −.443801 (P < .05)	N.S.	N.S.

Percentage weight changes versus change scores in the B.P.R.S. are shown using Spearman rank order correlations. Two clusters—thinking disturbance and paranoid reaction—show significant inverse correlations, and these during placebo administration, and when the drugs were given in combination.

placebo and combined treatment there was a significant correlation between percentage weight change and factor score changes for the thinking disturbance and paranoid reaction clusters. The results with chlordiazepoxide and thioridazine were not significant. The changes with both placebo and all drugs for the withdrawal and depressive clusters were also not significant (Table 29-III).

All the items in the thinking disturbance and paranoid reaction clusters of the BPRS are prominent in the schizophrenic illness, and the significant inverse relationships with weight change were in keeping with the results derived from our own rating scale.

Diagnostic Groupings and Weight Changes

Weight changes were examined in relation to diagnostic groupings. The only patients to show a gain in weight with chlordiazepoxide were those in the paranoid group (average gain of 4½ lb). The hebephrenic patients gained more weight with individual treatment than any other group, and this with combined treatment (average of 15½ lb). There were no other noteworthy relationships between diagnostic subgroups and weight change.

Variations in Weight with Age Group

The subjects were divided into three age groups: Group I, 19 to 27 years (seven patients); Group II, 28 to 35 years (six patients); and Group III, 36 years and over (nine patients). With chlordiazepoxide, Group I patients averaged a loss of 5½ lb, Group II, a loss of 2 lb; and Group III, a gain of 1 lb ($P < .01$). With thioridazine, all Group I patients gained weight (average 12½ lb), Group II had an average gain of 5 lb, and Group III an average gain of 3 lb. With combined treatment, all patients in Group I gained weight (average 10½ lb); all but one in Group II gained weight (average 11 lb); and all of Group III gained weight (average 7½ lb). These changes were not statistically significant. However, definite tendencies were demonstrated in this analysis. With chlordiazepoxide, the older the patient, the greater the tendency to gain weight. With thioridazine and combined treatment, however, the greater gains in weight occurred in the younger patients.

Hemoglobin Shifts and Weight Changes

There were no significant correlations during chlordiazepoxide treatment between hemoglobin shifts and changes in weight. Hemoglobin shifts with weight changes for thioridazine and combined treatment are shown in Table 29-IV. Complete serial values were obtained in eleven patients. In the placebo period prior to thioridazine, there was an increase of mean hemoglobin values for this group over the preceding drug period, and this was accompanied by a loss in weight in all instances except one.

TABLE 29-IV

WEIGHT CHANGES VERSUS HEMOGLOBIN CHANGES MEAN SCORES

Placebo		*Thioridazine*	*Placebo*
Weight change	–6½ lb	+10 lb	–0.3 lb
Hemoglobin change	+1.8 gm%	–1 gm%	+0.2 gm%
Placebo		*Combined Treatment*	*Placebo*
Weight change	–1 lb	+8½ lb	–7½ lb
Hemoglobin change	–0.1 gm%	–1.4 gm	+1.9 gm%

Spearman rank correlation: –.691727 for raw scores. Overall P value < .01.
Analysis of weight changes versus changes in hemoglobin concentration during placebo and drug administration using Spearman rank correlation. Inverse correlations between weight and hemoglobin changes are shown for placebo, thioridazine, and combined drug treatment.

With thioridazine, all but one patient had a drop in hemoglobin values and all but two had a corresponding gain in weight. During the following placebo period, there were again inverse shifts in hemoglobin and weight. A similar pattern occurred with the combination of drugs; only one patient who lost weight with the drug showed a decrease in hemoglobin values.

Hematocrit changes followed a similar sequence for both thioridazine and combined treatment.

Cholesterol Values and Weight Changes

Eleven of fourteen patients during thioridazine therapy had an average cholesterol decrease of 42 mg per cent with a corresponding average gain in weight of 9.8 lb. One patient had an increase in cholesterol with a gain in weight. With the combination therapy, eleven of twelve patients showed an average increase of 17 mg per cent cholesterol with an average gain in weight of 8 lb. The other patient showed a decrease in cholesterol with a gain in weight. The changes with chlordiazepoxide were small and inconsistent.

There were no correlations between other laboratory values and weight changes.

DISCUSSION

Obesity in psychiatric hospital populations on tranquilizers is well known and is considered to be a serious complication of psychotropic drug therapy.[6, 13, 22] Hospital diet, physical inactivity, and the psychological and physical shelter provided by hospitalization probably play some part in this. Length of illness and hospitalization and type of drug used prior to the study did not appear to have been important factors in differences in initial weight in this study. It is interesting to note that at the initiation of this study, ten of our twenty-two patients were within the desirable range of weight cited by the Metropolitan Life Insurance Company; and the average excess for the whole group was only 9½ lb, a figure probably comparable to that for a normal population at the present. The comparison of the initial and final weights is interesting because the group as a whole showed no gross changes. The results are in keeping with observations that lighter patients can show marked changes in weight as well as heavier patients. The overall weight variations suggest that pathological obesity in hospital populations is overstressed. Rather, the question why some patients become obese and others do not merit full biochemical investigation on an individual basis.

There are at least three possible explanations for weight changes in hospitalized schizophrenics. First, some workers have suggested that weight increase may be due to an improvement in well-being and appetite and reduced agitation and restlessness which often follow hospitalization, as well as hospital diet itself.[3, 4] It would, therefore, be a secondary phenomenon. Second, weight increase or decrease could be associated with alleviation or worsening of psychosis and thus be an expression of the basic pathological disease process.[7, 10, 12-15] Both Kraepelin and Bleuler supported this viewpoint.[8, 9] The studies by Crammer,[11] Gjessing,[12] and Rowntree and Kay[7] demonstrated a sensitive relationship between weight gain and loss and intensity of psychosis in individual patients with periodic catatonia. The controlled studies by Planansky in groups of schizophrenic patients led him to conclude that weight increase in these patients was at least partially dependent on psychiatric improvement and that the greater the clinical improvement, the greater the gain in weight.[13, 14] Alstrom's extensive studies of chronic schizophrenics of different diagnostic sub-types suggested that weight changes were an expression of the basic pathological process in those patients with catatonia or a "cerebral" type of illness.[10] It was speculated that water and ionic shifts during psychotic episodes could explain these fluctuations in weight.[11, 13] Third, where psychotropic drugs have been used in therapy, weight increase or decrease could be primarily due to psychotropic drug effect on certain central nervous or neuro-endocrine mechanisms and, if so, would occur irrespective of changes in the psychosis.[24, 25] Such mechanisms are obscure but may involve changes in the neuro-regulation of appetite,[23] or be due to hormone-induced shifts in sodium and water in the body.[24, 25]

The overall findings of this study suggest that variations in appetite, agitation, or motor behavior are not always solely responsible for variations in weight. There are limitations, however, in trying to correlate changes in appetite with weight variations. Appetite is a difficult factor to assess unless all food and fluid intake are measured. Absolute control of dietary intake over prolonged periods of time is an ideal situation difficult to apply in psychotic populations. The assessment of changes of appetite and intake in this study depended on simple observation on the part of the staff and the behavior and remarks of the patient. However, in a prolonged study of this nature, the staff got to know their patients well and were very sensitive to any change in patient behavior and habits. All observations were carefully noted on a standard rating scale at regular intervals on a blind basis.[19] Psychotherapy was always rated at the same time, thus eliminating the variable of a time discrepancy factor.

The clinical and weight correlations of our study are in keeping with previous observations that variations in weight may be an expression of the basic illness.[7-12, 15] The results with both our own rating scale and the BPRS scale support this. Studies have been reported in animals to show that the frontal and temporal lobes affect hunger and appetive drives, and that disturbances in both of these areas can produce psychotic symptoms.[26] Likewise, diencephalic lesions lead to appetite and weight changes.[26, 27] There were no significant changes in appetite in this study, but homeostatic changes of fronto-hypothalamic and temporo-hypothalamic connections with centers in the hypothalamus and hypothalamic pituitary axis could be responsible for changes in psychosis and metabolic and neuroendocrine changes at the same time.

On the other hand, psychotropic drug-induced sodium retention or increase in ADH production may be associated with water retention and weight increase, suggesting a mechanical mechanism for variations in weight.[24, 25] This may be dose-related, but this variable was minimized in this study by drug administration on a mg/kg body weight basis. It may be that psychotropic drugs affect centers regulating weight, water, salt, and glucose metabolism at the same time as they affect those pathways subserving the psychosis.[28-30] However, the most striking feature in this study was the high correlation between degree of weight change, global clinical change, and changes in both primary and florid schizophrenic symptomatology. With chlordiazepoxide treatment, both weight and clinical changes were small. More marked effects were seen with thioridazine, but combined treatment produced more changes in both global clinical improvement and weight than either of the other two. It is not plausible to assume weight increases were due to mechanical effects of thioridazine itself, since thioridazine and chlordiazepoxide were given in half doses when combined. Few significant relationships between weight changes and individual psychopathological items were seen when individual drugs were considered; the small population size was probably responsible for this since many reached near significance levels. When all drugs were considered together, significant relationship could then be seen. Likewise, many significant relationships between losses in weight and clinical deterioration were evident when all scores during placebo treatment were considered. These findings are indicative that weight changes are an expression of the basic disease process, irrespective of the influences of other factors.

Variations in blood hemoglobin concentration in untreated schizophrenics have been reported previously.[7, 31] They have also been reported with psychotropic drug therapy.[32, 33] According to Wintrobe, the hypothalamus may play some part in hematopoiesis, and changes in endocrine homeostasis are often effected in changes in the blood picture.[34] A direct drug influence on these systems could be responsible for hemoglobin and hematocrit shifts. A consistent correlation in this study between hemoglobin changes and variations in weight suggests that either a mechanical factor was involved in the form of water retention and hemodilution mediated by drug via neuroendocrine mechanisms, or that changes in hypothalamic homeostasis as part of the psychosis were responsible. Another possibility is that these changes were the result of drug action directly at marrow level. There was no conclusive evidence in this study that one of these mechanisms was operating to the exclusion of the others. However, changes in the homeostasis of the hypothalamic-pituitary axis could explain changes in weight psychopathology as well as the hemoglobin shifts.

The normal wide variation in serum cholesterol do not make cholesterol estimations a reliable index for comparative analysis unless the estimations cover a long observation period, and the results can only be accepted in this light. The only meaningful findings were the weight increases associated with cholesterol decreases during thioridazine treatment. These findings are contrary to the results of other investigations of psychotropic drug action.[35] Whether this association is due to the drug effect alone or to metabolic factors is not clear, for increase in weight itself is associated with increases in serum cholesterol.[36]

If the variations in weight and hematology in our study were an expression of the severity of psychosis, one would expect there to be correlations between the resting EEG and weight changes, clinical changes, and hematological and biochemical changes. A follow-up comparative analysis of clinical, weight, EEG, and laboratory changes in patients on placebo for prolonged periods of time is in progress.

SUMMARY

This study reports changes in weight patterns in relation to psychopathology, diagnosis, and age in a group of chronic schizophrenics treated over a prolonged period of time with placebo and chlordiazepoxide, thioridazine, alone and combined. Variations in appetite, motor activity, or agitation were not consistently associated with changes in weight. Significant relationships were shown between increases in weight and improvement of psychotic symptomatology and decreases in weight and worsening of symptomatology. Various mechanisms to explain weight changes with psychosis are discussed, but the findings of this study suggest that changes in weight are an expression of the basic illness. Only paranoid patients gained weight with chlordiazepoxide. The hebephrenic patients gained more weight with individual treatment than any other group, and this with chlordiazepoxide and thioridazine combined. With chlordiazepoxide, the older the patient, the greater the tendency to gain weight. With thioridazine and combined treatment, however, the greater gains in weight occurred in the younger patients. An additional observation of the study was that weight changes were correlated inversely with hemoglobin and hematocrit shifts. These variations could also have been associated with variations in intensity of psychosis.

Further studies will attempt to delineate the relationships between weight, psychopathology, EEG, and biochemical changes.

REFERENCES

1. Coppen, A.: The biochemistry of affective disorders. *J Psychiat*, 113:1237, 1967.
2. Russell, G. F. M.: Body weight and balance of water, sodium and potassium in depressed patients given electroconvulsive therapy. *Clin Sci*, 19:327, 1960.
3. Gordon, H. L. and Groth, C.: Weight change during and after hospital treatment. *Arch Gen Psychiat*, 10:187, 1964.
4. Kurland, A. A., Bethon, G. D., Michaux, M. H. and Agallianos, D. D.: Chlorpromazine-chlordiazepoxide and chlorpromazine-imipramine treatment: Side effects and clinical laboratory findings. *J New Drugs*, 6:80, 1966.
5. Caffey, E. M.: Experience with large scale interhospital cooperative research in chemotherapy. *Am J Psychiat*, 117:713, 1960-61.
6. Amdisen, A.: Drug-produced obesity, experience with chlorpromazine, perphenazine and clopenthixol. *Dan Med Bull*, 11:182, 1960.
7. Rowntree, D. W. and Kay, W. W.: Clinical biochemical and physiological studies in cases of recurrent schizophrenia. *J Ment Sci*, 98:100, 1952.
8. Bleuler, E.: *Textbook of Psychiatry.* New York, Macmillan, 1930.
9. Kraepelin, E.: *Dementia Praecox and Paraphrenia.* Edinburgh, Livingstone, 1919.
10. Alstrom, C. H.: *Uber Gewichtsschwankungen Bei Geisteskranken.* Copenhagen, E. Munksgaard, 1943.
11. Crammer, J. L.: Rapid weight changes in mental patients. *Lancet*, 2:259, 1957.
12. Gjessing, R.: Beitrage zur Somatologie der periodischen Katatonie VII. *Arch Psychiat Nerv Krankh*, 191:247, 1953.
13. Planansky, K.: Changes in weight in patients receiving a tranquilizing drug. *Psychiat Q*, 32:289, 1958.
14. Planasky, K. and Heilizer, F.: Weight changes in relation to the characteristics of patients on chlorpromazine. *J Clin Exp Psychopathol*, 20:53, 1959.
15. Rey, J. H., Willcox, D. R. C., Gibbons, J. L., Tait, H. and Lewis, D. J.: Serial biochemical and endocrine investigations in recurrent mental illness. *J Psychosom Res*, 5:155, 1961.

16. Holden, J. M. C., Itil, T. M., Keskiner, A. and Fink, M.: Thioridazine and chlordiazepoxide, alone and combined, in the treatment of chronic schizophrenia. *Comprehens Psychiat,* 9:633, 1968.
17. Holden, J. M. C. and Itil, T. M.: Laboratory changes with chlordiazepoxide and thioridazine alone and combined. *Can Psychiat Assoc J,* 14:299, 1969.
18. Itil, T., Holden, J. M. C., Fink, M., Shapiro, D. M. and Keskiner, A.: Treatment of chronic psychotic patients with combined medications. *Exc Med Int Cong Series No. 129,* Proc. 5th Int. Cong. Coll. Int. Neuropsychopharm., Washington, 1016, 1966.
19. Itil, T. and Keskiner, A.: Psychopathological and psychosomatic rating scales. *Psychiat Res Found Mo Pub No. 12,* 1966.
20. Overall, J. E. and Gorham, D. R.: The Brief Psychiatric Rating Scale. *Psychol Rep,* 10:799, 1962.
21. Statistical Bulletin. New weight standards for men and women. Metropolitan Life Ins. Co., 40:1, 1959.
22. Lassenius, A. B. and Osterman, E.: Komplikationer vid langvarig chlorpromazin— behandling. *Nordisk Medicin,* 7:789, 1956.
23. Mefferd, R. B., Labrosse, E. H., Gawienowski, A. M. and Williams, R. J.: Influence of chlorpromazine on certain biochemical variables of chronic male schizophrenics. *J Nerv Ment Dis,* 127:167, 1958.
24. Sletten, I. and Gershon, S.: The effect of chlorpromazine on water and electrolyte balance. *J Nerv Ment Dis,* 142:25, 1966.
25. Sletten, I., Mou, B., Cazenave, M. and Gershon, S.: The effects of caloric restriction on behavior and body weight in psychiatric subjects on chlorpromazine. *Dis Nerv Syst,* 28:519, 1967.
26. Andersson, B. and Larsson, S.: Physiological and pharmacological aspects of the control of hunger and thirst. *Pharmacol Rev,* 13:1, 1961.
27. Mayer, J.: The regulation of food intake and obesity. In *Weight Control: A collection of papers presented at the weight control colloquium,* Iowa State College Press, Ames, Iowa, 16, 1955.
28. Duchesne, P. Y. and Gerebtzoff, M. S.: Modification of hypothalamic neurosecretion by a neuroleptic. In *Prog Brain Res,* Bargmann and Schade (Eds.) Elsevier Pub. Co., Amsterdam, New York, 5:157, 1964.
29. Leading Articles, The Hypothalamus. *Brit Med J,* 2:844, 1966.
30. Leibowitz, S. F.: Mechanism of unexpected adrenergic effect from hypothalamic injection of chlorpromazine. In Proceedings of the 77th Annual Convention, American Psychological Association. Vol. 4, 1969.
31. Holden, J. M. C. and Itil, T. M.: The application of automated techniques in assessing psychotropic-drug-induced side effects. *Am J Psychiat,* 125:562, 1968.
32. Holden, J. M. C., Alvarez, U. C. and Itil, T. M.: Changes in laboratory values with butaperazine. *Curr Ther Res,* 10:304, 1968.
33. Holden, J. M. C., Itil, T. M. and Keskiner, A.: Comparison of perphenazine and P-5227 in chronic schizophrenics: clinical and EEG effects. *J Clin Pharmacol,* 9:163, 1969.
34. Wintrobe, M. M.: *Clinical Hematology.* Lea and Febiger, Philadelphia, 5th ed. 48, 1961.
35. Reinhardt, D. J., Tausig, T. and Alvarez, R.: Serum cholesterol evaluation with trifluoperazine (Stelazine) therapy. *Delaware St Med J,* 318, 1962.
36. Rifkind, B. M. and Begg, T.: Relationship between relative body weight and serum lipid levels. *Br Med J,* 2:208, 1966.

30

Rapid Treatment of Gross Obesity by Operant Techniques

John L. Bernard

A MERICAN society seems almost morbidly preoccupied with problems of real, or imagined, obesity (cf. consumer demand for such products as Metrecal, dietetic soft drinks, and "No-Cal Pizza"). Successful application of behavioristic techniques to the problem of anorexia nervosa has been reported by several writers, e.g. Ayllon, *et al.*,[2] Bachrach, *et al.*,[3] and Lang,[5] yet Ferster, *et al.*[4] have noted that the problem of obesity has received considerably less attention. Ayllon[1] does report one behavior modification program in which a hospitalized schizophrenic lost 17 per cent of her original body weight over a 14-month period when her chronic food stealing was established as a discriminative stimulus for her being removed from the dining room. Ferster, *et al.*[4] have reported what they describe as a "pilot program" for weight reduction, in which they note, however: "We cannot state whether the program we carried out is suitable for severely obese individuals (particularly those who have medical or psychiatric complications)."

This chapter describes the treatment of obesity in an individual who appears to meet all of Ferster's specifications; a) "severely obese" (the patient weighed 407 pounds at the beginning of the program), b) "medical complications" (she had been previously diagnosed as having a metabolic disturbance and was believed by the staff to have indications of endocrine disturbance as well), and c) "psychiatric complications" (she was hospitalized, and diagnosed as schizophrenic reaction, simple type). Ferster, *et al.* also note: "The central issue is the development of self-control in eating which will endure and become an available part of the individual's future repertoire."

This paper also reports the results of a six-week extinction period subsequent to the treatment procedure.

The patient, a white female in her mid-twenties, was first admitted to a psychiatric hospital in 1963. She was then diagnosed as chronic brain syndrome, associated with disturbance of metabolism, and discharged (against advice) six weeks later. While no record of her weight at that time is available, the writer recalls her as being grotesquely obese. Her second admission was in 1965, at which time her diagnosis was changed to schizophrenic reaction, simple type, and she was placed on a chronic ward. Her weight at that time was 350 lb.

In 1966, the writer established an experimental behavior modification ward in the hospital and arranged to have the patient transferred there. The treatment program to be described was not initiated until after she had been on the ward for several months, by which time her weight had risen to 407 lb, in spite of the fact that the ward physician had tried her on 1800-calorie and 1000-calorie diets. This was probably attributable (as noted by the ward personnel) to the fact that the patient's family brought her large amounts of "goodies" every time they visited, took her on outings that seemed to amount to nothing more than going from candy store to soda fountain to bakery to candy store (at the patient's request) and gave her a liberal allowance, most of which she spent on candy, cookies, cokes, etc.

PROCEDURE

In essence, the program involved controlling caloric intake. This was accomplished by placing her on an 1800-calorie diet, notifying the family that she would no longer be allowed to receive "goodies" (a restriction with which they complied after a token testing of limits), and restricting her "store privileges" in order to control her consumption of high-calorie sweets. It should be noted at this point that, while such tight controls are relatively easy to maintain on a behavior modification ward, one loophole remained to be plugged.

Experience on the ward had shown that, when a patient was restricted from a privilege (e.g. cigarettes and candy), she could often induce sympathetic friends to smuggle the restricted item to her or, if this failed, purchase it from other patients on a "black market" basis, using the ward's token currency. Thus, as an additional incentive for weight loss, the patient was told that she would be weighed regularly and paid ten tokens for each pound lost. While she was restricted from using these tokens at the ward store, they could be exchanged for such things as "walkout privileges," telephone calls, admission to dances, recreational events and movies, and for rent on a semi-private, or private room on the ward. During the months the ward had been in operation before the procedure was initiated, these tokens had gained clear status as a powerful secondary reinforcer, and the patient's earning power had thus far been relatively undistinguished.

The patient was weighed (a procedure that necessitated her standing on a board stretched across two 300-lb capacity medical scales) just prior to breakfast three days a week (Monday, Wednesday, and Friday) and paid on the spot for weight lost; payments often amounted to as much as fifty tokens at a time, on a ward where the average patient's "income" was about twenty-five tokens per day.

The extinction procedure involved returning her store privileges, while terminating payment for weight lost. The 1000-calorie diet initiated at Week 18 was continued, and the family was not informed that they might once more bring "goodies." (To have reinstated this aspect of the pre-treatment situation would have only served to confuse the family, and parenthetically, they had already informed the ward personnel that the patient no longer asked to be taken to candy stores, etc., when on outings.) Further, the patient was given a brief pep talk on the morning extinction began, informing her that she would continue to be weighed but would no longer be paid for weight lost. She was advised that her store privileges were being returned and encouraged to assume responsibility for controlling her own weight. This eliminated the most significant restrictions on caloric intake, and all reinforcement for weight loss, aside from the social reinforcement of compliments from ward personnel and other patients. The return of store privileges, while removing the patient's major source of income, may seem a hollow gesture, but it should be noted that she had accumulated several hundred tokens during the treatment period, and thus was one of the "wealthiest" patients on the ward.

RESULTS

During the first seventeen weeks of the procedure the patient's weight dropped from 407 to 337 lb, a loss of approximately 20 per cent of her initial body weight, at a rate of almost 4½ lb per week. It is notable that this matches the weight lost by Ayllon's patient over a 14-month interval. As no adverse physical reactions (e.g. dehydration) had been noted, her diet was reduced to 1000 calories per day, and the procedure continued. During the next three weeks she dropped to 318 lb; a loss of 19 lb at a rate of over 6 lb per week. This brought the total weight lost during the twenty-week treatment period to 89 lb; a loss of 22 per cent of initial body weight at a rate of 4½ lb per week.

Extinction began on the first Monday following the Friday on which the treatment procedure was terminated, by which time the patient's weight had risen from 318 to 323 lb. Over the subsequent six weeks she dropped to 305 lb, representing 18 lb lost over six weeks at a rate of 3 lb per week. While the rate during this period was more erratic than during the treatment period, there is no apparent tendency toward reversal of the trend.

The results obtained appear to indicate that the possibility of endocrine or metabolic dysfunction need not contraindicate a weight control program of this kind. Further, they reinforce Ayllon's[1] finding that severe obesity and "psychiatric complications" are not barriers to this approach. The fact that this patient lost weight at a rate almost four times that of Ayllon's patient may be attributable in part to the fact that her initial weight was considerably higher, but it also suggests that a program including positive reinforcement for weight loss is more effective than one which only controls caloric intake. Once this program was established, it required very little attention from staff or ward personnel. Since the diets in many state hospitals contain a preponderance of starchy foods, and weight control is a common problem, it seems that this sort of program might easily be adapted for larger populations (i.e. all patients on the ward who are overweight).

REFERENCES

1. Ayllon, T.: Intensive treatment of psychotic behavior by stimulus satiation and food reinforcement. *Behav Res Ther*, 1:53-61, 1963.
2. Ayllon, T., Haughton, E. and Osmond, H.: Chronic anorexia: A behavior problem. *Canad J Psychiat*, 9:147-154, 1964.
3. Bachrach, A. J., Erwin, W. J. and Mohr, J. P.: The control of eating behavior in an anorexic by operant techniques. In L. P. Ullmann and L. Krasner (Eds.): *Case Studies in Behavior Modification*. New York, Holt, Rinehart and Winston, p. 153-164, 1966.
4. Ferster, C. B., Nurnberger, J. I., and Levitt, E. B.: The control of eating. *J Math*, 1:87-109, 1962.
5. Lang, P. J.: Behavior therapy with a case of nervous anorexia. In L. P. Ullmann and L. Krasner (Eds.): *Case Studies in Behavior Modification*. New York, Holt, Rinehart and Winston, p. 217-222, 1966.

Bibliography

A S evidence of the massive effort bent in the direction of coping with obesity in humans, the bibliography prepared below deals with the relationship between obesity and psychiatry and psychology: dynamics, etiology, symptomatology, and therapy as it affects the lives of children, adolescents, adults, and psychotics.

Approximately 1,000 items are listed. While no presumption is made for completeness, every effort was directed to include all publications in the field printed between 1930-1971. Among the sources searched were the *Psychological Abstracts*, the *Index Medicus, Quarterly Index Medicus, The Index to Psychoanalytic Writings, Excerpta Medica (Psychiatry; Neurology and Psychiatry; Public Health, Social Medicine and Hygiene; Human Genetics; Physiology), Dissertation Abstracts, Sociological Abstracts, International Nursing Index, Abstracts for Social Workers, inter alia.*

The bibliography is divided into eleven categories, following the chapter order of the book, with one additional section, "Reviews of the Literature."

I must here express grateful thanks to Mrs. Shirley Schneer, a former graduate student in the School Psychology Program at Brooklyn College, for her help in retrieving the data and to her husband for his help in typing the first draft of the bibliography.

I. DYNAMICS AND ETIOLOGY

Abadi, M.: Nota acerca de algunos mecanismos en la psicogénesis de la obesidad. *Revista de Psicoanálisis*, 13:296-304, 1956.

Abadi, M.: *Del significado de algunas aspectos psicologicos en la obesidad.* Buenos Aires, Author, 1956.

Abraham, K.: The influence of oral eroticism on character formation. In *Selected Papers*. London, Hogarth, 1948.

Anand, B. K.: Nervous regulation of food intake. *Physiological Review*, 41:677-708, 1961.

Arné, L.: Obésité neurogène et psychogène. *Journal de Médecine de Bordeaux et du Sud-Ouest*, 134:78-81, 1957.

Babcock, C.: Food and its emotional significance. *Journal of the American Dietetic Association*, 24:390, 1948.

Bare, J. K.: *A detailed analysis of eating behavior*. U. S. Department of Health, Education and Welfare, Mental Health Research Grant, RO3-MH-0132901, 1963.

Bayer, L. M. and Reichard, S.: Androgyny, weight, and personality. *Psychosomatic Medicine*, 13:358-374, 1951.

Benedek, T.: Dominant ideas and their relationship to morbid cravings. *International Journal of Psycho-Analysis*, 17:1936.

Beneditte, G.: Obesity and thinness: Borderline between psychopathology and endocrinology, *Schweizerische Medizinische Wochenschrift*, 80:1129-1135, 1950.

Berblinger, K. W.: Obesity—Psychologic stress: A cause or a result. *Psychiatric Opinion*, 7:31-36; In N. L. Wilson (Ed.): *Obesity*. Philadelphia, Davis, 1969.

Bergler, E.: Psychoanalytic aspects of the personality of the obese. *Diseases of the Nervous System*, 18:196-198, 1957.

Bernhardt, H.: Nature of obesity: Contribution to energetics of human organism. *Deutsches Medizinisches Journal*, 6:40-42, 1955.

Berryman, G. H.: "Simple" obesity: Current review. *Journal of the American Dietetic Association*, 31:347-358, 1955.

Bigsby, F. L. and Muniz, C.: Medical management of the tension night eater. *Illinois Medical Journal*, 132:306-309, 1967.

Bigsby, F. L. and Muniz, C.: The varied role of motivation in obesity. *Illinois Medical Journal*, 121:632-635, 1962.

Blaise, E.: Inhibición de la expresión proyective de la agresión. Regresión. Obesidad. Análisis de la fantasía basica. *Revista de Psicoanálisis*, 13:53-57, 1956.

Blazer, A.: The obese character: Psychodynamics and psychotherapy as an adjunct to medical management. *International Record of Medicine*, 164:24-30, 1951.

Bleuler, M.: "Psychosomatik" fer Fettsucht. *Helvetica Medica Acta*, 19:293-308, 1952.

Blix, G. (Ed.): *Occurrence, causes and prevention of overnutrition*. Second Symposium of the Swedish Nutrition Foundation. Uppsala, Almqvist and Wiksells, 1964.

Block, R.: On the importance of the death wish in psychogenic disorders of the food instinct. *Zeitschrift für Psychosomatische Medizin und Psychoanalyse*, 13:63-69, 1967.

Bram, I.: Psychosomatic obesity, with comments on 924 cases. *Medical Record*, 157:673-676, 1944.

Brobeck, J. R.: Neural regulation of food intake. *Annals of the New York Academy of Science*, 63:6, 1955.

Brobeck, J. R., Winegrad, A., Feinstein, A. and Stunkard, A. J.: Obesity. *American Practitioner*, 12:543, 1961.

Brosin, H. W.: Psychiatric aspects of obesity. *Journal of the American Medical Association*, 155:1238-1239, 1954.

Brosin, H. W.: The psychology of overeating. In R. S. Goodhart (Ed.): *Overeating, Overweight and Obesity*. New York National Vitamin Foundation, 52-69, 1953.

Brosin, H. W.: Symposium on obesity. Psychology of overeating (including reference

398 *The Psychology of Obesity*

to a case of alternating anorexia and obesity). *New England Journal of Medicine*, 248:974-975, 1953.

Bruch, H.: Conceptual confusion in eating disorders. *Journal of Nervous and Mental Disease*, 133:46-54, 1961.

Bruch, H.: Discussion of obesity: Psychological and physiological aspects of marked obesity in a young adult female. *Journal of the Hillside Hospital*, 8:200-206, 1959.

Bruch, H.: Disturbed communication in eating disorders. *American Journal of Orthopsychiatry*, 33:99-104, 1963.

Bruch, H.: Eating disorders. *Forest Hospital Publications*, 1:9-15, 1962.

Bruch, H.: How psychology can help the overweight patient. *The Physician's Panorama*, 4:4-10, 1966.

Bruch, H.: Hunger and instinct. *Journal of Nervous and Mental Disease*, 149:91-114, 1969.

Bruch, H.: *The Importance of Overweight*. New York, Norton, 1957.

Bruch, H.: Neuro-psychological disturbances in obesity. *Psychiatry Digest*, 27:37-41, 1966.

Bruch, H.: Obesity. *Pediatric Clinics of North America*, 613-627, 1958.

Bruch, H.: Obesity. In *International Encyclopedia of the Social Sciences*. New York, Macmillan, 227-232, 1968.

Bruch, H.: Obesity and orality. *Contemporary Psychoanalysis*, 5:129-144, 1969.

Bruch, H.: Perturbations neuropsychiques et obésité, extrait de l'obésité. Paris, *Expansion Scientifique*, 176-179, 1963.

Bruch, H.: Psychiatric aspects of obesity. *Metabolism*, 6:461-467, 1957; *International Record of Medicine*, 171:8-9, 1958.

Bruch, H.: Psychological aspects of obesity. *Psychiatry*, 10:373-381, 1947.

Bruch, H.: Psychological aspects of obesity. *Bulletin of the New York Academy of Medicine*, 24:73-86, 1948.

Bruch, H.: Psychological aspects of obesity. *Borden's Review of Nutritional Research*, 19:57-73, 1958.

Bruch, H.: Psychological aspects of obesity. *Medical Record and Annals*, 58:187-192, 1958.

Bruch, H.: Psychological aspects of obesity. In *From Occurrence, Causes and Prevention of Overnutrition*. Stockholm, Almqvist and Wiksell, 1964, pp. 37-46.

Bruch, H.: Psychological aspects of obesity. *Psychosomatics*, 5:269-274, 1964.

Bruch, H.: Über die psychologischen Aspekte der Fettleibigkeit. *Medizinische Klinik*, 55:295-300, 1960.

Bruch, H.: The psychology of obesity. *Cincinnati Journal of Medicine*, 31:273-281, 1950.

Bruch, H.: Psychopathology of hunger and appetite. In S. Rado and G. E. Daniels (Eds.): *Changing Concepts of Psychosomatic Medicine*. New York, Grune and Stratton, 1956, pp. 180-191.

Bruch, H.: Psychophysiologic complaints and psychosomatic illnesses, Section III: Obesity. In *Tice's Practice of Medicine*, Vol. 10, New York, Harper and Row, 1970, pp. 15-19.

Bruch, H.: The psychosomatic aspects of obesity. *Journal of Mount Sinai Hospital*, 20:1-15, 1953.

Bruch, H.: Role of the emotions in hunger and appetite. *Annals of the New York Academy of Science*, 63:68-76, 1955.

Bruch, H.: Role of the emotions in obesity. *State of Mind*, No. 7/8, 1957.

Bruch, H.: Symposium on obesity. *Feelings*, 2, 1960.

Bruch, H., *et al.*: Adipositas: Panel discussion on the theory of Hilde Bruch. *Acta Psychiatrica et Neurologica Scandinavica*, 33:151-173, 1958.

Burner, M.: Psychological considerations on pathological excesses in modern civilization. *Praxis*, 53:661-664, 1964.

Bychowski, G.: On neurotic obesity. *Psychoanalysis and the Psychoanalytic Review*, 37:301-319, 1950.

Caldwell, J.: Lifelong obesity—A contribution to the understanding of recalcitrant obesity. *Psychosomatics*, 6:417-426, 1965.

Cameron, N.: *Personality Development and Psychopathology. A Diagnostic Approach*. Boston, Houghton Mifflin, 1963, 689-690.

Cantilo, E.: La adiposidad neurosomática. *Dia Médico*, 30:49-50, 1958.

Cappon, D.: Obesity. *Canadian Medical Association Journal*, 79:568-573, 1958.

Cappon, D.: *Toward an Understanding of Eating*. Toronto, University of Toronto Press, 1969.

Cassano, C.: Nosographic definition of essential obesity. *Giornale di Clinica Medica*, 34:201-232, 1953.

Cauffman, W. J. and Pauley, W. G.: Obesity and emotional status. *Pennsylvania Medical Journal*, 64:505-507, 1961.

Cautela, J. R.: Covert sensitization. *Psychological Reports*, 20:459-468, 1967.

Chirico, A. M. and Stunkard, A. J.: Physical activity and human obesity. *New England Journal of Medicine*, 263:935-940, 1960.

Cleghorn, R. A.: The interplay between endocrine and psychological dysfunction. In E. Wittkower and R. A. Cleghorn (Eds.): *Recent Developments in Psychosomatic Medicine*. Philadelphia, Lippincott, 1954.

Coddington, R. D., Sours, J. A. and Bruch, H.: Electrogastrographic findings associated with affective change. *American Journal of Psychiatry*, 120:357, 1963.

Conn, J. E.: Obesity: II. Etiological aspects. *Physiological Review*, 41:31, 1944.

Conrad, A.: The attitude toward food. *American Journal of Orthopsychiatry*, 7:360, 1937.

Conrad, E. H.: Psychogenic obesity: The effects of social rejection upon hunger, food craving, food consumption, and the drive-reduction value of eating for obese vs. normal individuals. *Dissertation Abstracts International*, 30(10-B):4787-4788, 1970.

Conrad, S. W.: The problem of weight reduction in obese women. *American Practitioner*, 5:38, 1954.

Conrad, S. W.: The management of obesity. In J. H. Nodine and J. H. Moyer (Eds.): *Psychosomatic Medicine*. Philadelphia, Lea and Febiger, 1962.

Conrad, S. W.: Phallic aspects of obesity. *Bulletin of the Philadelphia Association for Psychoanalysis*, 15:207-223, 1965.

Conrad, S. W.: The psychologic implications of overeating. *Psychiatric Quarterly*, 28:211-224, 1954.

Conrad, S. W.: The psychological causes and treatment of overeating and obesity. *American Practitioner*, 3:438-444, 1952.

Coriat, I. H.: Sex and hunger. *Psychoanalytic Review*, 8:375-381, 1921.

Covian, M. R.: Behavior and the nervous system. *Revista Paulista de Medicina*, 58:53-57, 1961.

Crisp, A. H., *et al.*: Sleep patterns, daytime activity, weight changes and psychiatric status: A study of three obese patients. *Journal of Psychosomatic Research*, 14:353-358, 1970.

Danowski, T. S. and Winkler, A. W.: Obesity as a clinical problem. *American Journal of Medical Science,* 208:622, 1944.

Darling, C. D. and Summerskill, J.: Emotional factors in obesity and weight reduction. *Journal of the American Dietetic Association,* 29:1204-1207, 1953.

deGennis, L.: Obesity: Of nervous origin. *La Revue du Prâcticien,* 2:1017-1021, 1952.

DeLa Fuente, R.: Psychological factors in obesity. Gaceta Medica de Mexico, 92:376-378, 1962.

Demole, M.: Question whether obesity is always due to overeating. *Revue Médicale de la Suisse Romande,* 71:649-659, 1951.

DeMoor, P.: Obesitas. *Belgisch Tijdschrift voor Geneeskunde,* 15:201-228, 1959.

Dempsey, J. A.: Relationship between obesity and treadmill performance in sedentary and active young men. *Research Quarterly for the American Association for Health, Physical Education, and Recreation,* 35:288-297, 1964.

Deri, S. K.: A problem in obesity. In A. Burton and R. E. Harris (Eds.): *Clinical Studies of Personality,* Vol. II, New York, Harper, 1955, pp. 525-581.

DeSousa, A., *et al.*: Obesity. Psychological aspects. *Journal of the Association of Physicians of India,* 16:245-246, 1968.

Deutsch, H.: Hysterical conversion symptoms—paralysis, speech defects, gluttony. In *Psychoanalysis of the Neuroses.* London, Hogarth, 1951.

Dick, A.: Psychological aspects of obesity. *Medical Arts and Sciences,* 15:95-98, 124-129, 1961.

Dorris, R. J. and Stunkard, A. J.: Physical activity: Performance and attitudes of a group of obese women. *American Journal of Medical Science,* 233:622, 1957.

Doumic, J. M.: Etiology and therapeutic aspects of obesity of neuropsychic origin. *Revue Médicale de France,* 41:249-251, 1960.

Dunbar, H. F.: *Emotions and Bodily Changes.* New York, Columbia University Press, 1946.

Editorial: Obesity: A continuing enigma. *Journal of the American Medical Association,* 211:492-493, 1970.

Einhorn, H. P.: A total approach to obesity. *Journal of Newark Beth Israel Hospital,* 12:101-107, 1961.

English, O. S. and Finch, S. M.: *Introduction to Psychiatry,* 3d ed., New York, Norton, 1964, 321-324.

Eppright, E. S., Swanson, P. and Iverson, C. A. (Eds.): *Weight Control: A Collection of Papers Presented at the Weight Control Colloquium.* Ames, Iowa, Iowa State College Press, 1955.

Epstein, S. and Levitt, H.: The influence of hunger and recall of food related words. *Journal of Abnormal and Social Psychology,* 64:130-135, 1962.

Evans, F. A.: Obesity. In G. G. Duncan (Ed.): *Diseases of Metabolism.* Philadelphia, Saunders, 1947, Ch. 10.

Fenichel, O.: *The Psychoanalytic Theory of Neurosis.* New York, Norton, 1945, 241, 381-382.

Ferster, C. B., Nurnberger, J. I. and Levitt, E. B.: The control of eating. *Journal of Mathetics,* 1:87-109, 1962.

Fertman, M. B.: Present status of our knowledge on pathogenesis. *Klinische Wochenschrift,* 34:665-669, 1956.

Finkler, R. S.: Endocrine and psychosomatic aspects. *Journal of the American Medical Women's Association,* 8:187-190, 1953.

Fink, G., Gottesfeld, H. and Glickman, L.: The "super-obese" patient. *Journal of Hillside Hospital*, 11:97-119, 1962.

Franco, F., *et al.*: Psychic aspects of obesity. *Rassegna di Studi Psichiatrici*, 54:361-365, 1965.

Frazier, S. H., Faubion, M. H., Giffin, M. E. and Johnson, A. M.: A specific factor in symptom choice. *Proceedings of Staff Meeting, Mayo Clinic*, 30:227, 1955.

Freed, S. C.: Psychic factors in the development and treatment of obesity. *Journal of the American Medical Association*, 133:369, 1947.

Freed, S. C. and Kroger, W. S.: Obesity. *Journal of Insurance Medicine*, 6:12-18, 1951.

Freud, S.: The interpretation of dreams. In *Complete Psychological Works of Sigmund Freud*, Vol. IV. London: Hogarth, 1953, 267-268.

Freyberger, H.: Depressive syndromes in chronic internal diseases, illustrated by obesity and ulcerative colitis. *Ärztliche Forschung*, 20:169-176, 1966.

Friedman, J.: Weight problems and psychological factors. *Journal of Consulting Psychology*, 23:524-527, 1959.

Fuchs, E.: Envy and gluttony. *Zeitschrift für Psychoanalytischer Pädagogik*, 7:222-231, 1933.

Garcia Reinoso, D.: Notas sobre la obesidad a través del estudio de Falstaff. *Revista de Psicoanálisis*, 13:170-177, 1956.

Garcia Vega, H.: Conflictos emocionales y regresión oral digestiva en una obesidad neurótica. *Revista de Psicoanálisis*, 13:305-311, 1956.

Garma, A.: Obesidad y dos tipos de alimentación. *Revista de Psicoanálisis*, 13:153-159, 1956.

Garma, A.: The psychosomatic shift through obesity, migraine, peptic ulcer, and myocardial infarction in a homosexual. *International Journal of Psycho-Analysis*, 49:241-245, 1968.

Gastineau, C. F. and Rynearson, E. H.: Obesity. *Annals of Internal Medicine*, 27:883, 1947.

Gelvin, E. P., McGavack, T. H. and Konigsberg, S.: Subjective impressions of 108 consecutive patients as to causes. *American Journal of Digestive Diseases*, 20:200-202, 1953.

Gilbert-Dreyfus, L.: Etiology and pathogenesis. *La Tunisie Médicale*, 38:43-61, 1950.

Gilbert-Dreyfus, L.: L'obésité paradoxale: Syndrome psychosomatique. *La Presse Médicale*, 56:249, 1948.

Gilbert-Dreyfus, L.: So-called endogenous obesity. *La Presse Médicale*, 61:321-322, 1953.

Gilbert-Dreyfus, L. and Held, R.: A propos des obésités. *Revue Française de Psychanalyse*, 22:59-82, 1950.

Gilbert-Dreyfus, L., Lamotte, M. and Job, J. C.: Obesity in relation to the central nervous system. La Semaine des Hôpitaux de Paris, 26:1423-1429, 1950.

Glass, D. C., *et al.*: Obesity and persuasibility. *Journal of Personality*, 37:407-414, 1969.

Gordon, E. S.: The present concept of obesity: Etiological factors and treatment. *Medical Times*, 97:142-155, 1969.

Grabovska, M. J.: Importance of mental factors in the occurrence of obesity. *Psychiatria Polska*, 4:301-305, 1970.

Graff, H.: Emotional aspects of weight loss in the cardiac patient. *Pennsylvania Medicine*, 70:68, 1967.

Graff, H.: Overweight and emotions in the obesity clinic. *Psychosomatics,* 6:89-94, 1965.

Gray, H.: Obesity: A challenge to the psychiatrist. *Stanford Medical Bulletin,* 1:195, 1943.

Greene, W. A.: *Psychologic Determinants of Organic Disease Survey of Twins.* U. S. Department of Health, Education and Welfare, Mental Health Research Grant MH-11668-04(12), 1969.

Grinberg, L.: La negación en el comer compulsive y en la obesidad. *Revista de Psicoanalisis,* 13:160-169, 1956.

Hamburger, W. W.: Appetite in man. *American Journal of Clinical Nutrition,* 8: 569-586, 1960.

Hamburger, W. W.: Emotional aspects of obesity. *Medical Clinics of North America,* 35:483-500, 1951.

Hecht, M. B.: Obesity in women: A psychiatric study. *Psychiatric Quarterly,* 29:203-231, 1955.

Hedderich, G., *et al.:* Unconscious self-assessment of obese patients. *Deutsche Medizinische Wochenschrift,* 96:784-789, 1971.

Hirsch, D. L. and Morse, W. J.: Emotional and metabolic factors in obesity. *Canadian Journal of Public Health,* 51:450-455, 1960.

Hjortzberg-Nordlund, H.: Obesity in 50-year-old-men: Genetic social and psychic aspects. *Lakartidningen,* 63:526-530, 1966.

Hochman, S.: Mental and psychological factors in obesity. *Medical Record,* 148:108-111, 1938.

Holland, B. C. and Ward, R. S.: Homeostasis and psychosomatic medicine. In S. Arieti (Ed.): *American Handbook of Psychiatry,* Vol. 3, New York, Basic Books, 1966, 344-361.

Hughes, R., *et al.:* Estimates of psychological time among obese and nonobese women. *Journal of Psychology,* 70:213-219, 1968.

Hunt, E. E., Peckos, P. S. and Fry, P. C.: *Factors in Human Obesity.* Symposium, Series 6. New York, National Vitamin Foundation, 1953.

Hurwitz, H. M.: *The Effect of Stress on Food Demand and Body Weight.* U. S. Department of Health, Education and Welfare. Mental Health Research Grant RO3-MH-02578 01, 1963.

Insua, J. A.: Aspectos psicologicos de la obesidad. *Prensa Medica Argentina,* 54:1164-1169, 1967.

Jones, A.: A study of the relationship between psychomotor performance and the physiological condition of obesity. *Dissertation Abstracts,* 17:1134-1135, 1957.

Jores, A.: Genesis: Psychosomatic aspects of obesity. *La Prensa Medica Argentina,* 38:3360-3361, 1951.

Jores, A.: Obesity, with special reference to its psychosomatic aspects. *Aesthetische Medizin; Medizinische Kosmetik,* 14:306-313, 1965.

Kaplan, H. I., Kaplan, H. S. and Leder, H.: Psychosomatic management of obesity. *New York State Journal of Medicine,* 57:2815, 1957.

Kaplan, S. D.: Obesity and the emotions. *Nebraska State Medical Journal,* 51:41-47, 1966.

Kasl, S. V., *et al.:* Some psychological factors associated with illness behavior and selected illnesses. *Journal of Chronic Diseases,* 325-345, 1964.

Kirschbaum, W. R.: Excessive hunger as a symptom of cerebral origin. *Journal of Nervous and Mental Disease,* 113:95, 1951.

Klotz, H. P., *et al.*: Neuropsychogenic forms of obesity: Study of antidiuretic activity of serum; Pathogenic significance. *La Semaine des Hôpitaux de Paris,* 32:3362-3371, 1956.

Koch, C. R. and Stunkard, A. J.: Obesity, age and the gastric "hunger" conditions. *Journal of Applied Physiology,* 15:133, 1960.

Kornhaber, A.: The stuffing syndrome. *Psychosomatics,* 11:580-584, 1970.

Kotkin, L.: Round number barrier in weight reduction. *New England Journal of Medicine,* 55:98-100, 1955.

Krotkiewski, M., *et al.*: Psychological problems of obesity; Some generalizations based on our experience in studies and treatment of obesity. *Polski Tygodnik Lekarski,* 23:720-723, 1968.

Krumbacher, K. and Meyer, J. E.: Das Appetitverhalten des Gesunden unter emotionalem Stress. *Zeitschrift für Psychosomatische Medizin,* 9:89, 1963.

Kurland, H. D.: Obesity: An unfashionable problem. *Psychiatric Opinion,* 7:20-24, 1970.

Lal, A. and Gandhi, J. S.: Aetiological importance of psychosomatic factors in the pathogenesis of obesity. *Journal of the Indian Medical Association,* 38:170-174, 1962.

Lanowski, T. W. and Winkler, A. W.: Obesity as a clinical problem. *American Journal of Medical Science,* 208:622, 1944.

LaRose, E. N., *et al.*: Mental health . . . psychiatric aspects of weight control. *Virginia Medical Monthly,* 90:425-427, 1963.

Leckie, E. V., *et al.*: Obesity and depression. *Journal of Psychosomatic Research,* 11:107-115, 1967.

Lefley, H. P.: Masculine-femininity in obese women. *Journal of Consulting and Clinical Psychology,* 7:180-186, 1971.

Liberman, D.: Humerismo en la transferencia e instinto de muerte, en un paciente obeso. *Revista de Psicoanálisis,* 14:292-306, 1957.

Losso, R. H.: La obesidad como expresión de una perturbación de la personalidad. *Acta Psiquiátrica y Psicológica América Latina,* 10:104-110, 1964.

McCance, C.: *Psychiatric Factors in Obesity.* Dissertation for diploma in psychological medicine, University of London, 1961.

McDonald, R. L.: Personality characteristics in patients with three obstetric complications. *Psychosomatic Medicine,* 27:383-389, 1965.

McKinnon, D. A.: Avoirdupois and the id. *McGill Medical Journal,* 29:88-94, 1960.

Maranon, G.: Psychologic factors of obesity according to a non-psychoanalytic physician. *Revista Ibérica de Endocrinología,* 3:7-23, 1956.

Martino, P.: Obesity. Some remarks on psychosomatic approach. *Bordeaux Médical,* 3:733-738, 1970.

Mayer, J.: Genetic factors in human obesity. *Annals of the New York Academy of Science,* 131:412-421, 1965.

Mayer, M.: The genetic factors in obesity. *Bulletin of the New York Academy of Medicine,* 36:323-343, 1960.

Mayer, J.: Genetic factors in obesity. *Postgraduate Medicine,* 37:A103-108, 1965.

Mayer, J.: Genetic, traumatic and environmental factors in the etiology of obesity. *Physiological Review,* 33:472-508, 1953.

Mayer, J.: *Overweight: Causes, Cost and Control.* Englewood Cliffs, N. J., Prentice-Hall, 1968.

Mayer, J.: Regulation of food intake and the multiple etiology of obesity. In E. S. Eppright, *et al.* (Eds.): *Weight Control.* Ames, Iowa, Iowa State College Press, 1955, 29-48.

Mendelson, M. J.: Psychological aspects of obesity. *Medical Clinics of North America,* 48:1373-1385, 1964.

Mendelson, M. J.: Psychological aspects of obesity studied by a clinic. *Dia Medico,* 35:807-808, 1963.

Mendelson, M. J.: Psychological aspects of obesity. *International Journal of Psychiatry,* 2:599-611, 1966.

Meyer, J. E. and Tuchelt-Gallwitz, A.: Psychiatrisch-psychologische Untersuchungen an weiblichen Fettsüchtigen. *Zeitschrift für Psychosomatische Medizin und Psychoanalyse,* 13:73-107, 1967.

Michaux, L. and Widlocher, D.: Problems posed by obesity and thinness in man. Psychological aspects. *Therapie,* 17:775-802, 1962.

Moll, R. P.: *Drive and Maturation Effects in Food Consumption.* U. S. Department of Health, Education and Welfare, Mental Health Research Grant, RO3-MH-06483 01, 1962.

Moore, M. E.: Obesity and mental health (letter). *Journal of the American Medical Association,* 183:807, 1963.

Morton, J. H.: Obesity and psychosomatic problems. *Psychosomatics,* 7:175-181, 1966.

Murphy, R.: The complexities of the problem of obesity. *Medical Clinics of North America,* 44:439, 1960.

Nicholson, W. M.: Emotional factors in obesity. *American Journal of Medical Science,* 211:443, 1946.

Nisbett, R. E.: Determinants of food intake in obesity. *Science,* 159:1254-1255, 1968.

Nisbett, R. E.: Taste, deprivation, and weight determinants of eating behavior. *Journal of Personality and Social Psychology,* 10:107-116, 1968.

Nisbett, R. E. and Kanouse, D. E.: Obesity, hunger, and supermarket shopping behavior. *Proceedings of the 76th Annual Convention of the American Psychological Association,* 3:683-684, 1968.

Noyes, A. P. and Kolb, L. C.: *Modern Clinical Psychiatry.* Philadelphia, Saunders, 1960, 461-465.

Obesity forum: *Psychosomatics,* 3:97-100, 1962.

Orbach, C. H.: Perceptual defense and somatization: A comparison of the perceptual thresholds of obese and peptic ulcer patients. *Dissertation Abstracts,* 20:4440, 1960.

Parson, W. and Crispell, K. R.: Obesity. *Medical Clinics of North America,* 36:385-392, 1952.

Pathe, G. and Morel, A.: Les obésités neurologique. *Concours Médical,* 80:1931-1932, 1958.

Patzer, H.: Cerebral obesity. *Acta Neurovegetativa,* 12:234-249, 1955.

Penick, S. B. and Stunkard, A. J.: Newer concepts of obesity. *Medical Clinics of North America,* 54:745-754, 1970.

Pennington, A. W.: Symposium on obesity; Reorientation on obesity. *New England Journal of Medicine,* 248:959-964, 1953.

Perestrello, D.: Psychosomatic aspects of obesity. *Arquivos Brasilieros de Medicine,* 51:219-224, 1961.

Perry, L. and Learnard, B.: Obesity and mental health (letter). *Journal of the American Medical Association,* 1963, 183:807-808.

Plauchu, M., Pommatau, E. and Vottero, R.: Etiologic factors and pathogenic aspects of obesity. *Le Journal de Médicine de Lyon,* 35:389-398, 1954.

Pomeranze, J.: Recurrent obesity. *New York State Journal of Medicine,* 56:3017-3020, 1956.

Quijada, H. and Manzanilla, L. M.: Contribucion al estudio de la obesidad a la luz del psicoanalisis. *Antioquia Medica,* Special number published for the Neuropsychiatric Congress of Medellin, 1955.

Rakoff, V.: The psychiatric aspects of obesity. *Modern Treatment,* 4:1111-1124, 1967.

Rakoff, V.: The psychiatric basis of obesity: An hypothesis of addiction. *Appied Therapeutics,* 7:103-107, 1965.

Rascovsky, A.: Estudio psicosomático del sindrome adiposogenital. In A. Rascovsky (Ed.), *Patología psicosomática.* Buenos Aires, El Ateneo, 1948, 573-596.

Rascovsky, A., Rascovsky, M. W. de and Schlossberg, T.: Basic psychic structure of the obese. *International Journal of Psycho-Analysis,* 31:144-149, 1950; *Revista de Psicoanálisis,* 8:141-151, 1951.

Ray, H. M.: The obese patient: A statistical study and analysis of symptoms, diagnosis, and metabolic abnormalities, sex difference-treatment. *American Journal of Digestive Diseases,* 14:153, 1947.

Reeve, G. H.: Psychological factors in obesity. *American Journal of Orthopsychiatry,* 12:674-678, 1942.

Rennie, T. A.: Obesity as a manifestation of a personality disturbance. *Diseases of the Nervous System,* 1:238-247, 1940.

Richardson, J. S.: Simple obesity. *Postgraduate Medical Journal,* 28:618-623, 1952.

Rodin, J.: *Effects of Distraction on Performance of Obese and Normal Subjects.* Unpublished doctoral dissertation, Columbia University, 1970.

Rome, H. P.: Obesity: Psychiatric aspects. *Proceedings of the Staff Meetings of the Mayo Clinic,* 35:131-135, 1960.

Rony, H. R.: *Obesity and Leanness.* Philadelphia, Lea and Febiger, 1940.

Rossier, P. H.: Die Fettsucht (obesitas) als psychosomatisches Geschehen. *Psyche,* 3: 18-25, 1949.

Rowland, C. V., Jr. (Ed.): Anorexia and obesity. *International Psychiatry Clinics,* 7: 231-360, 1970.

Rubin, T. I.: *Thin Book by a Formerly Fat Psychiatrist.* New York, Simon and Schuster, 1966.

Russell, G. F.: Is obesity really a psychological problem? *International Journal of Psychiatry,* 2:612-614, 1966.

Rynearson, E. H. and Gastineau, C. F.: *Obesity.* Springfield, Ill., Thomas, 1949.

Saffer, J. B.: Coping mechanisms of obese men. A psychometric and behavioral study. *Dissertation Abstracts,* 29(4-B):1511, 1968.

Salmon-Malebranche, A. R.: Psychic factor in obesity. *La Semaine des Hôpitaux de Paris,* 26:3489-3490, 1950.

Saucier, J. F.: The psychiatric aspect of obesity. *Laval Medical,* 36:154-163, 1965.

Scarpelli, P. T., *et al.*: Psychosomatic aspects of obesity in the evolutive age. I. General outline of the problem and case histories; Psycho-typology; Medico-social aspects. *Rassegna di Neurologia Vegetativa,* 19:496-512, 1965.

Schachter, S.: Cognitive effects on bodily functionings: Studies of obesity and eating. In D. C. Glass (Ed.): *Neurophysiology and Emotion.* New York, Rockefeller University Press, 1967.

Schachter, S.: Eat, eat. *Psychology Today,* 4:45-47, 78-79, 1971.

Schachter, S.: *Emotion, Obesity and Crime.* New York, Academy Press, 1971.

Schachter, S.: Obesity and eating. *Science,* 16:751-756, 1968.

Schachter, S.: Obesity and eating. In J. O. Whittaker (Ed.): *Recent Discoveries in Psychology.* Philadelphia, Saunders, 1972, Ch. 3.

Schachter, S.: Some extraordinary facts about obese humans and rats. *American Psychologist,* 26:129-144, 1971.

Schachter, S., Goldman, R. and Gordon, A.: Effects of fear, food deprivation, and obesity on eating. *Journal of Personality and Social Psychology,* 10:91-97, 1968.

Schachter, S. and Gross, L. P.: Manipulated time and eating behavior. *Journal of Personality and Social Psychology,* 10:98-106, 1968.

Schleimann, E.: *Sex and the Overweight Woman.* New York, Signet Press, 1970.

Schick, A.: Etiological aspects of psychosomatic conditions. In P. H. Hoch and J. Zubin (Eds.): *Current Problems in Psychiatric Diagnosis.* New York, Grune and Stratton, 1953, 231-243.

Schmallbach, K.: Family "in which obesity occurs at 40 years of age"; Psychosomatic aspects of obesity. *Schweizer Archiv für Neurologie and Psychiatrie,* 72:258-277, 1953.

Schneider, H.: Obesity: Psychosomatic aspects. *Schweizerische Medizinische Wochenschrift,* 86:675-680, 1956.

Schoenfeld, W. A.: *Psychosomatic Medicine.* New York, Hoeber, 1950, 49-54.

Schopbach, R. R. and Angel, J. L.: Obesity: An etiological study. *Psychiatric Quarterly,* 27:452-462, 1953.

Schopbach, R. R. and Matthews, R. A.: The psychological problems in obesity. *Archives of Neurology and Psychiatry,* 54:157, 1945.

Schwartz, R. A., Hershenson, D. B. and Shipman, W. G.: The sexual behavior of obese married women. *Proceedings of the Annual Convention of the American Psychological Association,* 6:445-446, 1971.

Selling, L. S.: Behavior problems in eating. *American Journal of Orthopsychiatry,* 16:163, 1946.

Seltzer, C. C. and Mayer, J.: A simple criterion of obesity. *Postgraduate Medicine,* 3:A101-A107, 1965.

Semen, E. I., *et al.:* Psychological aspects of obesity. *Studii si Cercetari de Endocrinologie,* 16:487-491, 1956.

Shipman, W. G. and Plesset, M. R.: Anxiety and depression in obese dieters. *Archives of General Psychiatry,* 8:530-535, 1963.

Shochet, B. B.: A comprehensive view of obesity. *Psychosomatics,* 3:223, 1962.

Shock, N. W.: Physiological factors in behavior. In J. McV. Hunt (Ed.): *Personality and Behavior Disorders,* Vol. I. New York, Ronald Press, 1944, 595-600.

Shorvon, J. H. and Richardson, J. S.: Sudden obesity and psychological trauma. *British Medical Journal,* 4634:951, 1949.

Simon, R. I.: Obesity as a depressive equivalent. *Journal of the American Medical Association,* 183:208-210, 1963.

Simonson, E., Brozek, J. and Keys, A.: Effect of meals on visual performance and fatigue. *Journal of Applied Physiology,* 1:270, 1948.

Simpon, S. L.: Causes of obesity. *Lancet,* 183:208-210, 1963.

Sjovall, T.: Obesity, VII. Psychodynamic aspects in etiology and therapy. *Svenska Lakartidningen,* 57:2490-2494, 1960.

Smith, W. F.: Obesity. *Connecticut State Medical Journal,* 12:735-738, 1948.

Stauder, K. H.: Studien zur Psychologie und Psychotherapie der Fettsüchtigen. *Psyche,* 12:641-686, 1959.

Stollreiter-Butzon, L.: Fettsucht also psychosomatische Symptombildung. *Psyche,* 4: 335-351, 1950.

Strauss, B. V.: Emotions and obesity. *New York State Journal of Medicine,* 55:2497-2501, 1955.

Stunkard, A. J.: Actividad fisica, emociones y obesidad humana. *Medicina Clinica,* 33: 421, 1959.

Stunkard, A. J.: *Clinical and Experimental Studies of Human Obesity.* U. S. Department of Health, Education and Welfare, Mental Health Research Grant MH-15383-1, 1968; MH-03684-04, 1961, 1962, 1963.

Stunkard, A. J.: "Dieting depression"; Incidence and clinical characteristics of untoward responses to weight reduction regimens. *American Journal of Medicine,* 23:77, 1957.

Stunkard, A. J.: The "dieting depression"; Untoward responses to weight reduction regimens among certain obese women. *Journal of Nervous and Mental Disease,* 123:194, 1956.

Stunkard, A. J.: Eating patterns and obesity. *Psychiatric Quarterly,* 33:284-295, 1959.

Stunkard, A. J.: Obesity. In *The Cyclopedia of Medicine, Surgery and Specialties.* Philadelphia, Davis, 1958, 558-562.

Stunkard, A. J.: Obesity. In A. Deutsch (Ed.): *Encyclopedia of Mental Health,* Vol. 4. Metuchen, N. J., Scarecrow Press, 1963, 1970, 1372-1385.

Stunkard, A. J.: Obesity. In A. M. Freedman, H. I. Kaplan and H. S. Kaplan (Eds.): *Comprehensive Textbook of Psychiatry.* Baltimore, Williams and Wilkins, 1967, 1059-1062.

Stunkard, A. J.: Obesity and the denial of hunger. *Psychosomatic Medicine,* 21:281-290, 1959.

Stunkard, A. J.: Obesity: Patterns and paradoxes. *Medical World News,* 64-65, 1970.

Stunkard, A. J.: The perception of hunger. In D. A. Hamburg, K. Pribham and A. J. Stunkard (Eds.): *Disorders of Perception.* Research publication, Association for Research in Nervous and Mental Disease, Vol. 48. Baltimore, Williams and Wilkins, 1970, 286-297.

Stunkard, A. J.: Physical activity, emotions and human obesity. *Psychosomatic Medicine,* 20:366-372, 1958.

Stunkard, A. J.: Research on a disease: Strategies in the study of obesity. In R. Roseler and N. S. Greenfield (Eds.): *Physiological Correlates of Psychological Disorder.* Madison, Wisc., University of Wisconsin Press, 1962, 211-220.

Stunkard, A. J., Grace, W. J. and Wolff, H. G.: The night-eating syndrome: A pattern of food intake among certain obese patients. *American Journal of Medicine,* 19: 78-86, 1955.

Stunkard, A. J. and Koch, C.: The interpretation of gastric motility: I. Apparent bias in the reports of hunger by obese persons. *Archives of General Psychiatry,* 11:74-82, 1964.

Stunkard, A. J. and Reader, J.: The management of obesity. *New York State Journal of Medicine,* 58:78-87, 1958.

Stunkard, A. J. and Wolff, H. G.: A mechanism of satiety: Function and disorder in human obesity. *Psychosomatic Medicine,* 18:515, 1956.

Stunkard, A. J. and Wolff, H. G.: Pathogenesis in human obesity: Function and disorder of a mechanism of satiety. *Psychosomatic Medicine,* 20:17, 1958.

Suchanek-Fröhlich, H.: Psychosomatische Aspekte zur Genese der Fettsucht, *Zeitschrift für Psycho-somatische Medizin,* 3:190-194, 1957.

Suczek, R. F.: The personality of obese women. *American Journal of Clinical Nutrition*, 5:197-202, 1957.

Suczek, R. F.: Psychological aspects of weight reduction. In E. S. Eppright, *et al.* (Eds.): *Weight Control.* Ames, Iowa, Iowa State College Press, 1955, 147-159.

Summers, L. D., Jr.: Goal-setting as a problem in the psychodynamics of obesity. *Dissertation Abstracts*, 17:1817, 1957.

Swanson, D. W. and Dinello, F. A.: Severe obesity as a habituation syndrome. *Archives of General Psychiatry*, 22:120-127, 1970.

Taille, J. de: Mental structure and obesity. *Gazette Medicale de France*, 38:328-331, 1961.

Tori, S.: Excessive obesity with early beginning. Case. *Revista di Clinica Pediatrica*, 54:33-55, 1954.

U. S. Department of Health, Education and Welfare, Public Health Service, National Center for Chronic Disease Control: *Obesity and Health*, Arlington, Va. 1967, 77 pp.

Voit, K.: Main symptom: Obesity *Münchener Medizinische Wochenschrift*, 92:1105-1114, 1950.

Waxler, S. H. and Leef, M. F.: Obesity . . . doctor's dilemma. *Geriatrics*, 24:98-106, 1969.

Weinberg, N., Mendelson, M. and Stunkard, A. J.: A failure to find distinctive personality features in a group of obese men. *American Journal of Psychiatry*, 117:1035, 1961.

Weintraub, W. and Aronson, M.: Application of verbal behavior analysis to the study of psychological defense-mechanisms. V. Speech pattern associated with overeating. *Archives of General Psychiatry*, 21:739-744, 1969.

Weiss, E. and English, O. S.: *Psychosomatic Medicine.* Philadelphia, Saunders, 1943, 335-349.

Withers, R. F. J.: Problems in the genetics of human obesity. *Eugenics Review*, 56:81-90, 1964.

Wolberg, L. R.: *Psychology of Eating.* New York, McBride, 1936.

Wulff, M.: Über einen interessanten oralen Symptomenkomplex und seine Bezeihung zur Sucht. *Internationale Zeitschrift für Psychoanalysis*, 18:281-302, 1932.

Young, C. M.: The prevention of obesity. *Medical Clinics of North America*, 48:1317-1333, 1964.

Yudkin, J.: The causes and cure of obesity. *Lancet*, 2:1135-1138, 1959.

Yudkin, J.: The cause and treatment of obesity. *Triangle*, 7:326-330, 1966.

II. BODY IMAGE

Alexander, W. R.: A study of body types, self-image, and environmental adjustment in freshmen college women. *Dissertation Abstracts*, 28:8A:3048, 1968.

Bruch, H.: Transformation of oral impulses (abstract). *Bulletin of the Association of Psychoanalytic Medicine*, 1:7-11, 1961.

Bruch, H.: Transformation of oral impulses in eating disorders: A conceptual approach. *Psychiatric Quarterly*, 35:458-481, 1961.

Cappon, D. and Banks, R.: Distorted body perception in obesity. *Journal of Nervous and Mental Disease*, 146:465-467, 1968.

Cappon, D. and Banks, R.: Orientational perception: II. Body perception in depersonalization. *Archives of General Psychiatry*, 13:375-379, 1965.

Collingwood, T. R. and Willett, L.: The effects of physical training upon self-concept and body attitude. *Journal of Clinical Psychology*, 27:411-412, 1971.

Fisher, S. and Cleveland, S. E.: *Body Image and Personality*. Princeton, N. J., Van Nostrand, 1958.

Fisher, S. and Cleveland, S. E.: The role of body image to psychosomatic symptom choice. *Psychological Monographs*, 69:402, 1955.

Fransella, F.: Measurement of conceptual change in accompanying weight loss. *Journal of Psychosomatic Research*, 14:347-351, 1970.

Freyberger, H.: Typologische Studien bei Fettsuchtskranken. *Ärtzliche Forschung*, 14: 293, 1960.

Glucksman, M. L. and Hirsch, J.: The response of obese patients to weight reduction. 3. The perception of body size. *Psychosomatic Medicine*, 31:1-7, 1969.

Hanley, C.: Physique and reputation of high-school boys. *Child Development*, 22: 247-260, 1951.

Hassan, I. N.: The body image and personality correlates of body type stereotypes. *Dissertation Abstracts*, 11A:4446, 1968.

Kretschmer, E.: *Physique and Character*. London, Kegan Paul, 1925.

Metropolitan Life Insurance Company: New weight standards for males and females. *Statistical Bulletin*, 40:2-3, 1959.

National Center for Health Statistics: *Weight by Age and Height of Adults: 1960-1962*. Washington, D. C., Vital and Health Statistics, Public Health Service Publication No. 1000, Series 11, No. 14, Government Printing Office, 1966.

Schilder, P.: *The Image and Appearance of the Human Body*. London, Paul, Trench, Trubner, 1935; New York, International Universities Press, 1950.

Schonbuch, S. S. and Schell, R. E.: Judgments of body appearance by fat and skinny male college students. *Perceptual and Motor Skills*, 24:999-1002, 1967.

Schonfeld, W. A.: Body-image disturbances in adolescents with inappropriate development. *American Journal of Orthopsychiatry*, 34:493-502, 1964.

Seltzer, C. C.: Bodily disproportion and dominant personality traits. *Psychosomatic Medicine*, 8:75-97, 1946.

Seltzer, C. C. and Mayer, J.: Body build and obesity: Who are the obese? *Journal of the American Medical Association*, 189:677-684, 1964.

Seltzer, C. C. and Mayer, J.: Body build (somatotype) distinctiveness in obese women. *Journal of the American Dietetic Association*, 55:454-458, 1969.

Seltzer, C. C. and Mayer, J.: How representative are the weights of measured men and women? *Journal of the American Medical Association*, 201:221-224, 1967.

Sheldon, W. H., Stevens, S. S. and Tucker, W. B.: *The Varieties of Human Physique*. New York, Hafner, 1963.

Shipman, W. G. and Sohlkhah, N.: Body image distortion in obese women (abstract). *Psychosomatic Medicine*, 29:540, 1967.

Staffieri, J. R.: A study of social stereotypes of body image in children. *Journal of Personality and Social Psychology*, 7:101-104, 1967.

Stunkard, A. J. and Burt, V.: Obesity and the body image. II. Age at onset of disturbances in the body image. *American Journal of Psychiatry*, 123:1443-1447, 1967.

Stunkard, A. J. and Mendelson, M.: Disturbances in body image of some obese persons. *Journal of the American Dietetic Association*, 38:328-331, 1961.

Stunkard, A. J. and Mendelson, M.: Obesity and the body image: I. Characteristics of disturbances in the body image of some obese persons. *American Journal of Psychiatry*, 123:1296-1300, 1967; In J. E. Jeffries (Ed.): *Psychosomatic Medicine*

Current Journal Articles. Flushing, N. Y., Medical Examination Publishing Company, 1971.

Witkin, H. A.: Psychological differentiation and forms of pathology. *Journal of Abnormal Psychology,* 70:317-336, 1965.

III. PSYCHOSOCIAL FACTORS

Ahmed, M. J., *et al.:* A sociological approach to a dietary survey and food habit study in an Andean community. *Tropical and Geographical Medicine,* 20:88-100, 1968.

Angel, J. L.: Constitution in female obesity. *American Journal of Physical Anthropology,* 7:433-471, 1949.

Bruch, H.: Social and emotional factors in diet changes. *Journal of the American Dental Association,* 63:461-465, 1961.

Bruch, H.: Social and emotional factors in diet changes. *Nutrition News,* 26:13-14, 1963.

Burnight, R. G. and Marden, P. G.: Social correlates of weight in an aging population. *Milbank Memorial Foundation Quarterly,* 45:75-92, 1967.

Chesler, J.: A study of attitudes and knowledge concerning obesity in an urban African community. *South African Medical Journal,* 35:129-131, 1961.

Cicheki, J.: Medicosocial problems of treatment of obesity. *Wiadomosci Lekarskie,* 18: 265-267, 1965.

Decourt, J. and Doumic, J. M.: Obesity: Anthropometric aspects. *La Semaine des Hôpitaux de Paris,* 28:844-854, 1952.

Fiumi, G., *et al.:* Obesity: A social problem. *Minerva Medica,* 62:1065-1069, 1971.

Gill, D. J.: The role of personality and environmental factors in obesity. *Journal of the American Dietetic Association,* 22:398, 1946.

Goldblatt, P. B., Moore, M. E. and Stunkard, A. J.: Social factors in obesity. *Journal of the American Medical Association,* 192:1039-1044, 1965.

Gomez Mont, F.: Medical, social and ethical aspects of obesity. *Gaceta Medica de Mexico,* 92:355-358, 1962.

Gray, H.: Mammoth obesity: Anthropometric study. *Stanford Medical Bulletin,* 8:106-109, 1950.

Günther, S.: Sociomedical significance of obesity. *Medizinische Welt,* 6:386-392, 1968.

Hawley, T. G. and Jansen, A. A. J.: Weight, height, body surface and overweight of Fijian adults from coastal areas. *New Zealand Medical Journal,* 74:18-21, 1971.

Henschel, A.: Obesity as an occupational hazard. *Canadian Journal of Public Health,* 58:491-493, 1967.

Holland, J., Masling, J. and Copley, D.: Mental illness in lower class normal, obese and hyperobese women. *Psychosomatic Medicine,* 32:351-357, 1971.

Howard, J. K.: Caloric intake and intelligence: A study among Bantu school-children. *Central Africa Journal of Medicine,* 12:63-64, 1966.

Käding, A.: Klinische und ernahrungsanamnestische Erhebungen bei Norm und Übergewichtigen. *Zeitschrift für die Gesamte Innere Medizin und Ihre Grenzgebiete,* 23:225-228, 1968.

Katz, M.: Obesity, race, body-cathexis, and self-confrontation on closed circuit television. *Dissertation Abstracts International,* 30(4-8):1899, 1969.

Kleevens, J. W.: Diets of urban Chinese households in Singapore in relation to income. *Singapore Medical Journal,* 7:202-208, 1966.

Klotz, H. P.: Reflexiones therapeutiques sur l'obésité. Aspect psycho-social. *Alimentation et la Vie,* 57:71-80, 1969.

Krebs, W.: Obesity, a therapeutic and social problem. *Deutsche Gesundheitswesen,* 15:2512-2515, 1960.

Lachnit, V.: Fettleibigkeit. Sozialmedizinische und praventive Aspekte. *Wiener Zeitschrift für Innere Medizin und Ihre Grenzgebiete,* 50:236-243, 1969.

McKenzie, J. C.: Profile on slimmers. *Journal of Market Research Society,* 9:77, 1967.

McKenzie, J. C.: Social and economic implications of minority food habits. *Proceedings of the Nutrition Society,* 26:197-205, 1967.

Maddox, G. L., Back, K. W. and Liederman, V. R.: Overweight as social deviance and disability. *Journal of Health and Social Behavior,* 9:287-298, 1968.

Maddox, G. L. and Liederman, V. R.: Overweight as a social disability with medical implications. *Journal of Medical Education,* 44:214-220, 1969.

Meyer, J. E.: The adipose patient in relation to his self concept and social image. *Psychotherapy and Psychosomatics,* 16:249-255, 1968.

Meyer, J. E. and Tuchelt-Gallwitz, A.: A study in social image, body image, and the problem of psychogenetic factors in obesity. *Comprehensive Psychiatry,* 9:148-154, 1968.

Montegriffo, V.: A survey of the incidence of obesity in the United Kingdom. *Postgraduate Medical Journal,* Supplement, 47:418-422, 1971.

Moore, M. E.: Obesity and mental health (letter). *Journal of the American Medical Association,* 183:807, 1963.

Moore, M. E., Stunkard, A. J. and Srole, L.: Obesity, social class, and mental illness. *Journal of the American Medical Association,* 181:962-966, 1962.

Muller, H.: Die Schul und Berufsentwicklung von fettsuchtigen Frauen. *Zeitschrift für die Gesamte Innere Medizin und Ihre Grenzgebiete,* 24:464-467, 1969.

Perry, L. and Learnard, B.: Obesity and mental health (letter). *Journal of the American Medical Association,* 183:807-808, 1963.

Pflanz, M.: Medizinische-soziologische Aspekte der Fettsucht. *Psyche,* 16:575-591, 1963.

Pflanz, M.: *Socialer Wandel und Krankheit.* Stuttgart, Thieme, 1962.

Powdermaker, H.: An anthropological approach to the problem of obesity. *Bulletin of the New York Academy of Medicine,* 36:286-295, 1962.

Rilliet, B.: The medico-social problems raised by alimentary diets. *Praxis,* 58:1017-1022, 1969.

Shack, W. A.: *The Analysis of Socio-Psychological Field Research Data (Ethiopia).* United States Department of Health, Education and Welfare, Mental Health Research Grant MH-16427-01, 1969.

Silverstone, J. T.: Psychosocial aspects of obesity. *Proceedings of the Royal Society of Medicine,* 61:371-375, 1968.

Silverstone, J. T., Gordon, R. P. and Stunkard, A. J.: Social factors in obesity in London. *Practitioner,* 220:682-688, 1969.

Sterkowicz, S.: Social and therapeutic problems of obesity. *Wiadomosci Lekarskie,* 20:1449-1453, 1967.

Stunkard, A. J.: Environment and obesity: Recent advances in our understanding of regulation of food intake in man. *Federation Proceedings,* 27:1367-1373, 1968.

Sussman, M. B.: Psycho-social correlates of obesity: Failure of "calorie-collectors." *Journal of the American Dietetic Association,* 32:423-428, 1956.

Vann, D. H.: Components of attitudes toward the obese including presumed responsibility for the condition. *Proceedings of the Annual Convention of the American Psychological Association*, 5:695-696, Part 2, 1970.

Zachowy, A. C.: *The Influence of Social Class on the Psychodynamics of Obesity.* Unpublished doctoral dissertation, State University of New York at Albany, 1969.

IV. CHILDHOOD AND ADOLESCENT OBESITY
Childhood

Apley, J. and MacKeith, R.: *The Child and His Symptoms: A Psychosomatic Approach.* Oxford, Blackwell, 1961.

Asher, P.: Obesity in children. *Developmental Medicine and Child Neurology*, 6:415-416, 1964.

Bakwin, H.: Obesity in children. *Journal de Pediatria*, 23:487-500, 1958.

Bartek, H.: On the psyche of the obese child. *Zeitschrift für Alternsforschung*, 19:317-324, 1966.

Battay, L.: Comparative studies on the mental and physical development of infants and children brought up in state institutions, nurseries, and at home. *Gyermekgyogyaszat*, 14:16-21, 1963.

Bentovin, A.: The clinical approach to feeding disorders of children. *Journal of Psychosomatic Research*, 14:313-320, 1970.

Berlin, J. N.: Some observations in child psychology. *Western Medicine*, 4:240-244, 1963.

Berry-Bertrand, N.: Intérêt théorique et practique de l'examen psychologique dans l'obésité infantile. *Psychologie Français*, 6:286-293, 1961.

Blaim, A.: Clinical and therapeutical problems in children with obesity and rheumatic fever. *Reumatologia*, 5:145-149, 1967.

Blaim, A.: Current views on the pathogenesis of obesity in children. *Pediatria Polska*, 35:1363-1367, 1960.

Boegner-Plichet, M. J.: Psychosomatic obesity in children. *Cahiers R.M.F.*, 77:57-59, 1963.

Bonnet, F. and Lozet, H.: Le context medicosocial de l'obésité chez l'enfant. *Acta Paediatrica Belgica*, 22:211-252, 1968.

Bronstein, L. F., Wexler, S., Brown, A. W. and Halpern, L. J.: Obesity in childhood: Psychologic studies. *American Journal of Diseases of Children*, 63:238, 1942.

Bruch, H.: Children who grow too fat. *Child Study*, 18:82-84, 1942.

Bruch, H.: Dietary treatment of obesity in childhood. *Journal of the American Dietary Association*, 20:361-364, 1944.

Bruch, H.: Disturbed communication in eating disorders. In F. Irving and M. Powell (Eds.): *Psychosomatic Ailments in Childhood and Adolescence.* Springfield, Ill., Thomas, 1967, 90-99.

Bruch, H.: Family background in eating disorders. In E. J. Anthony and C. Koupernik (Eds.): *The Child in His Family.* New York, Wiley, 1970, 285-309.

Bruch, H.: Fat children grown up. *American Journal of the Diseases of Children*, 90:201, 1955.

Bruch, H.: Food and emotional security. *Nervous Child*, 3:165-173, 1944.

Bruch, H.: The Fröhlich syndrome. *American Journal of Diseases of Children*, 58:1282-1289, 1939.

Bruch, H.: Juvenile obesity: Its course and outcome. *International Psychiatry Clinics*, 7:231-254, 1970.

Bruch, H.: The management of obesity in childhood. *Our Children's Health*, 3:8-12, 1942.

Bruch, H.: Obesity. In F. Irving and M. Powell (Eds.): *Psychosomatic Ailments in Childhood and Adolescence.* Springfield, Ill., Thomas, 1967, 103-123.

Bruch, H.: Obesity in childhood and endocrine treatment. *Journal of Pediatrics,* 18: 36-56, 1941.

Bruch, H.: Obesity in childhood: I. Physical growth and development of obese children. *American Journal of Diseases of Children,* 58:457-484, 1939.

Bruch, H.: Obesity in childhood: II. Basal metabolism and serum cholesterol of obese children. *American Journal of Diseases of Children,* 58:1001-1022, 1939.

Bruch, H.: Obesity in childhood: III. Physiologic and psychologic aspects of the food intake of obese children. *American Journal of Diseases of Children,* 59:739-781, 1940.

Bruch, H.: Obesity in childhood: IV. Energy expenditure of obese children. *American Journal of Diseases of Children,* 60:1082-1109, 1940.

Bruch, H.: Obesity in childhood and adolescence. *Postgraduate Medicine,* 22:246-251, 1957.

Bruch, H.: Obesity and overnutrition. In S. S. Gellis and B. M. Kagan (Eds.): *Current Pediatric Therapy.* Philadelphia, Saunders, 1964, 2-3.

Bruch, H.: Overnutrition and obesity. In L. E. Holt and R. McIntosh (Eds.): *Pediatrics.* New York, Appleton-Century-Croft, 1953, 1962, 255-258.

Bruch, H.: Overweight children. In *Your Weight and How to Control It.* New York, Doubleday, 1949, 83-101.

Bruch, H.: Psychiatric aspects of obesity in children. *American Journal of Psychiatry,* 99:752-757, 1943.

Bruch, H.: Psychosomatic approach to childhood disorders. In N. D. C. Lewis and B. L. Pacella (Eds.): *Modern Trends in Child Psychiatry.* New York, International Universities Press, 1946, 57-78.

Bruch, H.: Psychotherapie der kindlichen Fettsucht. In *Handbuch der Kinderpsychotherapie,* Vol. II. Münich, Reinhardt, 1969, 935-942.

Bruch, H. and Touraine, G.: Obesity in childhood: V. The family frame of obese children. *Psychosomatic Medicine,* 2:141-206, 1940.

Bruch, H. and Waters, I.: Benzedrine sulfate (Amphetamine) in the treatment of obese children and adolescents. *Journal of Pediatrics,* 20:54-64, 1942.

Burchinal, L. G. and Eppright, E. S.: Test of the psychogenic theory of obesity for a sample of rural girls. *American Journal of Clinical Nutrition,* 7:288-294, 1959.

Cacciaguerra, F.: Behavior changes of an intellectual, characterial, nutritional and neurotic type concurrent with rigorous and maintenance diet therapy of obese children. *Alti della Accademia Medica Lombarda,* 21:227-238, Supplement, 1966.

Cavalca, G. G., *et al.*: Clinical aspects and treatment of obesity in the evolutive age. Physiopathological and psychological contribution. *Rivista Sperimentale di Freniatria e Medicina Legale delle Alienazione Mentali,* 90:1059-1130, 1966.

Cazzullo, A. G., Cocchi, A., and Gemerali, I.: Obésité de l'enfance: Contribution a l'étude psychodynamique. *Acta Paedopsychiatrica,* 35:324-326, 1968.

Cazzullo, C. L.: Neuropsychological aspects of infantile obesity. *Atti della Accademia Medica Lombarda,* 21:267-280, Supplement.

Chandra, R. K.: Obesity in childhood and adolescence. *Indian Journal of Pediatrics,* 35:72-74, 1968.

Clayton, G. W. and Librik, L.: Therapy of exogenous obesity in childhood and adolescence. *Pediatric Clinics of North America,* 10:99-107, 1963.

Collipp, P., Schmierer, B., Greensher, J., Rezvani, I. and Halle, M.: Childhood obesity

—To treat or not to treat. *Medical Times,* 99:155-156, 159, 162, 166-167, 171, 175, 177, 1971.

Cornell, M. M.: Psychological variables in the mother related to infant feeding patterns. *Dissertation Abstracts,* 29(9B):3479, 1969.

Crawford, J. D.: Obesity. In S. S. Gellis and B. M. Kagan (Eds.): *Current Pediatric Therapy,* 3rd ed. Philadelphia, Saunders, 1968.

Crook, W. G.: Thoughts on obesity in children. *Clinical Pediatrics,* 9:3A-4A, 1970.

Dailly, R. and Bertrand, N.: Approche psychologique de l'obésité infantile. *Gazette Médicale de France,* 65:307-308, 1958.

Decourt, J.: Sur l'anorexie mentale de l'adolescence dans le sexe masculin. *Revue de Neuropsychiatrie Infantile et d'Hygiène Mentale de l'Enfance,* 12:499-503, 1964.

DiCagno, L., *et al.:* Importance of the psychogenic factors in the cause of essential infantile obesity. *Minerva Pediatrica,* 19:660-662, 1967.

Diedenhofen, H.: Psychologic aspects. *Medizinische Monatsschrift,* 7:178-179, 1953.

Ellis, R. W. B. and Tallerman, K. H.: Obesity in childhood; Study of 50 cases. *Lancet,* 2:615-620, 1934.

Faggioli: Aspetti genetici dell'obesita infantile. *Rivista Italiana di Medicina Igiene Scuola,* 15:267-274, 1969.

Frank, L.: On the therapy of obesity in children. *Clinica Pediatrica,* 50:208-216, 1968.

Fromm, E.: Dynamics in a case of obesity. *Journal of Clinical and Experimental Psychopathology,* 19:292-302, 1958.

Fry, P. C.: Comparative study of obese children selected on basis of fat pads. *Journal of Clinical Nutrition,* 1:453-467, 1953.

Generali, I.: Infantile obesity. Psychodynamic aspects. *Atti della Accademia Medica Lombarda,* 21:239-244, Supplement, 1966.

Giliberti Tincolini, V., *et al.:* The psychodynamics of obesity in childhood and adolescence. *Atti della Accademia Medica Lombarda,* 21:181-187, Supplement, 1966.

Goldbloom, R. B.: Obesity in childhood. *Borden's Review of Nutrition Research,* 29: 1-13, 1968.

Goldbloom, R. B.: The special problem of obesity in childhood. *Modern Treatment,* 4:1146-1161, 1967.

Gonzales, J. L.: Compensacíon y decompensacíon en una obesidad juvenil. *Revista de Psicoanalises,* 12:445, 1955.

Graham, H. B.: Corpulence or obesity in childhood and adolescence. *Medical Journal of Australia,* 2:648-659, 1950.

Haase, K. E. and Rosenfeld, H. A.: Zur Fettsucht im Kindesalter. *Zeitschrift für Kinderheilkunde,* 78:1, 1965.

Heimann, F. A. and Worthington-Foxley, S. B.: School health service, its history and future. *Revue d'Hygiene et Medecin Scolaires,* 18:88-98, 1965.

Herr, R.: "Worry bacon" in children and adolescents. A contribution from child-guidance and forensic-psychological practice. *Praxis der Kinderpsychologie unde Kinderpsychiatrie,* 14:147-148, 1965.

Hill, J.: Infant feeding and personality disorders: A study of early feeding in its relation to emotional and digestive disorders. *Psychiatric Quarterly,* 11:356, 1937.

Hill, L. F.: Obesity in children. *South Dakota Journal of Medicine and Pharmacy,* 11: 139-143, 1958.

Huber, E. G.: On the origin of juvenile obesity. *Wiener Medizinische Wochenschrift,* 111:367-374, 1961.

Huber, E. G.: Persönlichkeitsuntersuchungen in adipöser Kindern. *Neue Österreichische Zeitschrift für Kinderheilkunde,* 2:186-197, 1957.

Huber, E. G.: Psychologische Aspekte der kindlichen Fettsucht. *Acta Paedopsychiatrica,* 35:290-294, 1968.

Illingworth, R. S.: Childhood obesity. *Practitioner,* 205:210-212, 1970.

Illingworth, R. S.: Obesity. *Journal of Pediatrics,* 53:117-130, 1958.

Iversen, T.: Psychogenic obesity in children. *Acta Paediatrica,* 42:8-19, 1953.

Iversen, T., Juel-Nielsen, N., Quaade, F., Tolstrup, K. and Ostergaard, L.: On psychogenic obesity in children. *Acta Paediatrica,* 40:59-60, Supplement 83, 1951.

Iversen, T., Juel-Nielsen, N., Quaade, F., Tolstrup, K. and Ostergaard, L.: Psychogenic obesity in children with special reference to Hilde Bruch's theory. *Acta Paediatrica,* 41:574-576, 1952.

Josselyn, I.: *The Happy Child. A Psychoanalytic Guide to Emotional and Social Growth.* New York, Random House, 1955, 288-289.

Juel-Nielsen, N.: On psychogenic obesity in children. II. *Acta Paediatrica,* 42:130-146, 1953.

Kahn, E. J.: Obesity in children: Identification of a group at risk in a New York ghetto. *Journal of Pediatrics,* 77:771-774, 1970.

Kneebone, G. M.: Drug therapy: An effective treatment of obesity in childhood. *Medical Journal of Australia,* 2:663-665, 1968.

Kriesler, L.: L'abord psychosomatique de l'obésité commune de l'enfant. *Medicine de l'Enfant,* 74:309-326, 1967.

Laplane, R. and Etienne, M.: Child obesity; psychologic data; 100 cases. *Proceedings of the Royal Society of Medicine,* 46:1058-1059, 1953.

Laplane, R., Etienne, M. and Laplane, E.: Psychologic study of infantile obesity. *La Semaine des Hôpitaux de Paris,* 32:2793-3801, 1956.

Lauro, G. E.: *Aspects of Personality in Overweight and Underweight Preadolescent Girls.* Dissertation, New York University, 1958.

Lawrence, W. C.: A study of overweight schoolchildren. *Health Bulletin,* 28:44-46, 1970.

Leboeuf, G., *et al.:* Management of obesity in children. *Applied Therapeutics,* 7:32-37, 1965.

Levine, M. I. and Seligman, J. H.: Emotional reasons for obesity. In *Your Overweight Child.* New York, World, 1970, 27-44.

Lloyd, J. K. and Wolff, O. H.: Childhood obesity. *British Medical Journal,* 5245:145-148, 1961.

Lorber, J.: Obesity in childhood. *Clinical Pediatrics,* 6:325-326, 1967.

Lourie, R. S.: A pediatric-psychiatric viewpoint on obesity. *Pediatrics,* 20:553, 1957.

Lurie, O. R.: Psychological factors associated with eating difficulties in children. *American Journal of Orthopsychiatry,* 11:452, 1941.

Macaulay, D.: Obesity in infants and children. *Archives of Diseases in Childhood,* 26:539-542, 1951.

McHale, K.: *Comparative Psychology and Hygiene of the Overweight Child.* New York, Teachers College, Columbia University, Contributions to Education, No. 221, 1926.

McNaughton, J. W., *et al.:* A study of the energy expenditure and food intake of five boys and four girls. *British Journal of Nutrition,* 24:345-355, 1970.

McQuarrie, I.: Obesity in infants and children. *GP,* 2:35-37, 1950.

Maisch, H.: The intellectual achievement of a group of adipose children. An experimental contribution to the psychosomatic manifestations of adiposis in childhood. *Medizinische Klinik,* 43:1086-1091, 1965.

Maisch, H., Schönberg, D. and Wallis, H.: Psychosomatische Aspekte der einfachen Adipositas in Kindesalter. *Psyche,* 19:339-364, 1965.

Maisch, H. and Wallis, H.: Ein psychosomatisches Modell, gezeigt an der einfachen Adipositas der Kinder. II Sozial-psychologische und psychopathologische Befunde sowie psychologische Modellvorstelling. *Monatschrift für Kinderheilkunde,* 113: 219-222, 1965.

Maisch, H., *et al.*: The therapy of simple obesity in children. *Zeitschrift für Psychosomatische Medizine und Psychoanalyse,* 12:61-68, 1966.

Mayer, J.: Obesity in childhood and adolescence. *Medical Clinics of North America,* 48:1347-1358, 1964.

Mayer, J.: Some aspects of obesity in children. *Postgraduate Medicine,* 34:83-88, 1963.

Metzl, K., Keitges, P., Kantor, J. and Bordy, M.: The Pickwickian syndrome in a child. An extreme example of psychoneurotic obesity. *Clinical Pediatrics,* 8:49-53, 1969.

Moss, F. A.: Note on building likes and dislikes in children. *Journal of Experimental Psychology,* 7:475-478, 1924.

Mossberg, H. O.: Obesity in children: A clinical-prognostical investigation. *Acta Paediatrica Scandinavia,* 35:9, Supplement 2, 1948.

Obesity in Childhood: *Lancet,* 2:1353, 1966.

Ostergaard, L.: On psychogenic obesity in childhood. V. *Acta Paediatrica,* 43:507-521, 1954.

Posteraro, G.: Neuropsychological disorders in obesity in childhood. *Atti della Accademia Medica Lombarda,* 21:245-246, Supplement.

Prugh, D. E.: Some psychologic considerations concerned with the problem of over-nutrition. *American Journal of Clinical Nutrition,* 9:538-547, 1961.

Quaade, F.: *Obese Children: Anthropology and Environment.* Copenhagen, Danish Science Press, 1955.

Quaade, F.: On psychogenic obesity in children. III. *Acta Paediatrica,* 42:191-205, 1953.

Raimbault, G. and Vigy, M.: Aspects psychologiques de l'obésité de l'enfant. *Concours Médical,* 90:7421-7431, 1968.

Rascovsky, A.: Notas sobre la psicogénesis de la obesidad. *Prensa Medicale Argentina,* 15:1735-1739, 1948.

Rascovsky, A. and Rosquellas, A. R.: Estudio de la functión psicomotriz en el sindrome adiposogenital infantil. In A. Rascovsky (Ed.): *Patalogía psicomática.* Buenos Aires, El Ateneo, 1948, 597-604.

Rauh, J. L., Schumsky, D. A. and Witt, M. T.: Heights, weights, and obesity in urban school children. *Child Development,* 38:515-530, 1967.

Roger, R.: A "school phobia" in an obese girl. *Journal of Clinical Psychology,* 18:356-357, 1962.

Reilly, W. A.: Obesity in infants and children. *GP,* 4:41-46, 1951.

Reilly, W. A.: Treatment of obese children. *Southern Medical Journal,* 45:217-222, 1952.

Riedel, H.: Problem of obesity during childhood. *Medizinische Monatsschrift,* 7:146-149, 1953.

Romeo, G.: Character disorders in obesity in childhood. *Atti della Accademia Medica Lombarda*, 21:131-133, 1966.

Rony, H. R.: Juvenile obesity. *Endocrinology*, 16:601-610, 1932.

Rosenberg, D.: Juvenile obesity: Therapeutic problems in the light of a personal experience. *Lyon Médical*, 221:799-802 *passim*, 1969.

Rossini, R.: Neuro-psychological aspects of infantile obesity. *Atti della Accademia Medica Lombarda*, 21:127-143, Supplement, 1966.

Scanabissi, E., et al.: Electroencephalographic, psychological, endocrine and metabolic aspects of simple infantile obesity. *Minerva Pediatrica*, 22:2276-2282, 1970.

Schreier, K. and Spranger, J.: Obesity in childhood in the light of recent research. *Archiv für Kinderheilkunde*, 44:1-160, Supplement, 1961.

Schultz, F. W.: What to do about the fat child at puberty. *Journal of Pediatrics*, 19: 376, 1941.

Schwartz, A. S.: Eating problems. *Pediatric Clinics of North America*, 5:595-611, 1958.

Scrimshaw, N. S. and Gordon, J. E. (Eds.): *Malnutrition, Learning and Behavior: Proceedings of an International Conference.* Cambridge, Mass., Massachusetts Institute of Technology Press, 1968.

Seltzer, C. C. and Mayer, J.: An effective weight control program in a public school system. *American Journal of Public Health*, 60:679-689, 1970.

Selvini, M. P.: Die Bildung des Körperbewusstseins, die Ernährung des Kindes als Lernprocess. *Psychotherapy and Psychosomatics*, 15:293, 1967.

Sjovall, B.: Therapy: Obesity in infants and children. *Nordisk Medicin*, 51:871-873, 1954.

Soule, M.: Conflits dynamique de la psychologie et de la thérapeutique de l'enfant obese. *Médecine de l'Enfant*, 74:329-335, 1967.

Sperling, M.: The role of the mother in psychosomatic disorders in children. *Psychosomatic Medicine*, 11:377, 1949.

Spranger, J.: Significance of cerebral damage in childhood obesity. *Annales Paediatrici*, 197:39-61, 1961.

Spranger, J.: Therapy of obesity in childhood. *Internistische Praxis*, 5:89-93, 1965.

Spranger, J. and Dörken, J.: Kindliche Adipositas: Prüfung der Psychodynamik unter d-Norpseudophedrin. *Monatsschrift für Kinderheilkunde*, 114:394-396, 1966.

Spranger, J., et al.: Obesity in children. *Medizinische Monatsschrift*, 21:105-110, 1967.

Steiner, M. M.: Obesity in infants and children. *Pediatric Clinics of North America*, 2:553-565, 1955.

Steiner, M. M.: Symposium on pediatrics: Management of obesity in childhood. *Medical Clinics of North America*, 34:223-234, 1950.

Stuart, H. C.: Obesity in childhood. *Quarterly Review of Pediatrics*, 10:131-145, 1955.

Stunkard, A. J. and Pestka, J.: The physical activity of obese girls. *American Journal of Diseases of Children*, 103:812-817, 1962.

Tolstrup, K.: The necessity for differential eating disorders. Discussion of Hilde Bruch's paper on the family background. In E. J. Anthony and C. Koupernik (Eds.): *The Child in His Family.* New York, Wiley, 1970.

Tolstrup, K.: On psychogenic obesity in children. *Acta Paediatrica*, 42:289-304, 1953.

Tolstrup, K.: Psychosomatic aspects of obesity in childhood. *Psyche*, 16:592-599, 1963.

Vailati, G.: L'obesita nell'eta scolare. *Rivista Italiana di Medicina Igiene Scuola*, 15: 132-180, 1969.

Vamberová, M.: Therapeutic regimen in obese children. *Review of Czechoslovak Medicine*, 4:135-144, 1958.

Viani, F.: Neurological and electroencephalographic aspects of infantile obesity. *Atti della Accademia Medica Lombarda*, 21:159-180, Supplement, 1966.

Weill, J. and Bernfeld, J.: Obesity in infants and children. *La Semaine des Hôpitaux de Paris*, 27:3652-3659, 1951.

Weill, J. and Bernfeld, J.: Obesity in infants and children. *La Revue du Practicien*, 2:993-1001, 1952.

Whelen, W. S.: Childhood obesity. *British Medical Journal*, 5245:145-148, 1961.

Wilkes, E. T.: A survey of three hundred obese girls. *Archives of Pediatrics*, 77:441-451, 1960.

Willich, E.: Survey of therapy during childhood. *Die Medizinische*, 1382-1385, 1954.

Wolff, O. H.: Obesity in childhood. *Triangle*, 7:234-239, 1966.

Wolff, O. H.: Obesity in childhood and its effects. *Postgraduate Medical Journal*, 38: 629-632, 1962.

Wolff, P. H.: *Development of Affect Expressions in Small Children*. U. S. Department of Health, Education and Welfare, Mental Health Research Grant, MH-06034-7, 1968.

Wright, F. H.: Prevention of obesity in childhood. *Clinical Pediatrics*, 2:353-359, 1963.

Zhukovska, M. A.: Some clinical and diagnostic problems of obesity in children. *Pediatriia*, 45:72-79, 1966.

Adolescence

Bayles, S. and Ebaugh, F. G.: Emotional factors in eating and obesity. *Journal of the American Dietetic Association*, 26:430-434, 1950.

Berlin, J. N., Boatman, M. J., Sheimo, S. L. and Szurek, S. A.: Adolescent alternation of anorexia and obesity. *American Journal of Orthopsychiatry*, 21:387-419, 1951; In G. E. Gardner (Ed.): *Case Studies in Childhood Emotional Disabilities*. New York, American Orthopsychiatric Association, 1953.

Berryman, G. H.: Obesity in college students. *Journal of the American College Health Association*, 11:300-311, 1963.

Biener, K.: Übergewicht und Kostform Jugendlicher. *Internationale Zeitschrift für Vitaminforschung*, 39:323-333, 1969.

Bruch, H.: Eating disorders in adolescence. In J. Zubin and A. M. Freedman (Eds.): *The Psychopathology of Adolescence*. New York, Grune and Stratton, 1970, 181-196.

Bruch, H.: Family transactions in eating disorders. *Comprehensive Psychiatry*, 12: 238-248, 1971.

Bruch, H.: Obesity in adolescence. In G. Caplan and S. Lebovici (Eds.): *Adolescence: Psychosocial Perspectives*. New York, Basic Books, 1969, 213-225.

Bruch, H.: Obesity in relation to puberty. *Journal of Pediatrics*, 19:365-375, 1941.

Bruch, H.: Psychological aspects of obesity in adolescence. *American Journal of Public Health*, 48:1349-1353, 1958.

Bruch, H.: Puberty and adolescence; Psychologic considerations. In *Advances in Pediatrics*, Vol. 3. New York, Interscience Press, 1948, 219-296.

Bullen, B. A., Monello, L. F., Cohen, H. and Mayer, J.: Attitudes toward physical activity, food and family in obese and non-obese adolescent girls. *American Journal of Clinical Nutrition*, 12:1-11, 1963.

Bullen, B. A., Reed, R. B. and Mayer, J.: Physical activity of obese and nonobese adolescent girls appraised by motion picture sampling. *American Journal of Clinical Nutrition*, 14:211-223, 1964.

Canning, H. and Mayer, J.: Obesity: An analysis of attitudes, knowledge, and weight control in girls. *Research Quarterly*, 39:894-899, 1968.

Canning, H. and Mayer, J.: Obesity: An influence on high school performance. *American Journal of Clinical Nutrition*, 20:352-354, 1967.

Canning, H. and Mayer, J.: Obesity: Its possible effect on college acceptance. *New England Journal of Medicine*, 275:1172-1174, 1966.

Carrera, F.: Obesity in adolescence. *Psychosomatics*, 8:342-349, 1967.

Christiaens, L.: Obesities of the pubertal period. *Lille Médical*, 5:565-573, 1960.

Comolli, E.: Simple obesity of developmental age. *Minerva Medica*, 1:1555-1566, 1954.

DeNegri, M., *et al.*: Clinical and electroencephalographic correlations during disturbances in obese individuals. *Igiene Moderna*, 12:710-711, 1968.

Dudleston, A. K. and Bennion, M.: Effect of diet and/or exercise on obese college women. *Journal of the American Dietetic Association*, 56:126-129, 1970.

Dwyer, J. T., Feldman, J. J. and Mayer, J.: Adolescent dieters: Who are they? Physical characteristics, attitudes and dieting practices of adolescent girls. *American Journal of Clinical Nutrition*, 20:1045-1056, 1967.

Dwyer, J. T. and Mayer, J.: Variations in physical appearance during adolescence: Part I. Boys. *Postgraduate Medicine*, 41:99-107, 1967.

Dwyer, J. T. and Mayer, J.: Variations in physical appearance during adolescence: Part 2. Girls. *Postgraduate Medicine*, 41:91-97, 1967.

Easson, W. M.: *The Severely Disturbed Adolescent. Inpatient, Residential and Hospital Treatment.* New York, International Universities Press, 1969.

Frisk, M., *et al.*: Overweight in adolescents—a complex problem. *Annales Paediatriae Fenniae*, 12:234-245, 1966.

Friedman, J.: Psychological correlates of overweight, underweight and normal weight college women. *Dissertation Abstracts*, 19:3362, 1959.

Gallagher, J. R., Heald, F. P. and Masland, R. P.: Recent contributions to adolescent medicine. *New England Journal of Medicine*, 259:24-31, 1958.

Garell, D. C.: The obese person as an adolescent. *California Medicine*, 106:368-371, 1967.

Hammar, S. L.: The obese adolescent. *Journal of School Health*, 25:246-249, 1965.

Hammar, S. L.: A study of adolescent obesity. In A. Bandura and R. H. Walters (Eds.): *Social Learning and Personality Development.* New York, Holt, Rinehart and Winston, 1964.

Hammar, S. L., Holterman, V. and Campbell, M. M.: A study of adolescent obesity. *GP*, 28:78-85, 1963.

Heald, F. P.: Natural history and physiological bases of adolescent obesity. *Federation Proceedings*, 25:1-3, 1966.

Heald, F. P.: Obesity in the adolescent. *Pediatric Clinics of North America*, 7:207-220, 1960.

Heald, F. P. and Hollander, R. J.: The relationship between obesity in adolescence and early growth. *Journal of Pediatrics*, 67:35-38, 1965.

Huenemann, R. L.: Consideration of adolescent obesity as a public health problem. *Public Health Reports*, 83:491-495, 1968.

Huenemann, R. L., Hampton, M. C., Shapiro, L. R. and Behnke, A.: Adolescent food practices associated with obesity. *Federation Proceedings*, 25:4-10, 1966.

Huenemann, R. L., Shapiro, L. R., Hampton, M. C. and Mitchell, B. W.: Food and eating practices of teen-agers. *Journal of the American Dietetic Association,* 53: 17-24, 1968.

Huenemann, R. L., Shapiro, L. R., Hampton, M. C., Mitchell, B. W. and Behnke, A. R.: A longitudinal study of gross body composition and body conformation and their association with food and activity in a teenage population. Views of teenage subjects on body conformation, food, and activity. *American Journal of Clinical Nutrition,* 18:325-338, 1966.

Janson, P.: The pubertal slimness mania of young girls. *Landarzt,* 41:53-55, 1965.

Johnson, M. L., Burke, B. S. and Mayer, J.: Relative importance of inactivity and overeating in energy balance of obese high school girls. *American Journal of Clinical Nutrition,* 4:37-44, 1956.

Kannel, W. B., Pearson, G. and McNamara, P. M.: Obesity as a force of morbidity. In F. P. Heald (Ed.): *Adolescent Nutrition and Growth.* New York, Appleton-Century-Croft, 51-71, 1969.

Kline, A. J., Barron, J. and Roberts, M. M.: Comprehensive self-improvement program for inner city obese teenage girls. *Journal of School Health,* 39:21-28, 1969.

Klinke, E.: Etiology and pathogenesis during adolescence. (Adiposogigantism.) *Die Medizinische,* 749-751, 1952.

Lemieux, R. and Martel, A.: L'obésité de la puberté. *Laval Médical,* 13:60-73, 1948.

Lodi, G.: Adiposity and adolescence. *Minerva Pediatrica,* 22:2225-2227, 1970.

Lord, W. J.: Health education about obesity: The results of a two-year follow-up. *Journal of the College of General Practitioners,* 11:285-293, 1966.

McNaughton, J. W., *et al.*: A study of the food intake and activity of a group of urban adolescents. *British Journal of Nutrition,* 24:331-334, 1970.

Massengale, O. N. The obese adolescent. Observations on etiology, management, prevention. *Clinical Pediatrics,* 4:649-654, 1965.

Mayer, J.: Inactivity as a major factor in adolescent obesity. *Annals of the New York Academy of Sciences,* 131:502-506, 1965.

Mayer, J.: Obesity in adolescence. *Mental Clinics of North America,* 49:421-432, 1965.

Mayer, J.: *Obesity in Adolescents.* U. S. Department of Health, Education and Welfare, National Institutes of Health Research Grant, AM-02839-9, 1968.

Mayer, J.: Physical activity and anthropometric measurements of obese adolescents. *Federation Proceedings,* 25:11-14, 1966.

Medovy, H.: Problems of adolescence. *Canadian Medical Association Journal,* 90: 1354-1360, 1964.

Merrifield, H. H. and Caliel, R. J.: Effect of an "overload" concentric training of the quadriceps on strength and limb circumference in females. *Perceptual and Motor Skills,* 31:563-568, 1970.

Migdole, S. M.: An investigation of orality, depression, and denial in obese and non-obese adolescent females. *Dissertation Abstracts,* 4850-B, 1967.

Monello, L. F. and Mayer, J.: Obese adolescent girls: Unrecognized "minority" group? *American Journal of Clinical Nutrition,* 13:35-39, 1963.

Nathan, S. and Pisula, D.: Psychological observations of obese adolescents during starvation treatment. *Journal of the American Academy of Child Psychiatry,* 9: 722-740, 1970.

Obesity control for adolescents. *Roche Medical Image,* 32-34, 1967.

Pargman, D.: The incidence of obesity among college students. *Journal of School Health,* 39:621-627, 1969.

Payne, I. R., Rasmussen, D. M. and Shinedling, M.: Characteristics of obese university females who lose weight. *Psychological Reports*, 27:567-570, 1970.

Schachter, S.: Discussion of Dr. Bruch's paper (Eating disorders in adolescence). In J. Zubin and A. M. Freedman (Eds.): *The Psychopathology of Adolescence.* New York, Grune and Stratton, 1970, 197-202.

Schonfeld, W. A.: Management of male pubescence. *Journal of the American Medical Association*, 121:177-182, 1943.

Shapiro, L. R., Hampton, M. C. and Huenemann, R. L.: Teenagers: Their body size and shape, food, and activity. *Journal of School Health*, 37:166-170, 1967.

Shuttleworth, F. K.: The adolescent period: A pictorial atlas. *Monographs of the Society for Research in Child Development*, 14 (Ser. No. 50 Publ. 1951) 1949.

Sperling, M.: Psychosomatic disorders. In S. Lorand and H. Schneer (Eds.): *Adolescents: Psychoanalytic Approach to Problems and Therapy.* New York, Paul B. Hoeber, 1961, 202-216.

Stanley, E. J., Glaser, H. H., Levin, D. G., Adams, P. A. and Coley, I. L.: Overcoming obesity in adolescents. A description of a promising endeavor to improve management. *Clinical Pediatrics*, 9:29-36, 1970.

Stefanik, P. A., Heald, F. P. and Mayer, J.: Caloric intake in relation to energy output of obese and non-obese adolescent boys. *American Journal of Clinical Nutrition*, 7:55-62, 1959.

Steffenberg, M. L.: Overweight teenage girls. *Delaware Medical Journal*, 41:64, 1969.

Stolz, H. R. and Stolz, L. M.: *Somatic Development of Adolescent Boys.* New York, Macmillan, 1951.

Strear, S.: *A Comparison of Two Methods of Group Counseling With Obese Adolescents.* Doctoral dissertation, Yeshiva University, 1969.

Stuart, H. C.: Normal growth and development during adolescence. *New England Journal of Medicine*, 234:666-672, 693-700, 732-738, 1946.

Todd, R. L. and Siemers, D. P.: Results of reducing diet for overweight university students. *Lancet*, 69:429-430, 1949.

Unwin, J. R.: Biological growth during adolescence. In S. J. Shamsie (Ed.): *Adolescent Psychiatry.* New York, Schering Corporation, 1968, 25-33.

Vamberová, M., Parizkova, J. and Tejralova, J.: Effect of puberty on the development of obesity. *Ceskoslovenska Pediatrie*, 17:1057-1064, 1962.

Vamberová, M. and Tejralova, J.: Puberty in obesity. *Ceskoslovenska Pediatrie*, 15:1006-1013, 1960.

Werkman, S. L. and Greenberg, E. S.: Personality and interest patterns of obese adolescent girls. *Psychosomatic Medicine*, 29:72-80, 1967.

Witlers, R. F. J.: Problems in genetics of human obesity. *Eugenics Review*, 56:81-90, 1964.

Wolanski, N.: How to evaluate obesity in children and adolescents. *Pediatria Polska*, 45:101-106, 1970.

V. INDIVIDUAL THERAPY

Bayles, S.: Psychiatric contributions to the treatment of obesity. *American Journal of Medical Sciences*, 219:104-107, 1950.

Bernard, J. L.: Rapid treatment of gross obesity by operant techniques. *Psychological Reports*, 23:663-666, 1968.

Bigsby, F. L. and Muniz, C.: Surface psychotherapy in the treatment of obesity. *Medical Times*, 94:1161-1169, 1966.

Blancheton, C.: Psychological conditioning of the obese. *Clinique,* 59:671-673, 1964.

Bolding, O. T., *et al.:* Weight loss and psychological observations of gynecological patients. II. *Alabama Journal of Medical Science,* 7:87-91, 1970.

Bram, I.: Psychic factors in obesity; Observations in over 1,000 cases. *Archives of Pediatrics,* 67:543-552, 1950.

Bruch, H.: Effectiveness in psychotherapy or the constructive use of ignorance. *Psychiatric Quarterly,* 37:332-339, 1963.

Bruch, H.: Prognosis and treatment of obesity from a psychiatric point of view. *Problemes Actuels d'Endocrinologie et de Nutrition,* 7:319-326, 1963.

Bruch, H.: Prognosis and treatment of obesity from a psychiatrist's point of view. *Journal of the American Medical Women's Association,* 19:745-749, 1964.

Bruch, H.: Psychotherapeutic problems in eating disorders. *Psychoanalytic Review,* 50:573-587, 1963.

Bruch, H.: Psychotherapy and eating disorders. *International Psychiatry Clinics,* 7:335-351, 1970.

Bruch, H.: Psychotherapy in obesity. In J. H. Masserman (Ed.): *Current Psychiatric Therapies,* Vol. 8. New York, Grune and Stratton, 1968, 63-69.

Bruch, H.: Therapeutic problems in eating disorders. *Psychoanalytic Review,* 50:573-587, 1964.

Bruch, H.: Treatment of obesity (Overnutrition). In H. C. Shirkey (Ed.): *Pediatric Therapy.* St. Louis, Mosby, 1964, 235-240.

Cautela, J. R.: Treatment of compulsive behavior by covert sensitization. *Psychological Record,* 16:33-41, 1966.

Cohen, J. J.: Importance of unobtrusiveness in treating obesity. *GP,* 10:43-46, 1954.

Conrad, G.: Short-term casework treatment of obesity in two young women. *Israel Annals of Psychiatry and Related Disciplines,* 7:179-184, 1969.

Cornell Conference on Therapy: The management of obesity. *New York State Journal of Medicine,* 58:79-87, 1958.

Cornell Conference on Therapy: Treatment of obesity. *American Journal of Medicine,* 13:478-486, 1952.

Crider, B.: Psychotherapy in a case of obesity. *Journal of Clinical Psychology,* 2:50-58, 1946.

Dorfman, W.: Obesity: Psychosomatic treatment. *New York State Journal of Medicine,* 51:2655-2656, 1951.

Duncan, G. G., *et al.:* Correction and control of intractable obesity. *Journal of the American Medical Association,* 181:309, 1962.

Erlande, G.: Functional obesity. *Le Progrès Médical,* 80:307-312, 1952.

Fazekas, J. F. and Alman, R. W.: Neuropsychological aspects of hyperorexia and anorexogenic agents. *Practitioner,* 187:566-573, 1961.

Foreyt, J. P.: Control of overeating by aversion therapy. *Dissertation Abstracts International,* 30(12-B):5688, 1970.

Foreyt, J. P. and Kennedy, W. A.: Treatment of overweight by aversion therapy. *Behaviour Research and Therapy,* 9:29-34, 1971.

Freed, S. C.: Obesity: Newer concepts. *GP,* 14:63-68, 1953.

Freyberger, H. and Strube, K.: On the psychodynamics and psychotherapy of increased eating needs in obese patients. *Schweizerische Medizinische Wochenschrift,* 93:559-563, 1963.

Freyberger, H. and Strube, K.: Psychosomatic aspects of obesity. *Psyche,* 16:561-578, 1963.

Freyberger, H. and Strube, K.: On the psychosomatics and the psychotherapy of obesity. *Deutsche Medizinische Wochenschrift,* 87:199-203, 1962.

Gained, R.: Fenfluramine (Ponderax) in the treatment of obese psychiatric out-patients. *British Journal of Psychiatry,* 115:963-964, 1969.

Genevard, G.: Psychothérapie et obésité. *Praxis,* 48:413-417, 1959.

Glenn, M. B.: Education and motivation in the treatment of obesity. *Journal of the American College Health Association,* 13:521-531, 1965.

Goldiamond, I.: Self-control procedures in personal behavior problems. *Psychological Reports,* 17:851-868, 1965.

Hamburger, W. W.: The occurrence and meaning of dreams of food and eating: I. Typical food and eating dreams of four patients in analysis. *Psychosomatic Medicine,* 20:1-16, 1958.

Harris, M. B.: Self-directed program for weight control: A pilot study. *Journal of Abnormal Psychology,* 74:263-270, 1969.

Hashim, S. A. and Van Itallie, T. B.: Studies in normal and obese subjects with a monitored food dispensary device. *Annals of the New York Academy of Science,* 131:654-661, 1965.

Hochrein, M. and Schleicher, I.: Zur Beurteilung, Begutachtung und Behandlung der Fettleibigkeit. *Medizinische Monatsschrift,* 9:649-656, 730-734, 1955.

Hochrein, M. and Schleicher, I.: Zur Therapie der Adipositas. *Münchener Medizinische Wochenschrift,* 93:1395-1404, 1951.

Huckel, H.: More than bread: 6 cases of compulsive eating. *Psychoanalysis,* 4:53-62, 1955.

Hutton, J. H. and Creticos, A. P.: Obesity and its treatment. *Industrial Medicine and Surgery,* 35:355-360, 1966.

Jolliffe, N. and Alpert, E.: Symposium on prolonged illness; "Performance index" as therapeutic tool in the management of obesity. *Medical Clinics of North America,* 37:733-746, 1953.

Jonas, A. D.: Obesity: Psychologic approach to the problem. *American Practitioner,* 1:933-937, 1950.

Kennedy, W. A. and Foreyt, J. P.: Control of eating behavior in an obese patient by avoidance conditioning. *Psychological Reports,* 22:571-576, 1968.

Kessler, P.: Zur Behandlung der exogenen Fettsucht. *Medizinische Monatsschrift,* 5: 96-97, 1951.

Kleine, H. O.: Die Psychotherapie in der Behandlung Fettsüchtiger. *Münchener Medizinische Wochenschrift,* 100:265-268, 1958.

Kroger, W. S.: Psychologic factors in obesity and anorexic drugs. *American Practitioner,* 10:2169-2171, 1959.

Lee, A. R., Bruch, H. and Stunkard, A. J.: Clinical symposium: Psychological and physiological aspects of marked obesity in a young adult female. *Journal of Hillside Hospital,* 8:190-215, 1959.

Lindner, R.: Solitaire, the story of Laura. In *The Fifty-Minute Hour, a Collection of True Psychoanalytic Tales.* New York, Rinehart, 1954, 79-118.

Macdonald, I.: Trends in the treatment of obesity. *Guy's Hospital Reports,* 119:329-336, 1970.

Mann, W. N.: Obesity and its treatment. *Practitioner,* 164:436-440, 1950.

Mayer, J.: Obesity: Psychologic aspects and therapy. *Postgraduate Medicine,* 25:739-746, 1959.

Mendelson, M., Weinberg, N. and Stunkard, A. J.: Obesity in men: A clinical study of twenty-five cases. *Annals of Internal Medicine,* 54:660, 1961.

Meynen, G. E.: A comparative study of three treatment approaches with the obese: Relaxation, covert sensitization and modified systematic desensitization. *Dissertation Abstracts International,* 31(5-B):2998, 1970.

Netto, L. F.: Treatment of obesity. *Resenha Clinico-Cientifica,* 38:195-199, 1969.

Penick, S. B.: The use of amphetamines in obesity. *Psychiatric Opinion,* 7:26-30, 1970.

Pennington, A. W.: Obesity. Therapy: Developments of the past 150 years. *American Journal of Digestive Diseases,* 21:65-69, 1954.

Proksch, N.: Differential diagnosis and therapy of female obesity. *Zeitschrift für die gesamte innere Medizin und ihre Grenzgebiete,* 11:381-383, 1956.

Psychologic management in a patient with morbid obesity. *Journal of the Tennessee Medical Association,* 64:122-126, 1971.

Richardson, H. B.: Obesity as a manifestation of neurosis. *Medical Clinics of North America,* 30:1187-1202, 1946; 29:1217, 1945.

Richardson, H. B.: Obesity and neurosis: A case report. *Psychiatric Quarterly,* 20: 400-424, 1946.

Richardson, H. B.: Psychotherapy of the obese patient. *New York State Journal of Medicine,* 47:2574-2578, 1947.

Riss, W.: *CNS Control of Food Intake, Energy Output and Emotion.* U. S. Department of Health, Education and Welfare, Mental Health Research Grant RO3-MH-0239 01, 1963.

Robinson, S., *et al.:* Motivation for the addiction to amphetamine and reducing drugs. *Israel Annals of Psychiatry and Related Disciplines,* 7:213-232, 1969.

Rosenberg, P.: Use of mood ameliorating agents (d-amphetamine-amobarbital combination) in psychogenic obesity. *American Practitioner,* 4:818-823, 1953.

Schmidt, S. C.: Treatment of obesity. *Medical Record,* 163:118-126, 1950.

Settel, E.: Combined d-amphetamine and chlordiazepoxide therapy in the emotionally disturbed obese patient. *Clinical Medicine,* 70:1077-1088, 1963.

Silverstone, J. T. and Solomon, T.: Psychiatric and somatic factors in the treatment of obesity. *Journal of Psychosomatic Research,* 9:249-255, 1965.

Solomon, N.: The study and treatment of the obese patient. *Hospital Practice,* 4:90-94, 1969.

Solow, C.: *Effects of Intestinal By-pass Surgery for Obesity.* U. S. Department of Health, Education and Welfare, National Institute of Mental Health Research Grant RO3-MH-17294-01, 1970.

Stellar, E.: *Neurological Mechanisms Underlying Behavior.* U. S. Department of Health, Education and Welfare, National Institute of Mental Health Research Grant, MH-03571-9, 1968.

Stollak, G. E.: Weight loss obtained under different experimental procedures. *Psychotherapy: Theory, Research and Practice,* 4:61-64, 1967.

Stuart, R. B.: Behavioral control of overeating. *Behavior Research and Therapy,* 5: 357-365, 1967.

Stuart, R. B.: Situational versus self control. In R. D. Rubin (Ed.): *Advances in Behavior Therapy.* New York, Academy Press, 1971.

Stuart, R. B. and Davis, B.: *Slim Chance in a Fat World, Behavioral Control of Obesity.* Champaign, Ill., Research Press, 1972.

Stuart, R. B.: A three-dimensional program for the treatment of obesity. *Behavior Research and Therapy,* 9:177-186, 1971.

Stunkard, A. J.: Psychological aspects of obesity—Summary. "Progress to uncertainty." *International Journal of Psychiatry,* 2:614-616, 1966.

Stunkard, A. J.: Untoward reactions to weight reduction among certain obese persons. *Annals of the New York Academy of Sciences,* 63:4-5, 1955.

Tyler, V. O. and Straughan, J. H.: Coverant control and breath holding as techniques for the treatment of obesity. *Psychological Record,* 20:473-478, 1970.

Wang, R. I. H. and Sandoval, R.: Current status of drug therapy in management of obesity. *Wisconsin Medical Journal*, 68:219-220, 1969.

Weil, J. N.: Psicoanálisis de una obesa con perversiones sexuales. *Revista de Psicoanálisis*, 14:389-500, 1957.

Weinhaus, R. S.: The management of obesity. Some recent concepts. *Missouri Medicine*, 66:719-723, 730, 1969.

Wolpe, J.: *Psychotherapy by Reciprocal Inhibition.* Stanford, Stanford University Press, 1958.

Wolpe, J.: Reciprocal inhibition as the main base of psychotherapeutic effects. *Archives of Neurology and Psychiatry*, 72:205-226, 1954.

Young, C. M.: Helping the overweight individual. In E. S. Eppright, *et al.* (Eds.): *Weight Control.* Ames, Iowa, Iowa State College Press, 1955, 188-198.

Young, C. M., Moore, N. S., Berresford, K. K. and Einret, B. M.: What can be done for the obese patient? Report of a study in an experimental clinic. *American Practitioner*, 6:685-695, 1955.

VI. GROUP THERAPY

Becker, B. J.: The obese patient in group psychoanalysis. *American Journal of Psychotherapy*, 14:322-337, 1960.

Bowser, L. J., Trulson, M. F., Bowling, R. C. and Stare, F. J.: Methods of reducing: Group therapy versus individual clinic interview. *Journal of the American Dietetic Association*, 29:1193-1196, 1953.

Brown, W. A.: Obesity: A solution, group action. *Nursing Outlook*, 6:456-457, 1958.

Chapman, A. L.: An experiment with group conferences for weight reduction. *Public Health Report*, 68:439-440, 1953.

Chapman, A. L.: Weight-control—Simplified concept (psychological basis and group psychotherapy). *Public Health Reports*, 66:725-731, 1951.

Cornacchia, A.: A layman's view of group therapy in weight control. *Canadian Journal of Public Health*, 58:505-507, 1958.

Dorfman, W.: The challenge of obesity. *New York State Journal of Medicine*, 56: 1642-1645, 1956.

Dorfman, W., Slater, S. and Gottlieb, N.: Drug and placebo in group treatment of obesity. *International Journal of Group Psychotherapy*, 9:345-351, 1959.

Feiner, A. H.: A study of certain aspects of the perception of parental figures and sexual identification of an obese adolescent female group. *American Journal of Digestive Diseases*, 21:298-299, 1954; *Dissertation Abstracts*, 14:868-869, 1954.

Ford, M. J.: Group approach to weight control. *American Journal of Public Health*, 43:997-1000, 1953.

Freyberger, H. and Kark, B.: Gruppentherapie bei Fettsuchtskranken. *Münchener Medizinische Wochenschrift*, 100:268-271, 1958.

Glaser, K.: Group discussions with mothers of hospitalized children. *Pediatrics*, 26: 132, 1960.

Glomset, D. A.: Group therapy for obesity. *Journal of the Iowa State Medical Society*, 47:496-498, 1957.

Grant, M.: The group approach for weight control: Report of a pilot study in Boston, 1949-50. *Group Psychotherapy*, 4:156-165, 1951.

Hagen, R. L.: Group therapy versus biblio-therapy in weight reduction. *Dissertation Abstracts International*, 31(5-B): 2985-2986, 1970.

Harmon, A. R., Purhonen, R. A. and Rasmussen, L. P. S.: Obesity: A physical and emotional problem. *Nursing Outlook*, 6:452-456, 1958.

Harvey, H. I. and Simmons, W. D.: Weight reduction; Group methods; Preliminary report. *American Journal of Medical Sciences*, 225:623-625, 1953.

Harvey, H. I. and Simmons, W. D.: Weight reduction; A study of the group method: Report on progress. *American Journal of Medical Sciences*, 227:521-525, 1954.

Heyden-Stucky, S.: Gewichtszunahmen, Übergwicht, Gewichtsreduktion. *Schweizerische Medizinische Wochenschrift*, 97:78-81, 1967.

Holt, H. and Winick, C.: Group psychotherapy with obese women. *Archives of General Psychiatry*, 5:156-168, 1961.

Jenkins, B. W.: Group therapy without group. *GP*, 17:110-112, 1956.

Karvinen, E. and Kotilainen, M.: Group therapy for obesity: A study of results obtained at weight reducing courses in Finland. *Annales Medicinae Internae Fenniae*, 52:155-161, 1963.

Keneally, H. J., Jr.: A group approach to weight control. *American Journal of Public Health*, 48:208-218, 1958.

Kornhaber, A.: Group treatment of obesity. *GP*, 38:116-120, 1968.

Kosofsky, S.: An attempt at weight control through group psychotherapy. *Journal of Individual Psychology*, 13:58-71, 1957.

Kotkov, B.: Experiences in group psychotherapy with the obese. *International Record of Medicine*, 164:566-576, 1951.

Kotkov, B.: Experiences in group psychotherapy with obese women. *Psychosomatic Medicine*, 15:243-251, 1953.

Krotkiewski, M., *et al.*: Group therapy for obesity in a sanitorium. *Wiadomosci Lekarskie*, 18:1845-1847, 1965.

Kurlander, A. B.: Group therapy in reducing; 2 year follow-up of Boston pilot study. *Journal of the American Dietetic Association*, 29:337-339, 1953.

Linder, L.: Group therapy in the treatment of obesity. *Svenska Lakartidningen*, 60: 2612-2619, 1963.

Louden, A. M. and Schreiber, E. D.: A controlled study of the effects of group discussions and an anorexiant in out-patient treatment of obesity with attention to the psychological aspects of dieting. *Annals of Internal Medicine*, 65:80, 1966.

Mährlein, W., Schnabl, S. and Bothe, E.: Psychotherapeutic aspects of the treatment of obesity. *Deutsche Gesundheitswesen*, 16:194-197, 1961.

Mees, H. L. and Keutzer, C. S.: Short term group psychotherapy with obese women. A pilot project. *Northwest Medicine*, 66:548-550, 1967.

Munves, E. D.: Dietetic interview or group discussion-decision in reducing? *Journal of the American Dietetic Association*, 29:1197-1203, 1953.

Naumberg, M.: The use of art in analytically oriented group therapy of obese women. *Proceedings of the International Group Therapy Association*, 1959.

Naumberg, M. and Caldwell, J.: The use of spontaneous art in analytically oriented group therapy of obese women. *Acta Psychotherapeutica et Psychosomatica*, 7: 254-287, Supplement, Part 2, 1959.

Penick, S. B., Filion, R., Fox, S. and Stunkard, A. J.: Behavior modification in the treatment of obesity. *Psychosomatic Medicine*, 33:49-55, 1971; *Mental Health Digest*, 3:14-15, 1971.

Penick, S. B., Filion, R., Fox, S. and Stunkard, A. J.: A day hospital approach to the treatment of human obesity. *Journal of the American Medical Association*, 212: 865-866, 1970.

Powers, R.: A pilot study in group weight control. *Journal of the Florida Medical Association*, 45:791-793, 1959.

Reivich, R. S., Ruiz, R. A. and Lapi, R. M.: Extreme obesity—psychiatric, psychometric and psychotherapeutic aspects. *Journal of the Kansas Medical Society,* 67:134-140, 146, 1966.

Schwartz, E. and Goodman, J. I.: Group therapy of obesity in elderly diabetics. *Geriatrics,* 7:280-283, 1952.

Schwobel, G.: Zur analytischen Gruppenpsychotherapie der Adipositas. *Praxis,* 58: 1033-1039, 1969.

Simmons, W. D.: The group approach to weight reduction. *Journal of the American Dietetic Association,* 30:437-449, 1954.

Simmons, W. D.: Group methods in weight reduction. In E. S. Eppright, *et al.* (Eds.): *Weight Control.* Ames, Iowa, Iowa State College Press, 1955, 219-231.

Slawson, P. F.: Group psychotherapy with obese women. *Psychosomatics,* 6:206-209, 1965.

Stunkard, A. J., Levine, H. and Fox, S.: The management of obesity: Patient self-help and medical treatment. *Archives of Internal Medicine,* 125:1067-1072, 1970.

Stunkard, A. J., Levine, H. and Fox, S.: Self-help groups: TOPS is tops among ways to lose weight. *Journal of the American Medical Association,* 209:1989, 1969.

Stunkard, A. J., Levine, H. and Fox, S.: A study of a patient self-help group for obesity. *Proceedings of the 8th International Congress for Nutrition,* Prague, 1969.

Suczek, R. F.: Psychological aspects of obesity: Group weight reduction. *Journal of the American Dietetic Association,* 30:442-446, 1954.

Wagonfeld, S. and Wolowitz, H. M.: Obesity and the self-help group: A look at TOPS. *American Journal of Psychiatry,* 125:249-252, 1968.

Wine, D. B., *et al.:* Group psychotherapy with 27 starving men. *Psychiatry Digest,* 29:17-20, 1968.

Wollersheim, J. P.: Effectiveness of group therapy based upon learning principles in the treatment of overweight women. *Journal of Abnormal Psychology,* 76:462-474, 1970; *Dissertation Abstracts International,* 30(1-B):396, 1969.

Wool, M. L., Kanter, S. K. and Gray, W.: Group psychotherapy in preventive psychiatry: A preliminary report. *International Journal of Group Psychotherapy,* 5:404-414, 1955.

VII. HYPNOTHERAPY

Brodie, E. I.: A hypnotherapeutic approach to obesity. *American Journal of Clinical Hypnosis,* 6:211-215, 1964.

Browne, S. E.: Brief hypnotherapy with passive children. *Medical World,* 100:384-386, 1964.

Cantilo, E.: Endocrine disorders and hypnosis. *Dia Medico,* 33:2849-2852, 1961.

Clawson, T. A., Jr.: Hypnosis in medical practice. *American Journal of Clinical Hypnosis,* 6:232-236, 1964.

Coppolino, C. A.: *Get Slim and Stay Slim with Hypnosis.* New York, Power Publications, 1966.

Erickson, M. H.: The utilization of patient behavior in the hypnotherapy of obesity: Three case reports. *American Journal of Clinical Hypnosis,* 3:112-116, 1960.

Fogelman, M. J. and Crasilneck, H. B.: Food intake and hypnosis. *Journal of the American Dietetic Association,* 32:519-523, 1956.

Glover, F. S.: Use of hypnosis for weight reduction in a group of nurses. *American Journal of Clinical Hypnosis,* 3:250-251, 1961.

Grabovska, M. J., *et al.:* Hypnosis in complex treatment of obesity of alimentary origin. *Sovetskaia Meditsina,* 31:54-56, 1968.

Grabovska, M. J., *et al.:* The significance of hypnotherapy in complexive treatment of obesity. *Polskie Archivum Medycyny Wewnetrznej,* 42:383-387, 1969.

Hanley, F. W.: The treatment of obesity by individual and group hypnosis. *Canadian Psychiatric Association Journal,* 12:549-551, 1967.

Hershman, S.: Hypnosis in the treatment of obesity. *International Journal of Clinical and Experimental Hypnosis,* 3:136-139, 1955.

Hypnose gegen Adipositas: *Arztliche Praxis,* 21:1203, 1969.

Kamens, I. M.: Hypnosis as an adjunct in obesity—case histories. *Journal of the American Society of Psychosomatic Dentistry and Medicine,* 13:5-11, 1966.

Kroger, W. S.: Comprehensive management of obesity. *American Journal of Clinical Hypnosis,* 12:165-176, 1970.

Kroger, W. S.: Systems approach for understanding obesity: Management by behavioral modification through hypnosis. *Psychiatric Opinion,* 7:6-19, 1970.

Mann, H.: Group hypnosis in the treatment of obesity. *American Journal of Clinical Hypnosis,* 1:114-116, 1959.

Morton, J. H.: Hypnosis and psychosomatic illness. *American Journal of Clinical Hypnosis,* 3:67-74, 1960.

Oakley, R. P.: Hypnosis with a positive approach in the management of "problem" obesity. *Journal of the American Society of Psychosomatic Dental Medicine,* 7: 28-40, 1960.

Owen-Flood, A.: Slimming under hypnosis: The obese adolescent. *Medical World,* 93:310-312, 1960.

Petrie, S. and Stone, R.: *Programmed Course on How to Reduce and Control Your Weight Through Self Hypnosis.* Englewood Cliffs, N. J., Prentice-Hall, 1967.

Shibata, J. L.: Hypnotherapy of patients taking unbalanced diets. *American Journal of Clinical Hypnosis,* 10:81-83, 1967.

VIII. DIET

Anand, B. K.: Nervous regulation of food intake. *American Journal of Clinical Nutrition,* 8:529, 1960.

Anderson, I. R., *et al.*: Eating patterns of obesity. A study of recorded diets of obese patients in an out-patient clinic. *Maryland Medical Journal,* 15:60-61, 1966.

Andriasov, A. N. and Braksh, T. A. (Eds.): *Nutrition and Behavior.* Leningrad, Meditsina, 1966.

Aretz, H. H., *et al.*: Mental changes in obese patients during out-patient weight reduction. *Deutsche Medizinische Wochenschrift,* 96:778-784, 1971.

Ballantyne, D. A.: Starvation therapy in obesity. *British Medical Journal,* 3:370, 1971.

Barnes, M. J.: Some emotional factors related to obesity and dieting. *Smith College Studies in Social Work,* 11:131 (abstract), 1940.

Barnes, M. J.: Some reasons why obese children find dieting difficult. *Smith College Studies in Social Work,* 11:342-375, 1941.

Bauer, J.: Appetite and overeating in their relation to obesity. *American Journal of Digestive Diseases,* 14:397-400, 1947.

Beaudoin, R. and Mayer, J.: Food intakes of obese and non-obese women. *Journal of the American Dietetic Association,* 29:29-33, 1953.

Biggers, W. H.: Obesity. Affective changes in the fasting state. *Archives of General Psychiatry,* 14:218-221, 1966.

Bloom, W. L.: Fasting as an introduction to the treatment of obesity. *Metabolism,* 8: 214-220, 1959.

Brook, C. Mc.: Appetite and obesity. *New Zealand Medical Journal,* 46:243-254, 1947.

Brosin, H. W.: The psychology of appetite. In M. G. Wohl and R. S. Goodhart

(Eds.): *Modern Nutrition in Health and Disease: Dietotherapy.* Philadelphia, Lea and Febiger, 1955, 76-89.

Brown, J. D. and Pulsifer, D. H.: Outpatient starvation in normal and obese subjects. *Aerospace Medicine,* 267-269, 1965.

Brozek, J.: Experimental investigation on nutrition and human behavior: A postscript. *American Scientist,* 51:139, 1963.

Brozek, J.: Food as essential: Experimental studies on behavioral fitness. In S. M. Farber, N. L. Wilson and R. H. L. Wilson (Eds.): *Food and Civilization—A Symposium.* Springfield, Ill., Thomas, 1966.

Brozek, J.: Psychological performance. In H. Spector, M. S. Peterson and T. E. Friedeman (Eds.): *Methods for Evaluation of Nutritional Adequacy and Status: A Symposium.* Chicago, University of Chicago Press, 1954.

Brozek, J.: Research on diet and behavior. *Journal of the American Dietetic Association,* 57:321-325, 1970.

Brozek, J.: *Symposium on Nutrition and Behavior.* New York, National Vitamin Foundation, 1957.

Brozek, J., Guetzkow, H. and Baldwin, M. V.: A quantitative study of perception and association in experimental semi-starvation. *Journal of Personality,* 19:245-264, 1951.

Brozek, J. and Vaes, G.: Experimental investigation of the dietary deficiencies on animal and human behavior. *Vitamins and Hormones,* 19:43, 1961.

Bruch, H.: The allure of food cults and nutrition quackery. *Journal of the American Dietetic Association,* 57:316-320, 1970.

Bruch, H.: The emotional significance of the preferred weight. *American Journal of Clinical Nutrition,* 5:192-196, 1957.

Bruch, H.: Psychological aspects of reducing. *Psychosomatic Medicine,* 14:337-346, 1952.

Bruch, H.: The psychology of reducing. *Quarterly Journal of Child Behavior,* 3:350-363, 1951.

Bruch, H.: What makes people food cultists or victims of nutrition quackery. In G. Blix (Ed.): *Food Cultism and Nutrition Quackery.* Stockholm, Almqvist and Wiksells, 1970, 82-92.

Bruch, H. and Janis, M.: Adjustment to dietary changes in various somatic disorders. *National Research Council Bulletin,* 108:66-73, 1943.

Brull, L.: Dietetics: Weight reduction. *Revue Médicale de Liège,* 10:685-687, 1955.

Cavagnini, F., Peracchi, M. and Bianchi Porro, G.: Starvation therapy in obesity. *British Medical Journal,* 2:527, 1957.

Cohen, S.: Psychosomatic reflections on the zero calorie diet. *Western Medicine,* 7: 14-15, 1966.

Conrad, S. W.: Resistance of the obese to reducing. *Journal of the American Dietetic Association,* 30:381, 1954.

Conradi, M. L., *et al.*: Indications of clinical fasting therapy. *Zeitschrift für Ärztliche Forbildung,* 63:1284-1288, 1969.

Cooperman, W. L.: Food as reinforcer for obese versus normals. *Dissertation Abstracts International,* 31(7-B):4306, 1971.

Crisp, A. H.: The possible significance of some behavioral correlates of weight and carbohydrate intake. *Journal of Psychosomatic Research,* 11:117-131, 1967.

Crumpton, E., Wine, D. B. and Drenick, E. J.: Starvation: Stress or satisfaction? *Journal of the American Medical Association,* 196:394-396, 1966.

The Psychology of Obesity

Damm, G.: Limitations of dietetic therapy. *Deutsche Medizinische Wochenschrift*, 81: 1408-1410, 1956.

Dibold, H.: Diet as an experience. *Hippokrates*, 31:14-19, 1960.

Drenick, E. J. and Smith, R.: Weight reduction by prolonged starvation: Practical management. *Postgraduate Medicine*, 36:95-100, 1964.

Drenick, E. J., Swendseid, M. E., Blahd, W. H. and Tuttle, S. G.: Prolonged starvation as treatment for severe obesity. *Journal of the American Medical Association*, 187:100-105, 1964.

Duncan, G. G., Cristofori, F. C., Yue, J. K. and Murthy, M. S. S.: The control of obesity by intermittent fasts. *Medical Clinics of North America*, 48:1359-1372, 1964.

Duncan, G. G., Jensen, W. K., Cristofori, F. C. and Schless, G. L.: Intermittent fasts in the correction and control of intractable obesity. *American Journal of Medical Science*, 245:515-520, 1963.

Duncan, G. G., Jensen, W. K., Fraser, R. I. and Cristofori, F. C.: Correction and control of intractable obesity. *Journal of the American Medical Association*, 181:309-312, 1962.

Dwyer, J. T., Feldman, J. J. and Mayer, J.: The social psychology of dieting. *Journal of Health and Social Behavior*, 11:269-287, 1970; *Mental Health Digest*, 3:1-13, 1971.

Fábry, P. and Tepperman, J.: Meal frequency—A possible factor in human pathology. *American Journal of Clinical Nutrition*, 23:1059-1068, 1970.

Fischer, N.: Obesity, affect, and therapeutic starvation. *Archives of General Psychiatry*, 17:227-233, 1967.

Forbes, G. B.: Weight loss during fasting: Implications for the obese. *American Journal of Clinical Nutrition*, 23:1212-1219, 1970.

Formica, E.: Diet in relation to the physiology of adolescence. *Minerva Pediatrica*, 22:2208-2211, 1970.

Franklin, R. E. and Rynearson, E. H.: An evaluation of the effectiveness of dietary instruction for the obese. *Staff Meetings of the Mayo Clinic*, 35:123-131, 1960.

Friedhoff, A. J.: Biochemical effects of experimental diets. *Journal of Psychiatric Research*, 5:265-271, 1967.

Fuller, R.: Psychological results in treated phenylketonuria. I. Gesell findings. *Proceedings of the American Psychopathological Association*, 56:153-180, 1967.

Glass, D. C. (Ed.): *Biology and Behavior: Studies of Obesity and Eating.* New York, Rockefeller University Press, 1967.

Glatzel, H.: Psychological consequences of prolonged dietary investigations. Possible sources of physiological misinterpretation? *Nutritio et Dieta*, 5:3-11, 1963.

Glucksman, M. L. and Hirsch, J.: The response of obese patients to weight reduction: A clinical evaluation of behavior. *Psychosomatic Medicine*, 30:1-11, 1968.

Glucksman, M. L., Hirsch, J., McCully, R. S., Barron, B. A. and Knittle, J. L.: The response of obese patients to weight reduction. II. A quantitative evaluation of behavior. *Psychosomatic Medicine*, 30:359-373, 1968.

Goldman, R. L.: The effects of the manipulation of the visibility of food on the eating behavior of obese and normal subjects. *Dissertation Abstracts International*, 30 (2-A):807, 1969.

Goodhart, R. S.: *Overeating, Overweight and Obesity.* New York, National Vitamin Foundation, 1953.

Graff, H. and Stellar, E.: Hyperphagia, obesity and finickiness. *Journal of Comparative and Physiological Psychology*, 55:418, 1962.

Grossman, M. I.: Integration of current views on the regulation of hunger and appetite. *Annals of the New York Academy of Science,* 63:76, 1955.

Harris, M. B.: The portly psychologist, or on the perils of using a control group. *Psychological Reports,* 29:557-558, 1971.

Harris, M. B. and Bruner, C. G.: A comparison of a self-control and a contract procedure for weight control. *Behaviour Research and Therapy,* 9:347-354, 1971.

Hickox, A. C.: What is psychodietetics? *Hospital Progress,* 42:100-102, 1961.

Isrig, F. A., *et al.:* Some behavioral effects of two experimental synthetic nutrients. *Psychopharmacologia,* 12:227-235, 1968.

Johnson, W. G.: The effect of prior-taste and food visibility on the food-directed instrumental performance of obese individuals. *Dissertation Abstracts International,* 31(3-B):1539-1540, 1970.

Johnson, W. G. and Wunderlich, R. A.: Effect of prior taste and food visibility on the food-directed instrumental performance of the obese. *Proceedings of the Annual Convention of the American Psychological Association,* 5:485-486, 1970.

Jones, G. M.: Obesity and reduction diet. *Postgraduate Medicine,* 20:451-456, 1956.

Jordan, H.: Voluntary intragastric feeding: Oral and gastric contributions to food intake and hunger in man. *Journal of Comparative and Physiological Psychology,* 68:498-508, 1969.

Jordan, H., Wieland, W. F., Zebley, S. P., Stellar, E. and Stunkard, A. J.: Direct measurement of food intake in man: A method for the objective study of eating behavior. *Psychosomatic Medicine,* 28:836-842, 1966.

Kermorgant, Y.: Personalization of the dietary regime of the obese. *Concours Medical,* 87:3769-3770, 1965.

Keys, A., Brozek, J., Henschel, A., Mickelson, O. and Taylor, H. L.: *The Biology of Human Starvation.* Minneapolis, University of Minnesota Press, 1950.

Kollar, E. J. and Atkinson, R. M.: Responses of extremely obese patients to starvation. *Psychosomatic Medicine,* 28:227-246, 1966.

Kollar, E. J., Atkinson, R. M. and Albin, D. L.: The effectiveness of fasting in the treatment of superobesity. *Psychosomatics,* 10:125-135, 1969.

Kollar, E. J., Slater, G. R., Palmer, J. O., Docter, R. F. and Mandell, A. J.: Measurement of stress in fasting man. *Archives of General Psychiatry,* 11:113-125, 1964.

Krosnick, A.: Medical implications of weight reduction programs. *Public Health News,* 50:195-198, 1969.

Kutland, H. D.: Extreme obesity: A psychophysiological disorder. *Psychosomatics,* 8:107-111, 1967.

Lange, E.: Critical situation during therapeutic reducing diet; Problem of central nervous disorders during therapy. *Ärztliche Wochenschrift,* 11:822-825, 1956.

Laszlo, J.: Changes in the obese patient and his adipose tissue during prolonged starvation. *Southern Medical Journal,* 58:1099-1108, 1965.

Lausa, R. D.: Efforts to lose weight in 414 young men. *Archives of Environmental Health,* 17:366-371, 1968.

Leconte des Floris, R., Paquette, J. P. and Grandmottet, P.: Le traitement dietetique de l'obésité. *Guide Medical,* 22/23:25-32, 1968.

Leon, G. R.: *Maintenance of Weight Loss Over a One-Year Period.* National Institute of Mental Health Research Grant RO3-MH-18658-01, 1970.

Liebermeister, H.: Weight reduction by diet, drugs, and operative method in obesity. *Klinische Wochenschrift,* 49:125-134, 1971.

McCann, M. and Trulson, M. F.: Long-term effect of weight-reducing programs. *Journal of the American Dietetic Association,* 31:1108-1110, 1955.

McCarthy, M. C.: Dietary and activity patterns of obese women in Trinidad. *Journal of the American Dietetic Association,* 48:33-37, 1966.

MacCuish, A. C., Munro, J. F. and Duncan, L. S. P.: Follow-up study of refractory obesity treated by fasting. *British Medical Journal,* 1:91-92, 1968.

Mathis, J. L.: Obesity—Sin or savior? *Psychosomatics,* 6:171-172, 1965.

Maxfield, J. and Konish, F.: Patterns of food intake and physical activity in obesity. *Journal of the American Dietetic Association,* 49:406-408, 1966.

Mayer, J.: Appetite and obesity. *Atlantic Monthly,* 195:58-62, 1955.

Mayer, J.: Satiety and weight control. *American Journal of Clinical Nutrition,* 5:180-185, 1957.

Mayer, J.: Some aspects of the problem of regulating food intake and obesity. *International Psychiatry Clinics,* 7:255-334, 1970.

Meerloo, J. A. M. and Klauber, L. D.: Clinical significance of starvation and oral deprivation. *Psychosomatic Medicine,* 14:491, 1952.

Miéville, C.: Reducing cures. For whom? Why? How? *Praxis,* 60:266-271, 1971.

Miller, C. H.: Current understanding of eating and dieting. *Psychosomatics,* 5:119-126, 1964.

Miller, D. S., *et al.*: Obesity: Physical activity and nutrition. *Proceedings of the Nutrition Society,* 25:100-107, 1966.

Miroux, M.: A charming and disastrous tradition: "The snack." *Clinique,* 59:667-669, 1964.

Monello, L. F., Seltzer, C. C. and Mayer, J.: Hunger and satiety sensations in men, women, boys and girls: A preliminary report. *Annals of the New York Academy of Science,* 131:593-602, 1965.

Munro, J. F., *et al.*: Further experience with prolonged therapeutic starvation in gross refractory obesity. *British Medical Journal,* 4:712-714, 1970.

Pliner, P. L.: Internal regulation of food intake by normal and obese subjects as a function of various preloads. *Dissertation Abstracts International,* 31(6-A):3042-3043, 1970.

Reunanen, A.: Treatment of obesity by total or subtotal fasting. A review. *Duodecim,* 85:1259-1268, 1969.

Rodgers, W. L.: Specificity of specific hungers. *Journal of Comparative and Physiological Psychology,* 64:49-58, 1967.

Rosenstock, I. M.: Psychological forces, motivation, and nutrition education. *American Journal of Public Health,* 59:1992-1997, 1969.

Ross, L. D.: Cue-controlled and cognition-controlled eating among obese and normal subjects. *Dissertation Abstracts International,* 31(6-B):3693-3694, 1970.

Rowland, C. V., Jr.: Psychotherapy of six hyperobese adults during total starvation. *Archives of General Psychiatry,* 18:541-548, 1968.

Ruedi, B., *et al.*: Treatment of obesity by prolonged complete fasting. *Therapeutische Umschau,* 27:560-565, 1970.

Schiele, B. C. and Brozek, J.: Experimental neurosis resulting from semi-starvation in man. *Psychosomatic Medicine,* 10:31, 1948.

Schrub, J. C., *et al.*: Obesity and fast therapy. Immediate and long-term reducing. *Semaine des Hôpitaux de Paris,* 47:217-227, 1971.

Schultz, A. L., Werner, L. A. and Kerlow, A.: The use of total starvation in the management of chronic obesity. *Minnesota Medicine,* 48:441-447, 1965.

Schur, S.: Simplified diet planning for the patient. *Bulletin of the New York Academy of Medicine,* 36:399-406, 1960.

Seaton, D. A. and Rose, K.: Defaulters from a weight reduction clinic. *Journal of Chronic Diseases,* 18:1007-1011, 1965.

Shipman, W. G. and Plesset, M. R.: Predicting the outcome for obese dieters. *Journal of the American Dietetic Association,* 42:383, 1963.

Silverstone, J. T. and Lascelles, B. D.: Dieting and depression. An assessment of affective disturbance occurring during the clinical trial of a new anorectic preparation. *British Journal of Psychiatry,* 112:513-519, 1966.

Simon, J.: Psychologic factors in dietary restriction. *Journal of the American Dietary Association,* 37:109-114, 1960.

Slabochová, Z., *et al.:* Some aspects of pathogenesis and therapy of obesity. *Voprosy Pitaniia,* 24:36-42, 1965.

Spencer, I. O. B.: Death during therapeutic starvation for obesity. *Lancet,* 1/7555: 1288-1290, 1968.

Strang, J. M., McClugage, H. B. and Evans, F. A.: Further studies in the dietary correction of obesity. *American Journal of Medical Science,* 179:687, 1930.

Stunkard, A. J.: Hunger and satiety. *American Journal of Psychiatry,* 118:212-217, 1961.

Swanson, D. W. and Dinello, F. A.: Follow-up of patients starved for obesity. *Psychosomatic Medicine,* 32:209-214, 1970.

Swanson, D. W. and Dinello, F. A.: Severe obesity as a habituation syndrome: Evidence during a starvation study. *Archives of General Psychiatry,* 22:120-127, 1970.

Swanson, D. W. and Dinello, F. A.: Therapeutic starvation in obesity. *Diseases of the Nervous System,* 30:669-674, 1969.

Thompson, T. J., Runcie, J. and Miller, V.: Treatment of obesity by total fasting up to 249 days. *Lancet,* 2:992-996, 1966.

Tremolières, J., Klotz, H. P., Farquet, J. and Cros, J.: Effects of the emotional state, of agents modifying it and of diuretics, upon weight changes in obesity. *Nutritio et Dieta,* 4:98-106, 1962.

Tycowa, M., *et al.:* Late results of hunger therapy. *Polski Tygodnik Lekarski,* 26: 479-482, 1971.

Vetter, K. and Lisewski, G.: Obesity, its pathogenesis, symptomatology, and therapy. *Zeitschrift für Ärztliche Forbildung,* 56:1233-1238, 1962.

Watson, G.: *Nutrition and Your Mind: The Psychochemical Response.* New York, Harper and Row, 1972.

Weiss, E.: Psychosomatic aspects of dieting. *Journal of Clinical Nutrition,* 1:140-148, 1953.

Wilson, W. P., Schleuse, L. W. and Johnson, J. E.: Early effects of a formula diet on mood of psychologically normal, obese patients. *Diseases of the Nervous System,* 23:20-22, 1962.

Wittigstein, G.: The psychic factor in the diet. *Hippokrates,* 30:625-628, 1959.

Wooley, O. W.: Long term food regulation in the obese and non-obese. *Dissertation Abstracts International,* 31(2-B):922, 1970.

Wooley, S. C.: Real and imaginary calories: Their effects on subsequent food intake in the obese and nonobese. *Dissertation Abstracts International,* 30(3-B):1390, 1969.

Young, C. M., Berresford, K. and Moore, N. S.: Psychologic factors in weight control. *American Journal of Clinical Nutrition,* 5:188-191, 1957.

Young, C. M., *et al.*: Problem of the obese patient. *Journal of the American Dietetic Association,* 31:1111-1115, 1955.

Young, P. T.: Psychologic factors regulating the feeding process. *American Journal of Clinical Nutrition,* 5:154-161, 1957.

IX. TESTS

Atkinson, R. M. and Ringuette, E. L.: A survey of biographical and psychological features in extraordinary fatness. *Psychosomatic Medicine,* 29:121-133, 1967.

Bailey, W. L., Shinedling, M. M. and Payne, I. R.: Obese individuals' perception of body image. *Perceptual and Motor Skills,* 31:617-618, 1970.

Bruch, H.: Obesity in childhood and personality development. *American Journal of Orthopsychiatry,* 11:467-475, 1941.

Cacciaguerra, F.: "Self-image" of obese children at the beginning of and during treatment, studied by means of a sentence completion test. *Atti della Accademia Medica Lombarda,* 21:247-256, Supplement, 1966.

Cacciaguerra, F., *et al.*: Contribution to the study of the personality of the mothers of obese children with the Rorschach psychodiagnostic test. *Atti della Accademia Medica Lombarda,* 21:189-197, Supplement, 1966.

Colombo, G. and Bono, G.: Valutazione psicologica dei soggetti disendocrini; Nota preventiva. *Minerva Pediatria,* 3:33-35, 1951.

Crumpton, E., Wine, D. B. and Groot, H.: MMPI profiles of 7 obese men and 6 other diagnostic categories. *Psychological Reports,* 19:1110, 1966.

DeRenzis, G., *et al.*: Body representation in a group of obese and lean children analyzed by means of the Human Pattern Design technique. *Pediatria,* 76:539-541, 1968.

D'Errico, A.: Human figure drawings of obese children. *Atti della Accademia Medica Lombarda,* 21:199-209, Supplement, 1966.

Feiner, A. H.: A study of certain aspects of the perception of parental figures and sexual identification of an obese adolescent female group. *American Journal of Digestive Diseases,* 21:298-299, 1954; *Dissertation Abstracts,* 14:868-869, 1954.

Goodman, M. and Kotkov, B.: Predictions of trait ranks from Draw-a-Person measurements of obese and non-obese women. *Journal of Clinical Psychology,* 9:365-367, 1953.

Gottesfeld, H.: Body and self-cathexis of super-obese patients. *Journal of Psychosomatic Research,* 6:177-183, 1962.

Grundig, M. H.: Comparison of MMPI profiles of developmental and reactive overweight college students: An analysis of important personality factors. *Dissertation Abstracts,* 27(9-A):2880-2881, 1967.

Karp, S. A. and Pardes, H.: Psychological differentiation (field dependence) in obese women. *Psychosomatic Medicine,* 27:238-244, 1965.

Klar, H.: Color psychology and medicine. 1. Adiposity in the light of the color test. *Medico Boehringer,* 2:43-47, 1963.

Klar, H.: On the prevention of psychogenic obesity. The Chi-square method in the Lüscher color test. *Medizinische Welt,* 3:150-155, 1965.

Kotkov, B. and Goodman, M.: The Draw-a-Person tests of obese women. *Journal of Clinical Psychology,* 9:362-364, 1953.

Kotkov, B. and Murawski, B.: A Rorschach study of the personality structure of obese women. *Journal of Clinical Psychology,* 8:391-396, 1952.

Levitt, H. and Fellner, C.: MMPI profiles on three obesity sub-groups. *Journal of Consulting Psychology,* 29:91, 1965.

McCully, R. S., Glucksman, M. L. and Hirsch, J.: Nutrition imagery in the Rorschach materials of food-deprived obese patients. *Journal of Projective Techniques,* 32:375-382, 1968.

Masling, J., Rabie, L. and Blondheim, S. H.: Obesity, level of aspiration, and Rorschach and TAT measures of oral dependence. *Journal of Consulting Psychology,* 31:233-239, 1967.

Sarnoff, I.: *Testing Freudian Concepts. An Experimental Social Approach.* New York, Springer, 1971, 135-136, 219-221.

Schneider, J. A.: Use of the Lüscher test in medical practice. *Medizinische Welt,* 21: 1171-1172, 1965.

Sparer, P. I. and Gottesfeld, H.: Psychologic factors in overweight individuals on a special weight reduction program. *Memphis Mid-S. Medical Journal,* 44:343-344, 1969.

Spence, D. and Ehrenberg, B.: Effects of oral deprivation on responses to subliminal and supraliminal verbal food stimuli. *Journal of Abnormal and Social Psychology,* 69:10-18, 1964.

Wolfgang, A. and Wolfgang, J.: Exploration of attitudes via physical interpersonal distance toward the obese, drug users, homosexuals, police and other marginal figures. *Journal of Clinical Psychology,* 27:510-512, 1971.

Wolowitz, H.: Food preferences as an index of orality. *Journal of Abnormal and Social Psychology,* 69:650-654, 1964.

Zucker, L.: A case of obesity: Projective techniques before and during treatment. *Rorschach Research Exchange,* 12:202-215, 1948.

X. PSYCHOSES

Allyon, T.: Intensive treatment of psychotic behavior by stimulus satiation and food reinforcement. *Behaviour Research and Therapy,* 1:53-61, 1963.

Allyon, T. and Haughton, E.: Control of behavior of schizophrenic patients by food. *Journal of the Experimental Analysis of Behavior,* 5:343-352, 1962.

Bachet, M.: *Études des troubles causes par la denutrition dans un asile d'alienes.* Paris, Arnette, 1943.

Bernard, J. L.: Rapid treatment of gross obesity by operant techniques. *Psychological Reports,* 23:663-666, 1968.

Biasci, G.: Obesity and mental disease. A study of 40 obese patients in the Psychiatric Hospital of Volterra. *Rassegna di Studi Psichiatrici,* 57:842-854, 1968.

Binswanger, L.: The case of Ellen West. In R. May, E. Angel and H. F. Ellenberger (Eds.): *Existence: A New Dimension in Psychiatry and Psychology.* New York, Basic Books, 1958, 237-364.

Binswanger, L.: Der Fall Ellen West. *Schweitzer Archiv für Neurologie und Psychiatrie,* 53:255-257, 1944; 54:69-117, 330-360; 55:16-40, 1945.

Bruch, H.: Developmental obesity and schizophrenia. *Psychiatry,* 21:65-70, 1958.

Bruch, H.: Eating disorders and schizophrenic development. In *Psychoneuroses and Schizophrenia.* Philadelphia, Lippincott, 1966, 113-124.

Bruch, H.: Falsification of bodily needs and body concepts in schizophrenia. *Archives of General Psychiatry,* 6:18-24, 1962.

Bruch, H.: Studies in schizophrenia. *Acta Psychiatrica et Neurologica Scandinavica,* Supplement 130, Copenhagen, 1959, 34.

Caffey, E. M. and Klett, C. J.: Side effects and laboratory findings during combined drug therapy of chronic schizophrenia. *Diseases of the Nervous System,* 22:370-375, 1961.

Casey, J. F., Hollister, L. E., Klett, C. J., Lasky, J. J. and Caffey, E. M., Jr.: Combined drug therapy of chronic schizophrenia. *American Journal of Psychiatry*, 117:997-1003, 1961.

Catalono, F.: Familial aspects of schizophrenic disorders and dystrophic (adipose or adipose-genital) disorders. *Acta Neurologica*, 19:807-814, 1964.

Coddington, R. D. and Bruch, H.: Gastric perceptivity in normal, obese and schizophrenic patients. *Psychosomatics*, 11:571-579, 1970.

Dehu, J.: Results of the use of M-634 as a corrective of the secondary effects of neuroleptics in a psychiatric service for women. *Annales Medico-Psychologiques*, 120:619-622, 1962.

Dohan, F. C., *et al.*: Relapsed schizophrenics: More rapid improvement on a milk and cereal free diet. *British Journal of Psychiatry*, 115:595-596, 1969.

Dorfman, W.: Depression and psychosomatic illness. *Southwestern Medicine*, 43:195-197, 1962.

Duquay, R. and Flach, F. F.: An experimental study of weight changes in depression. *Acta Psychiatria Scandinavia*, 40:1-9, 1964.

Gordon, H. L. and Groth, C.: Weight changes during and after hospital treatment. *Archives of General Psychiatry*, 10:187-191, 1964.

Gordon, H. L., Law, A., Hohman, K. E. and Groth, C.: The problem of overweight in hospitalized psychotic patients. *Psychiatric Quarterly*, 34:69-82, 1960.

Harmatz, M. G. and Lapuc, P.: Behavior modification of overeating in a psychiatric population. *Journal of Consulting and Clinical Psychology*, 32:583-587, 1968.

Haward, L. R. C.: The inadequacy of anorexogenic drugs in the treatment of obese psychiatric patients. *Psychiatria et Neurologia*, 149:129-135, 1965.

Holden, J. M. C. and Holden, U. P.: Weight changes with schizophrenic psychosis and psychotropic drug therapy. *Psychosomatics*, 11:551-561, 1970.

Kalinowsky, L.: Variations of body weight and menstruation in mental illness and their relation to shock treatment. *Journal of Nervous and Mental Disease*, 108:423-430, 1948.

Klett, C. J. and Caffey, E. M.: Weight changes during treatment with phenothiazine derivatives. *Journal of Neuropsychiatry*, 2:102-108, 1960.

Kraepelin, E.: *Ein Lehrbuch für Studierende und Ärzte*. Leipzig, Barth, 1913.

Lederer, W.: Uprooting depression without depression. Obesity and other psychosomatic equivalents of depression. *Nervenarzt*, 36:118-122, 1965.

Maslow, A. H. and Mittelmann, B.: *Principles of Abnormal Psychology: The Dynamics of Psychic Illness*. New York, Harper, 1951, 383-387.

Modell, W. and Husser, A. E.: Failure of dextroamphetamine to influence eating and sleeping patterns in obese schizophrenic patients. Clinical and pharmacological significance. *Journal of the American Medical Association*, 193:275-278, 1965.

Moore, C. H.: Weight reduction in a chronic schizophrenic by means of operant conditioning procedures: A case study. *Behaviour Research and Therapy*, 7:129-131, 1969.

Nobel, W.: *Das Verhalten des Körpergewichts bei Manisch-Depressiven und Schizophren*. Basel, 1936.

Orlovskaia, D. D.: Clinical features of endocrine disorders arising during the course of schizophrenia. *Zhurnal Nevropatologii i Psikhiatrii imeni S.S. Korsakova*, 68:735-742, 1968.

Perez, M., *et al.*: Overweight and senile age. Observations on 2,682 subjects, residents in geriatric institutes. *Giornale di Gerontologia*, 12:267-281, 1964.

Planansky, K.: Changes in weight in patients receiving a "tranquilizing" drug. *Psychiatric Quarterly*, 32:289-303, 1958.

Poire, R., Crance, J. P. and Rombach, F.: Results of a three-year experience with prolonged, supervised use of an anorexigenic agent, Fenfluramine, in a psychiatric hospital, without special diet and irrespective of patients' cooperation. *Annales de Medicine*, 5:575-601, 1966.

Rudenko, G. M.: Clinical features of schizophrenia associated with endocrine disorders—obesity, hirsutism. *Zhurnal Nevropotologii i Psikhiatrii imeni S. S. Korsakova*, 69:1708-1715, 1969.

Singh, M. M., DeDios, L. V. and Kline, N. S.: Weight as a correlate of clinical response to psychotropic drugs. *Psychosomatics*, 11:562-570, 1970.

Slettin, I. W., Mou, B., Cazenave, M. and Gershon, S.: The effects of caloric restriction on behavior and body weight during chlorpromazine therapy. *Diseases of the Nervous System*, 28:519-522, 1967.

Slettin, I. W., Viamontes, G., Hughes, D. D. and Korol, B.: Total fasting in psychiatric subjects: Psychological, physiological and biochemical changes. *Canadian Psychiatric Association Journal*, 12:553-558, 1967.

Thorpe, J. G., Schmidt, E., Brown, P. T. and Casrell, D.: Aversion relief therapy: A new method for general application. *Behaviour Research and Therapy*, 2:71-82, 1964.

Ueda, M., *et al.*: Study on obesity in hospitalized psychotic patients. *Bulletin of the Seishin-Igaku Institute, Institute of Psychiatry*, 15:1-14, 1968.

Verbizier, J. de, Guillon, A. and Benkhoucha, M.: Apropos of slimming cures by RP-8,228 in a psychiatric hospital. *Toulouse Médical*, 63:437-443, 1962.

Waitzkin, L.: Weight gain among hospitalized, mentally ill men. *Behavioral Neuropsychiatry*, 1:15-18, 1969.

Waitzkin, L. and Carbonell, F.: Overweight among hospitalized psychotic men. *Psychiatric Quarterly Supplement*, 40:91-96, 1966.

XI. REVIEWS OF LITERATURE

Bett, W. R.: Obesity: A survey of the recent literature. *Irish Journal of Medical Science*, 6:183-187, 1951.

Brooks, C.: The hypothalamus and obesity. *Medical Journal of Australia*, 1:327-331, 1948.

Burdon, A. P. and Paul, L.: Obesity: A review of the literature, stressing the psychosomatic approach. *Psychiatric Quarterly*, 25:568-580, 1951.

Iafusco, F. and Stoppoloni, G.: Developmental, clinical and metabolic aspects of obesity in childhood. *Pediatria*, 76:479-534, 1968.

Izar, G.: Obesity. Review of the literature. *Minerva Medica*, 2:33-54, 1954.

Feinstein, A. R.: The treatment of obesity: An analysis of methods, results and factors which influence success. *Journal of Chronic Diseases*, 11:349-393, 1960.

Kalb, S. W.: Review of group therapy in weight reduction. *American Journal of Gastroenterology*, 26:75-80, 1956.

Kaplan, H. I. and Kaplan, H. S.: The psychosomatic concept of obesity. *Journal of Nervous and Mental Disease*, 125:181-189, 1957.

Lehman, E.: Feeding problems of psychogenic origin: Survey of the literature. In R. S. Eissler, *et al.* (Eds.): *Psychoanalytic Study of the Child*, Vols. 3/4. New York, International Universities Press, 1948, 461-488.

Lopez-Ibor, J.: Obesity and thinness as forms of life; Review of the literature. *Actas Luso-Espanadas de Neurologia y Psiquiatria,* 14:279-287, 1955.

Mayer, J.: Appetite and the many obesities. *Australian Annals of Medicine,* 13:282-305, 1964.

Mayer, J.: Obesity: A review of the literature. *Annual Review of Medicine,* 14:111, 1963.

Salvioli, G.: Essential obesity: Review of the literature. *Giornale di Clinica Medica,* 34:388-392, 1953.

Seltzer, C. C., *et al.*: A review of genetic and constitutional factors in human obesity. *Annals of the New York Academy of Science,* 134:688-695, 1966.

Short, J. J.: Obesity: Review of studies in etiology, metabolism, complications of treatment (with special reference to woman who weighed 489 pounds). *Medical Arts and Sciences,* 6:10-17, 1952.

Soforenko, H.: Obesity, a brief general review. *General Practitioner,* 8:9, 1950.

Stunkard, A. J. and McLaren, M.: The results of treatment for obesity. A review of the literature and report of a series. *Archives of Internal Medicine,* 103:79-85, 1959.

Biographical Sketches

Pauline Austin Adams, Ph.D., is a psychologist at Children's Hospital at Stanford in Palo Alto, California. She is also in private practice. Dr. Adams has been a research associate in psychology at Swarthmore College, the University of California, the V.A. Hospital at Palo Alto and Stanford University, as well as a Postdoctoral Fellow, National Institute of Mental Health, at the latter institution. She is the author of nearly two dozen articles on learning, perception, and intellectual functioning in learning disability children.

John L. Bernard, Ph.D., received his doctorate from the University of Alabama in 1962 and his diplomate in psychology in 1967. He is currently Associate Professor and Director of Clinical Training at Memphis State University's Department of Psychology.

Carol G. Bruner, B.A., is a doctoral candidate at the University of New Mexico in the field of Educational Foundations. She has studied at Cornell and the University of Southern California.

Robert G. Burnight, Ph.D., was Professor of Sociology at Brown University and training director of the Population Studies and Training Center from 1961 to 1971. Since then, Dr. Burnight is Adjunct Professor of Sociology and Director of East Asian Studies in the Carolina Population Center of the University of North Carolina. His duties have sent him to Thailand, where he is Population Advisor to the Rector of Mahidol University in Bangkok.

Gustav Bychowski, M.D., studied medicine in Zurich and went on to Vienna for psychiatry and psychoanalysis. He practiced and taught in Warsaw until 1939. He has been in the United States since 1941, teaching at New York University, Down State Medical Center, the Institute of Psychiatry of Mt. Sinai Medical School, and maintaining private practice. He has published numerous articles and books. Among the latter are: *Psychotherapy of Psychoses; Dictators and Disciples; Evil in Man: Anatomy of Hate and Violence;* and *Specialized Techniques in Psychotherapy.*

Frank Carrera, III, M.D., is Associate Professor of Psychiatry at the University of Florida in Gainesville. He was a member of the Florida Committee to the 1971 White House Conference on Children and Youth and is President of the Northeast Florida Psychiatric Society.

Ida Lou Coley, O.T.R., graduated from San Jose State College and is Head of the Occupational Therapy Department at Children's Hospital, a specialized hospital and rehabilitation center for children at Stanford University, Palo Alto, California.

Frank A. Dinello, Ph.D., is Associate Professor in the Department of Psychology, DePaul University and Director of its Mental Health Clinic.

439

Johanna T. Dwyer, D.Sc., Assistant Professor in the Department of Nutrition and Lecturer in the Department of Maternal and Child Health, Harvard School of Public Health, is also Associate Editor of the *Journal of Nutrition Education.* Her research interests are in the areas of weight control behavior, the psychological aspects of bodily appearance, and the nutrition knowledge of various groups.

Milton H. Erickson, M.D., is a diplomate, American Board of Psychiatry and Neurology and the Founding President of the American Society of Clinical Hypnosis; he was the Editor of the *American Journal of Clinical Hypnosis* for its first ten years and is now Editor Emeritus; and he is a Life Fellow of both the American Psychiatric and American Psychological Associations.

Jacob J. Feldman, Ph.D., specializes in the field of health survey methodology. He is Professor of Biostatistics at the Harvard School of Public Health. His book, *The Dissemination of Health Information,* was published in 1966.

Helen H. Glaser, M.D., has a strong interest in the psychological problems of the child and his family, especially in such areas as failure to thrive, hospitalization and chronic illness. She has held faculty appointments in departments of pediatrics and psychiatry at the Universities of Colorado, Harvard, and Stanford. After training and working as a pediatrician and writing intensively in that field, Dr. Glaser decided to further her interest in psychiatry and is currently a psychiatric resident at the New York State Psychiatric Institute in New York City.

Myron L. Glucksman, M.D., is Director of the Danbury Hospital Mental Health Clinic in Danbury, Connecticut and also on the clinical faculty of the Department of Psychiatry at Yale University.

Phillip B. Goldblatt, M.D., has been connected with the Department of Psychiatry at Yale University since 1967. In his first three years there, Dr. Goldblatt was a post-doctoral fellow and subsequently project coordinator of the Psychiatric Utilization Review and Evaluation Project, working on psychiatric evaluation research in the area of community mental health. He is also in private practice in New Haven.

Harry Gottesfeld, Ph.D., is a diplomate in clinical psychology and Director of Mental Health, New York City Health and Hospitals Corporation.

Frederick W. Hanley, M.D., is in the full-time practice of psychiatry as well as on the Visiting Staff of the Vancouver General Hospital Clinical Institute of Psychiatry, University of British Columbia. He is one of the leading exponents of hypnotherapy in Canada.

Mary B. Harris, Ph.D., grew up in St. Louis, went east to Radcliffe for her B.A. and west to Stanford for her Ph.D. She is now on the faculty of the University of New Mexico in the College of Education. She is a frequent contributor to the journals on the subject of behavior modification. Her first book, *Classroom Uses of Behavior Modification,* was published in 1972.

Jules Hirsch, M.D., has been associated with Rockefeller University and Hospital since 1954 and is now Professor at the university and Senior Physician to the hospital. He is a diplomate in the American Boards of Internal Medicine and of Nutrition. For five years he was Editor of the *Journal of Nutrition* and is on the editorial boards of four other journals. He has contributed forty-five articles to various publications.

J. M. C. Holden, MRC Psych, MRCP (Glasgow), is consultant psychiatrist at Middlewood Hospital, Sheffield, England and previously held the posts of Physician Superintendent, St. Louis State Hospital, and Clinical Associate Professor of Psychiatry at the Missouri Institute of Psychiatry, University of Missouri School of Medicine.

U. P. Holden, B.A. (Hon.), University of Manchester, has served as Senior Clinical Psychologist, Winwick Hospital, Lancaster, England and as Clinical Research Psychologist with the Missouri Institute of Psychiatry, St. Louis and also the Division of Mental Health of Missouri.

Herbert Holt, M.D., Ph.D., is Dean of the School of Clinical Education, Southeastern University and Director of the Herbert Holt Institute for Psychoanalysis and Psychotherapy in New York City.

Norman Kiell, Ed.D., the editor of this volume, is Professor, Psychological Services Center, Department of Student Affairs and Services, Brooklyn College. He has written several dozen articles and book reviews as well as two books: *The Universal Experience of Adolescence* and *The Adolescent Through Fiction: A Psychological Approach.* The University of Wisconsin Press has published two bibliographies he has edited: *Psychoanalysis, Psychology and Literature* and *Psychiatry and Psychology in the Visual Arts and Aesthetics.*

Eric J. Kahn, M.D., received his medical education in South Africa and England. He is a Fellow of the Royal College of Physicians (Edinburgh) and a Fellow of the American Academy of Pediatrics. His present appointment is that of Director of Pediatrics, Harlem Hospital Center, New York and he is also Clinical Professor of Pediatrics, Columbia University.

William S. Kroger, M.D., is the author of numerous books and has produced several motion pictures which are circulated to medical schools throughout the world. He is Executive Director of the Institute for Comprehensive Medicine and Director of the Psychosomatic and Hypnotherapy Center in Beverly Hills, California, where he is engaged in the private practice of psychiatry and psychosomatic medicine.

Ruth M. Lapi, M.D., has been staff physician at the Massillon (Ohio) State Hospital, the Winnetka (Illinois) North Shore Health Resort, and the public schools of Denver and Jackson County, Missouri. She is a member of the American Board of Psychiatry and Neurology and Associate Professor, Kansas University Medical Center.

A. Russell Lee, M.D., is Chief of Community Consultation and Education at the Emanuel Mental Health Center, Turlock, California.

Dorothy G. Levin, P.S.W., was Director of Social Work at Children's Hospital, Stanford and is now a Counselor at the University of California at Santa Cruz. She is also engaged in the private practice of psychotherapy.

Veronica Liederman, B.A., graduated from Pomona College and was a candidate for the Ph.D. at Harvard. From 1967 to 1968, she was an instructor in sociology and research associate in medical sociology at Duke University. She has co-authored several articles which deal primarily with geriatrics.

Robert S. McCully, Ph.D., is Professor and Head of the Division of Psychology, Medical University of South Carolina in Charleston. He is also a member of the faculty of the New York Institute, C. G. Jung Foundation. He has authored *Rorschach Theory and Symbolism: A Jungian Approach to Clinical Materials* (1971).

George L. Maddox, Ph.D., Professor of Sociology and Chief, Division of Medical Sociology, Duke University Medical School, is also Program Coordinator of the Duke Center for the Study of Aging and Human Development.

Parker G. Marden, Ph.D., is an Associate Professor of Sociology at Cornell University, Program Associate in the International Population Program, and Co-Director of Cornell's Comprehensive Health Planning Program. He received his doctorate in sociology from Brown University in 1966 and was a research associate there in the Institute for Health Sciences.

Jean Mayer, D.Sc., Professor of Nutrition at Harvard University, is the author of over five hundred articles and several books on various aspects of nutrition. He is especially well-known for his studies on the physiological mechanism of the regulation of food intake and the etiology of various types of obesity in experimental animals and in man. Dr. Mayer has served as special consultant to President Nixon on hunger and as Chairman of the White House Conference on Nutrition and Hunger in 1969.

Myer Mendelson, M.D., holds the rank of Professor of Clinical Psychiatry in the University of Pennsylvania School of Medicine and is also Attending Psychiatrist at the Institute of the Pennsylvania Hospital in Philadelphia. He is the author of *Psychoanalytic Concepts of Depression* (1960) and numerous articles relating to depression and to obesity.

Mary E. Moore, M.D., was getting her Ph.D. in experimental psychology from Rutgers University at the time she was working on the obesity study found in Chapter 5. Since then, she has received her M.D. from Temple University School of Medicine, where she has done a straight medical internship and residency and is currently an instructor in the Section of Rheumatology at Temple University Hospital,

Susan Nathan, Ph.D., is on the psychology staff at Children's Hospital of Pittsburgh. Her B.A. was obtained at Vassar and her doctorate at the University of Chicago's School of Human Development.

Sidnor B. Penick, M.D., is Bond Certified in internal medicine and Board eligible in psychiatry. Dr. Penick is Director of Research at the Carrier Clinic Foundation in Belle Mead, New Jersey and Associate Professor of Psychiatry, Rutgers Medical School.

Dorothy Pisula, Ph.D., is interested in developmental problems of children. Dr. Pisula is Chief Psychologist at Children's Hospital of Pittsburgh. Her B.A. comes from Seton Hill College in Pennsylvania and her Ph.D. from Catholic University.

Hortense Powdermaker, Ph.D. (1903-1970), was Professor of Anthropology at Queens College of the City University of New York and the author of *After Freedom; A Cultural Study in the Deep South; Copper Town: Changing Africa; Probing Our Prejudices;* and *Stranger and Friend: the Way of an Anthropologist.*

Ronald S. Reivich, M.D., a National Institute of Mental Health Career Scientist awardee (1967-1972), is also a National Institute of Mental Health Career Teacher awardee (1964-1966). Currently, he is serving as Associate Professor of Psychiatry at the University of Kansas Medical Center, Visiting Lecturer in psychopharmacology at the Menninger School of Psychiatry, and is a candidate in the Topeka Psychoanalytic Institute.

Rene A. Ruiz, Ph.D., received his doctorate in psychology from the University of Nebraska and has taught at the University of Kansas School of Medicine and the University of Arizona. He is now Professor of Psychology at the University of Missouri. He is co-author of *The Normal Personality: Issues and Insights* and has published numerous articles in related areas.

Stanley J. Schachter, Ph.D., is Professor of Psychology, Columbia University. The American Psychological Association presented its Distinguished Scientific Contribution Award to him in 1969. Dr. Schachter has recently published *Emotion, Crime and Obesity,* is the author of many articles on obesity, and is the advisor to a host of doctoral candidates and graduates in the field.

J. Trevor Silverstone is Consultant Psychiatrist and Senior Lecturer at St. Bartholomew's Hospital, London. He has been interested in the study of weight disorders for many years and has spent a year with Dr. A. J. Stunkard at the University of Pennsylvania studying certain aspects of the psychophysiology of hunger. In addition to his psychiatric post, Mr. Silverstone is Consultant-in-Charge at the Weight Reduction Clinic at Hackney Hospital, where he is continuing his research.

E. James Stanley, M.D., was an intern in pediatrics at the Stanford University Medical Center during the beginning of the study in Chapter 14. In 1970, he served as a Child Psychiatry Fellow in the Department of Psychiatry at the University of

Colorado Medical Center in Denver and was last reported to be on military tour of duty.

Richard B. Stuart, D.S.W., is Professor at the School of Social Work at the University of Michigan in Ann Arbor. He has long been interested in treating obesity through behavior therapy and has written considerably on the subject. *Slim Chance in a Fat World* was published in 1972.

Albert J. Stunkard, M.D., has been since 1962 Professor and Chairman of the Department of Psychiatry at the University of Pennsylvania. He has also taught at Cornell University Medical College. In 1971-1972, he was on sabbatical leave at the Center for Advanced Study in the Behavioral Sciences at Stanford. Dr. Stunkard has worked in the field of obesity since 1953 and the majority of his seventy-five publications are in this area.

David W. Swanson, M.D., was, when he collaborated on Chapter 24, with Dr. Dinello, Associate Professor of Psychiatry, Loyola University of Chicago. At the present time, he is Consultant, Section of Psychiatry, Mayo Clinic and Associate Professor, Mayo Graduate School.

Charles Winick, Ph.D., has been Director of the national program in drug dependence and abuse of the American Social Health Association since 1961, is a founding director of the National Advisory Council on Narcotics, and is research director of the New York State Joint Legislative Committee on Narcotics. He has taught at Columbia University, Postgraduate Center for Mental Health, University of Rochester, City University of New York and elsewhere. He is the author of three books and over two-hundred articles. His latest book is *The Lively Commerce. Prostitution in the United States* (1971).

Janet P. Wollersheim, Ph.D., is Assistant Professor of Psychology at the University of Montana. Her major interests lie in adult and child clinical psychology. For the past three years she has been concentrating her research in the area of psychological treatment outcome studies. Present research activities involve continued studies of obesity, studies on eliminating incontinence in mental patients, and research in milieu therapy in a psychiatric clinic.

Author Index

445

Subject Index

A

Academic record, of adolescent, 141, 144-145
Acculturation, 63
Acting out, 235
Activity, physical, *see* Exercise
Actuarial table, 93
Addiction, to eating, 181
Adjective Check-List, 146, 148
Adolescent obesity, 44-45, 113, 124
   see also Juvenile obesity
Adolescent
   academic record, 141, 144-145
   anxiety, 143
   attitude of, to obesity, 301, 304-305
      to psychiatrist, 113
   body image, 44-45, 145-146, 147
   characteristics, 139-150
   control of, by parent, 144
   delusion, 130
   diagnosis, 114
   diet, 140, 315-317
      starvation, 112-138
   exercise, 143
   family of, 120, 141-142
   hallucination of, 130
   hospitalization, 139-150
   incidence of obesity, 113
   in Iowa, 116
   mood alteration, 130
      apathy, 129-130
      passivity, 126
   pathology, 130
   peer relations, 148
   psychodynamics, 117
   self-concept, 146
   self-esteem, 143
   social adjustment, 141, 144-145
   therapy, 112-138, 139-150
      failure in, 130
      group, 141, 143-144
      occupational, 147
   weight change, 142
Adoption, 112
Aerobics, 175
Affect, *see* Emotion
Age, at onset of obesity, *see* Onset, age at, of
   obesity

Aging, eating habits of, 73
   incidence of obesity among, 92-105
Aggression, eating as, 202
   as identification, 216
   introjected, 236
   masculine, 191
   oral, 77, 182, 349
   of superobese, 368
Agoraphobia, 183, 187
   see also Phobia
Alcoholism, 141, 143
Alcoholics Anonymous, 367
Amenorrhea, 183, 184, 185, 187, 200, 214
Amnesia, post-hypnotic, 286
Amphetamine, 270, 310
Anal libido, 194
Anesthesia, glove, 274-275, 279
Anger, in group therapy, 233
   as stimulus to eating, 156
Anorexia nervosa, 43, 121, 153, 154-155, 214,
   215-216, 217, 220, 392
Anorexogens, 270
Anthropology, as approach to obesity, 75-83
Anthropomorphic measurement, 115-116
Antidepressant, 121
Anxiety, 127, 169, 234, 259, 280, 285, 374
   adolescent, 143
   castration, 185, 192
   in dieting, 73, 79
   about failure, 203
   neurosis, 229
   separation, 110-112, 120, 127, 182, 197,
      202, 372
   of superobese, 366, 367
   symbolism of, 182
   as symptom, 181
Apathy, of adolescent, 129-130
Aphorism, ix, 76, 281
Apparatus, body-sizing, 48-50
Appetite, control, 274-275, 279
   suppressant, 161
Arab, attitude to weight, 304
Asthma, onset of obesity with, 142
Attitude
   adolescent, to obesity, 301, 304-305
   Arab, 304
   to body weight, 63
   of child psychiatrist, 122

449